Inborn Errors of Metabolism

Editors

AYMAN W. EL-HATTAB
V. REID SUTTON

PEDIATRIC CLINICS OF NORTH AMERICA

www.pediatric.theclinics.com

Consulting Editor
BONITA F. STANTON

April 2018 • Volume 65 • Number 2

ELSEVIER

1600 John F. Kennedy Boulevard • Suite 1800 • Philadelphia, Pennsylvania, 19103-2899

http://www.theclinics.com

THE PEDIATRIC CLINICS OF NORTH AMERICA Volume 65, Number 2
April 2018 ISSN 0031-3955, ISBN-13: 978-0-323-58411-1

Editor: Kerry Holland
Developmental Editor: Casey Potter

The Pediatric Clinics of North America (ISSN 0031-3955) is published bimonthly by Elsevier Inc., 360 Park Avenue South, New York, NY 10010-1710. Months of issue are February, April, June, August, October, and December. Periodicals postage paid at New York, NY and additional mailing offices. Subscription prices are $216.00 per year (US individuals), $613.00 per year (US institutions), $292.00 per year (Canadian individuals), $816.00 per year (Canadian institutions), $338.00 per year (international individuals), $816.00 per year (international institutions), $100.00 per year (US students and residents), and $165.00 per year (international and Canadian residents and students). To receive students/resident rare, orders must be accompanied by name of affiliated institution, date of term, and the signature of program/residency coordinator on institution letterhead. Orders will be billed at individual rate until proof of status is received. Foreign air speed delivery is included in all *Clinics* subscription prices. All prices are subject to change without notice. **POSTMASTER:** Send address changes to *The Pediatric Clinics of North America*, Elsevier Health Sciences Division, Subscription Customer Service, 3251 Riverport Lane, Maryland Heights, MO 63043. **Customer Service: 1-800-654-2452 (US and Canada). From outside of the US and Canada: 1-314-447-8871. Fax: 1-314-447-8029. For print support, E-mail: JournalsCustomerService-usa@elsevier.com. For online support, E-mail: JournalsOnlineSupport-usa@elsevier.com.**

Reprints. For copies of 100 or more, of articles in this publication, please contact the Commercial Reprints Department, Elsevier Inc., 360 Park Avenue South, New York, NY 10010-1710. Tel.: 212-633-3874; Fax: 212-633-3820; E-mail: reprints@elsevier.com.

The Pediatric Clinics of North America is also published in Spanish by McGraw-Hill Inter-americana Editores S.A., Mexico City, Mexico; in Portuguese by Riechmann and Affonso Editores, Rua Comandante Coelho 1085, CEP 21250, Rio de Janeiro, Brazil; and in Greek by Althayia SA, Athens, Greece.

The Pediatric Clinics of North America is covered in *MEDLINE/PubMed (Index Medicus), Excerpta Medica, Current Contents, Current Contents/Clinical Medicine, Science Citation Index, ASCA, ISI/BIOMED,* and *BIOSIS.*

PROGRAM OBJECTIVE

The goal of the *Pediatric Clinics of North America* is to keep practicing physicians and residents up to date with current clinical practice in pediatrics by providing timely articles reviewing the state-of-the-art in patient care.

TARGET AUDIENCE

All practicing pediatricians, physicians and healthcare professionals who provide patient care to pediatric patients.

LEARNING OBJECTIVES

Upon completion of this activity, participants will be able to:

1. Review inborn errors of metabolism including pathophysiology, manifestations, evaluation, and management
2. Discuss complex molecules and phenotypes in inborn errors of metabolism
3. Recognize inborn errors of metabolism with hypoglycaemia, myopathy, hepatopathy and other related diseases.

ACCREDITATION

The Elsevier Office of Continuing Medical Education (EOCME) is accredited by the Accreditation Council for Continuing Medical Education (ACCME) to provide continuing medical education for physicians.

The EOCME designates this enduring material for a maximum of 15 *AMA PRA Category 1 Credit*(s)™. Physicians should claim only the credit commensurate with the extent of their participation in the activity.

All other healthcare professionals requesting continuing education credit for this enduring material will be issued a certificate of participation.

DISCLOSURE OF CONFLICTS OF INTEREST

The EOCME assesses conflict of interest with its instructors, faculty, planners, and other individuals who are in a position to control the content of CME activities. All relevant conflicts of interest that are identified are thoroughly vetted by EOCME for fair balance, scientific objectivity, and patient care recommendations. EOCME is committed to providing its learners with CME activities that promote improvements or quality in healthcare and not a specific proprietary business or a commercial interest.

The planning committee, staff, authors and editors listed below have identified no financial relationships or relationships to products or devices they or their spouse/life partner have with commercial interest related to the content of this CME activity:

Mohammed Almannai, MD; Cinzia Maria Bellettato, PhD; Gerard T. Berry, MD; William J. Brucker, MD, PhD; Carolina F.M. De Souza, MD, PhD; Suzanne D. DeBrosse, MD; Didem Demirbas, PhD; Areeg El-Gharbawy, MD; Ayman W. El-Hattab, MD, FAAP, FACMG; Àngels Garcia-Cazorla, MD, PhD; Thatjana Gardeitchik, MD; Kerry Holland; Leroy Hubert, PhD; Trishna Kantamneni, MD; Alison Kemp; Uta Lichter-Konecki, MD, PhD; Rajkumar Mayakrishnan; Shawn E. McCandless, MD; Nicholas Ah Mew, MD; Lileth Mondok, MD; Eva Morava, MD, PhD; Sumit Parikh, MD; Jean-Marie Saudubray, MD; Maurizio Scarpa, PhD, MD; Lori-Anne P. Schillaci, MD; Evgenia Sklirou, MD; Bonita F. Stanton, MD; Ulrike Steuerwald, MD; Marshall L. Summar, MD; V. Reid.Sutton, MD, FACMG; Michael F. Wangler, MD; Jeroen Wyckmans, MD.

The planning committee, staff, authors and editors listed below have identified financial relationships or relationships to products or devices they or their spouse/life partner have with commercial interest related to the content of this CME activity:

Terry G.J. Derks MD, PhD has received a research grant for the Glyde trial; Vitaflo International, Ltd
Jerry Vockley MD, PhD has received a research grant from Ultragenyx Pharmaceuticals
David A. Weinstein MD, MMSc has received a research grant for the Glyde trial; Vitaflo International, Ltd

UNAPPROVED/OFF-LABEL USE DISCLOSURE

The EOCME requires CME faculty to disclose to the participants:

1. When products or procedures being discussed are off-label, unlabelled, experimental, and/or investigational (not US Food and Drug Administration [FDA] approved); and
2. Any limitations on the information presented, such as data that are preliminary or that represent ongoing research, interim analyses, and/or unsupported opinions. Faculty may discuss information about pharmaceutical agents that is outside of FDA-approved labelling. This information is intended solely for CME

and is not intended to promote off-label use of these medications. If you have any questions, contact the medical affairs department of the manufacturer for the most recent prescribing information.

TO ENROLL

To enroll in the *Pediatric Clinics of North America* Continuing Medical Education program, call customer service at 1-800-654-2452 or sign up online at http://www.theclinics.com/home/cme. The CME program is available to subscribers for an additional annual fee of USD 301.60.

METHOD OF PARTICIPATION

In order to claim credit, participants must complete the following:
1. Complete enrolment as indicated above.
2. Read the activity.
3. Complete the CME Test and Evaluation. Participants must achieve a score of 70% on the test. All CME Tests and Evaluations must be completed online.

CME INQUIRIES/SPECIAL NEEDS

For all CME inquiries or special needs, please contact elsevierCME@elsevier.com.

Contributors

CONSULTING EDITOR

BONITA F. STANTON, MD
Founding Dean, Seton Hall-Hackensack Meridian School of Medicine, President, Academic Enterprise, Hackensack Meridian Health Robert C. and Laura C. Garrett Endowed Chair for the School of Medicine, Dean Professor of Pediatrics, Seton Hall University, South Orange, New Jersey, USA

EDITORS

AYMAN W. EL-HATTAB, MD, FAAP, FACMG
Consultant, Pediatrics Department, Division of Clinical Genetics and Metabolic Disorders, Tawam Hospital, Al-Ain, United Arab Emirates

V. REID SUTTON, MD, FACMG
Professor, Department of Molecular and Human Genetics, Baylor College of Medicine, Texas Children's Hospital, Houston, Texas, USA

AUTHORS

MOHAMMED ALMANNAI, MD
Department of Molecular and Human Genetics, Baylor College of Medicine, Texas Children's Hospital, Houston, Texas, USA

CINZIA MARIA BELLETTATO, PhD
Brains for Brain Foundation, Department of Women and Children Health, Padova, Italy

GERARD T. BERRY, MD
Professor of Pediatrics, Division of Genetics and Genomics, Boston Children's Hospital, Harvard Medical School, Boston, Massachusetts, USA

WILLIAM J. BRUCKER, MD, PhD
Clinical Fellow in Pediatrics, Division of Genetics and Genomics, Boston Children's Hospital, Harvard Medical School, Boston, Massachusetts, USA

CAROLINA F.M. DE SOUZA, MD, PhD
Medical Genetics Service, Hospital de Clínicas de Porto Alegre, Porto Alegre, Rio Grande do Sul, Brazil

SUZANNE D. DEBROSSE, MD
Assistant Professor, Department of Genetics and Genome Sciences, Case Western Reserve University, Center for Human Genetics, University Hospitals Cleveland Medical Center, Cleveland, Ohio, USA

DIDEM DEMIRBAS, PhD
Research Fellow in Pediatrics, Division of Genetics and Genomics, Boston Children's Hospital, Harvard Medical School, Boston, Massachusetts, USA

TERRY G.J. DERKS, MD, PhD
Section of Metabolic Diseases, University of Groningen, University Medical Center Groningen, Beatrix Children's Hospital, Groningen, The Netherlands

AREEG EL-GHARBAWY, MD
Assistant Professor of Pediatrics, University of Pittsburgh School of Medicine, Children's Hospital of Pittsburgh of UPMC, Pittsburgh, Pennsylvania, USA; Faculty of Medicine, Cairo University, Cairo, Egypt

AYMAN W. EL-HATTAB, MD, FAAP, FACMG
Consultant, Pediatrics Department, Division of Clinical Genetics and Metabolic Disorders, Tawam Hospital, Al-Ain, United Arab Emirates

ÀNGELS GARCIA-CAZORLA, MD, PhD
Neurology Department, Neurometabolic Unit, Hospital Sant Joan de Deu and CIBERER-ISCIII, Barcelona, Spain

THATJANA GARDEITCHIK, MD
Department of Human Genetics, Radboud University Medical Center, Nijmegen, The Netherlands

LEROY HUBERT, PhD
Research Fellow, Department of Molecular and Human Genetics, Baylor College of Medicine, Houston, Texas, USA

TRISHNA KANTAMNENI, MD
Neurological Institute, Center for Pediatric Neurology, Cleveland Clinic, Cleveland, Ohio, USA

UTA LICHTER-KONECKI, MD, PhD
Division of Medical Genetics, Department of Pediatrics, Children's Hospital of Pittsburgh of UPMC, University of Pittsburgh, University of Pittsburgh Medical Center, Pittsburgh, Pennsylvania, USA

SHAWN E. MCCANDLESS, MD
Professor, Department of Genetics and Genome Sciences, Case Western Reserve University, Director, Center for Human Genetics, University Hospitals Cleveland Medical Center, Cleveland, Ohio, USA

NICHOLAS AH MEW, MD
Rare Disease Institute, Children's National Health System, Washington, DC, USA

LILETH MONDOK, MD
Neurological Institute, Center for Pediatric Neurology, Cleveland Clinic, Cleveland, Ohio, USA

EVA MORAVA, MD, PhD
Department of Pediatrics, University Hospitals Leuven, Leuven, Belgium; Hayward Genetics Center, Tulane University School of Medicine, New Orleans, Louisiana, USA

SUMIT PARIKH, MD
Associate Professor of Neurology, Neurological Institute, Center for Pediatric Neurology, Cleveland Clinic, Cleveland Clinic Lerner College of Medicine of Case Western Reserve University, Cleveland, Ohio, USA

JEAN-MARIE SAUDUBRAY, MD
Department of Neurology, Neurometabolic Unit, Hopital Pitié Salpétrière, Paris, France

MAURIZIO SCARPA, PhD, MD
Professor, Brains for Brains Foundation, Department of Women and Children Health, University of Padova, Padova, Italy; Center for Rare Diseases, Department of Pediatric and Adolescent Medicine, Helios Dr. Horst Schmidt Klinik, Wiesbaden, Germany

LORI-ANNE P. SCHILLACI, MD
Assistant Professor, Department of Genetics and Genome Sciences, Case Western Reserve University, Center for Human Genetics, University Hospitals Cleveland Medical Center, Cleveland, Ohio, USA

EVGENIA SKLIROU, MD
Division of Medical Genetics, Department of Pediatrics, Children's Hospital of Pittsburgh of UPMC, University of Pittsburgh, University of Pittsburgh Medical Center, Pittsburgh, Pennsylvania, USA

ULRIKE STEUERWALD, MD
Medical Center, National Hospital System, Torshavn, Faroe Islands

MARSHALL L. SUMMAR, MD
Rare Disease Institute, Children's National Health System, Washington, DC, USA

V. REID SUTTON, MD, FACMG
Professor, Department of Molecular and Human Genetics, Baylor College of Medicine, Texas Children's Hospital, Houston, Texas, USA

JERRY VOCKLEY, MD, PhD
Professor of Pediatrics and Human Genetics, Chief of Medical Genetics, Director of the Center for Rare Disease Therapy, University of Pittsburgh School of Medicine, Children's Hospital of Pittsburgh of UPMC, Pittsburgh, Pennsylvania, USA

MICHAEL F. WANGLER, MD
Assistant Professor, Department of Molecular and Human Genetics, Baylor College of Medicine, Jan and Dan Duncan Neurological Research Institute, Texas Children's Hospital, Program in Developmental Biology, Baylor College of Medicine, Houston, Texas, USA

DAVID A. WEINSTEIN, MD, MMSc
Professor, University of Connecticut School of Medicine, Farmington, Connecticut, USA; Director, Glycogen Storage Disease Program, Connecticut Children's Medical Center, Hartford, Connecticut, USA

JEROEN WYCKMANS, MD
Department of Pediatrics, University Hospitals Leuven, Leuven, Belgium

Contents

> The specialty of inherited metabolic disease is at the forefront of progress
> in medicine, with new methods in metabolomics and genomics identifying
> the molecular basis for a growing number of conditions and syndromes.
> This article presents an updated pathophysiologic classification of inborn
> errors of metabolism and a method of clinical screening in neonates, late-
> onset emergencies, neurologic deterioration, and other common clinical
> scenarios. When and how to investigate a metabolic disorder is presented
> to encourage physicians to use sophisticated biochemical investigations
> and not miss a treatable disorder.

> When a child presents with high-anion gap metabolic acidosis, the pedia-
> trician can proceed with confidence by recalling some basic principles.
> Defects of organic acid, pyruvate, and ketone body metabolism that pre-
> sent with acute acidosis are reviewed. Flowcharts for identifying the under-
> lying cause and initiating life-saving therapy are provided. By evaluating
> electrolytes, blood sugar, lactate, ammonia, and urine ketones, the pro-
> vider can determine the likelihood of an inborn error of metabolism.
> Freezing serum, plasma, and urine samples during the acute presentation
> for definitive diagnostic testing at the provider's convenience aids in the
> differential diagnosis.

> The urea cycle disorders are a group of inherited biochemical diseases
> caused by a complete or partial deficiency of any one of the enzymes or
> transport proteins required to convert toxic ammonia into urea and to pro-
> duce arginine and citrulline. The clinical manifestations of these disorders
> are mostly the result of acute or chronic hyperammonemia, which affects

the central nervous system. Affected individuals can also develop hepatic dysfunction. These disorders can present at any age from the immediate newborn to later in life. Early diagnosis and treatment are key to improving outcomes.

Although hyperinsulinism is the predominant inherited cause of hypoglycemia in the newborn period, inborn errors of metabolism are the primary etiologies after 1 month of age. Disorders of carbohydrate metabolism often present with hypoglycemia when fasting occurs. The presentation, diagnosis, and management of the hepatic glycogen storage diseases and disorders of gluconeogenesis are reviewed.

Phenylketonuria is a defect in phenylalanine metabolism resulting in the excretion of phenylketones and severe intellectual disability. The principle of eliminating the offending amino acid from the diet as a successful treatment strategy was demonstrated. The development of a low-methionine diet to treat homocysteinuria was established after identifying the transsulfuration pathway, resulting in cysteine synthesis. Both conditions are examples of disorders of amino acid metabolism. Lesch-Nyhan syndrome, a rare disorder of purine metabolism resulting in intellectual disability and self-injurious behavior, is a classical inborn error of metabolism. Disorders of creatine biosynthesis are relatively newly described and less known diseases.

Inborn errors of metabolism (IEMs) are relatively uncommon causes for seizures in children; however, they should be considered in the differential diagnosis because several IEMs are potentially treatable and seizures can be resolved if appropriate treatment is initiated. Clues from clinical presentation, physical examination, laboratory tests, and brain imaging can raise the possibility of IEM. Several IEMs can present with seizures, either as the main presenting finding or as a part of a more complex phenotype. These include cofactor-related disorders, glycine and serine metabolism defects, and other disorders.

Movement disorders in the pediatric age group are largely of the hyperkinetic type. Metal ion accumulation in the central nervous system presents predominantly with movement disorders and over time leads to psychomotor decline. Abnormalities in monoamine and amino acidergic neurotransmitter metabolism present in individuals with a combination of abnormal movements, epilepsy, and cognitive and motor delay. Detailed clinical history, careful examination, appropriate diagnostic workup with metabolic screening, cerebrospinal fluid neurotransmitters, and targeted genetic testing help with accurate diagnosis and appropriate treatment. This article provides an overview on movement disorders present in childhood secondary to inborn errors of metal transport and neurotransmitter metabolism.

Fatty acid oxidation disorders (FAODs) and carnitine shuttling defects are inborn errors of energy metabolism with associated mortality and morbidity due to cardiomyopathy, exercise intolerance, rhabdomyolysis, and liver disease with physiologic stress. Hypoglycemia is characteristically hypoketotic. Lactic acidemia and hyperammonemia may occur during decompensation. Recurrent rhabdomyolysis is debilitating. Expanded newborn screening can detect most of these disorders, allowing early, presymptomatic treatment. Treatment includes avoiding fasting and sustained extraneous exercise and providing high-calorie hydration during illness to prevent lipolysis, and medium-chain triglyceride oil supplementation in long-chain FAODs. Carnitine supplementation may be helpful. However, conventional treatment does not prevent all symptoms.

The liver is one of the most essential organs in metabolism and is responsible for metabolizing a wide variety of molecules from amino acids to sugars. Although it is responsible for many essential metabolic processes, it is one of the most severely affected by metabolic disease because, in many cases, it is the first to be exposed to the toxic intermediates. The metabolism of galactose, fructose, and tyrosine involve the liver, and although there are systemic findings in metabolic disease involved with these substrates, severe hepatopathy is a common presenting aspect of galactosemia, hereditary fructose intolerance, and tyrosinemia type I.

Peroxisomes and lysosomes are distinct subcellular compartments that underlie several pediatric metabolic disorders. Knowledge of their function and cell biology leads to understanding how the disorders result from genetic defects. Diagnostic and therapeutic approaches for the disorders take advantage of the cell biology mechanisms. Peroxisomal disorders are characterized by enzymatic defects in peroxisomal pathways leading to metabolic and lipid changes, whereas lysosomal storage disorders are marked by accumulation of substrates of lysosomal pathways inside the lysosome. The human diseases related to these two organelles are reviewed, focusing on general disease patterns and underlying diagnosis and treatment principles.

Congenital disorders of glycosylation (CDG) and mitochondrial disorders have overlapping clinical features, including central nervous system, cardiac, gastrointestinal, hepatic, muscular, endocrine, and psychiatric disease. Specific abnormalities orienting the clinician toward the right diagnostic approach include abnormal fat distribution, coagulation abnormalities, together with anticoagulation abnormalities, hyperinsulinism, and congenital malformations in CDG. Diabetes, sensorineural deafness, and depression are very rare in CDG but common in mitochondrial disease. Chronic lactic acidosis is highly suggestive of mitochondrial dysfunction. Serum transferrin isoform analysis is specific for glycosylation abnormalities but not abnormal in all types of CDG.

Newborn screening programs aim to achieve presymptomatic diagnosis of treatable disorders, allowing for early initiation of medical care to prevent or reduce significant morbidity and mortality. Many of the conditions included in the newborn screening panels are inborn errors of metabolism; however, screening for endocrine, hematologic, immunologic, and cardiovascular diseases and hearing loss is also included in many panels. Newborn screening tests are not diagnostic, and therefore, diagnostic testing is needed to confirm or exclude the suspected diagnosis. Further advancement in technology is expected to allow continuous expansion of newborn screening.

PEDIATRIC CLINICS OF NORTH AMERICA

THE CLINICS ARE AVAILABLE ONLINE!
Access your subscription at:
www.theclinics.com

Erratum

In the September 2017 issue of *Pediatric Clinics of North America* 64 (2017), in the article 'Transfusion Decision Making in Pediatric Critical Illness' (pages 991–1015) by Chris Markham, MD, Peter Hovmand, PhD, and Allan Doctor, MD. Sara Small, MSW (Social Systems Design Laboratory, Brown School of Social Work, Washington University, Campus Box 1196, 1 Brookings Drive, St Louis, MO 63130, USA) should be listed as the article's second author.

Pediatr Clin N Am 65 (2018) xv
https://doi.org/10.1016/j.pcl.2018.01.003
0031-3955/18

Foreword

New Understanding of Mechanisms and New Hope for Treatments

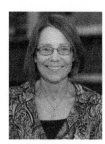

Bonita F. Stanton, MD
Consulting Editor

Inborn errors of metabolism (IEM) are defined by the National Institutes of Health as "a group of disorders that causes a block in a metabolic pathway leading to clinically significant consequences."[1] The 500+ IEMs identified to date are generally classified into six groups: urea cycle disorders, organic acidemias, fatty acid oxidation defects, amino acidopathies, carbohydrate disorders, and mitochondrial disorders. As also noted by Ayman W. El-Hattab, MD and V. Reid Sutton, MD, the Guest Editors of this issue of *Pediatric Clinics of North America*, while individually most IEM are rare, in aggregate, an estimated 1/1000 persons have an IEM.[2] Therefore, it is important for child health providers to remain informed about the many advances in the field of IEM in recent years.

The manifestations of an IEM result from a range of mechanisms typically resulting in either the production of excessive amounts of toxic substances or the inadequate production of critical substances. Disease manifestations, once viewed as resulting from single gene defects, are now understood to result from a host of factors, including interactions with other genes, interactions between the impacted gene and the environment, epigenetic factors, and the hosts' microbiome. Recognition of the contribution of these multiple ramifications and interactions beyond the impact of the genetic mutation itself has greatly increased our understanding of the mechanisms of the gene mutation and possible treatment approaches.[3] Indeed, our growing recognition that the interactions within a cell or organ and between the impacted individual and his/her environment produce results far greater than would be expected from a simple additive process has led to a new appreciation of the manifestations of IEM.[4,5]

This greater appreciation of the complexity of IEMs has led to the development of many new ways to diagnose, evaluate, and approach the mutations and the

Pediatr Clin N Am 65 (2018) xvii–xviii
https://doi.org/10.1016/j.pcl.2018.01.002
0031-3955/18/© 2018 Published by Elsevier Inc.

pediatric.theclinics.com

deliberating disease effects. These advances have been accompanied by substantial improvements in survival, resulting in new challenges and opportunities for treatment approaches.[2] In this issue of *Pediatric Clinics of North America*, Professors El-Hattab and Sutton and the distinguished clinicians and scientists they have assembled summarize and explain advances made in the field as a whole as well as those specific to individual categories of disorders. The multiple manifestations and the speed at which diagnostic and treatment advances have been made over the last decade for the IEM assure the relevance of this issue for all pediatric care providers regardless of specialties or areas of focus.

Bonita F. Stanton, MD
Seton Hall-Hackensack Meridian School of Medicine
Seton Hall University
400 South Orange Street
South Orange, NJ 07079, USA

E-mail address:
bonita.stanton@shu.edu

REFERENCES

1. National Institutes of Health (NIH). Available at: https://www.genome.gov/27551373/the-nih-mini-study-general-information-about-inborn-errors-of-metabolism/. Accessed December 24, 2017.
2. Alfadhel M, Al-Thihli K, Moubayed H, et al. Drug treatment of inborn errors of metabolism: a systematic review. Arch Dis Child 2013;98(6):454–61.
3. Argmann CA, Houten SM, Zhu J, et al. A next generation multiscale view of inborn errors of metabolism. Cell Metab 2016;23(1):13–26.
4. Scriver CR, Waters PJ. Monogenic traits are not simple: lessons from phenylketonuria. Trends Genet 1999;15:267–72.
5. Dipple KM, McCabe ER. Modifier genes convert "simple" Mendelian disorders to complex traits. Mol Genet Metab 2000;71:43–50.

Preface

Approach to Inborn Errors of Metabolism in Pediatrics

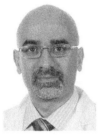
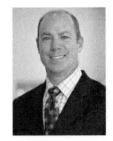

Ayman W. El-Hattab, MD, FAAP, FACMG   V. Reid Sutton, MD, FACMG

Editors

Inborn errors of metabolism (IEM) are a group of disorders that result from impairment in normal metabolic processes, most often due to an enzyme or transporter deficiency. More than 500 IEM have been recognized with the vast majority presenting during childhood. Although IEM are individually rare, they are collectively common, with an overall incidence of around 1/1000 live births. This number is double the incidence of the commonest cancer in children, leukemia, which is 1/2000. Therefore, IEM are not uncommon, and all pediatricians are expected to encounter many children with these diseases throughout their practice.

Many IEM present with metabolic decompensation that can be life threatening. Early recognition and prompt initiation of appropriate treatment are critical in reducing morbidity and mortality. It is therefore important for the pediatrician to recognize signs and symptoms of various IEM, know how to request and interpret the appropriate metabolic tests, initiate basic medical treatment, and know when to refer to a metabolic specialist. This is important as these children often see their pediatrician first for general complaints such as developmental delay or vomiting. In addition, because of the shortage of specialists in medical biochemical genetics worldwide, it is critical that pediatricians, alone or in consultation with metabolic specialists, become able to initiate treatments that can significantly reduce morbidity and mortality.

Individuals with IEM are currently living longer because of early diagnosis with the expansion of newborn screening programs and significant improvements in therapies and management for these conditions. With such prolonged survival, many more children with IEM are in need of continuous primary care provided by pediatricians. It is therefore important for pediatricians, as primary care providers for the children with IEM, to understand the natural history of these disorders and be able to identify early signs of metabolic decompensation.

Pediatr Clin N Am 65 (2018) xix–xx
https://doi.org/10.1016/j.pcl.2018.01.001
0031-3955/18/© 2018 Published by Elsevier Inc.   **pediatric.theclinics.com**

With the expanded newborn screening, more affected children can be identified early, and knowing what confirmatory testing to do and what initial treatments are indicated is critical to ensure that newborn screening programs indeed improve and save children's lives.

IEM have been classically categorized according to the affected metabolic pathway, such as amino acid, fatty acid, and carbohydrate metabolism defects. In this issue, however, IEM are grouped based upon presenting symptoms, which is more relevant to how we all approach a clinical problem. The first article in this issue, by Saudubray, presents an overview of pathophysiology and manifestations of IEM. Acidosis, hyperammonemia, and hypoglycemia, the common metabolic derangements observed in IEM, are then discussed. The next article, by Schillaci and colleagues, presents IEM with acidosis (organic acidemias and defects of pyruvate and ketone body metabolism) and is followed by an article by Summar and Ah Mew that discusses IEM presenting with hyperammonemia (urea cycle defects). The article by Weinstein and colleagues presents IEM with hypoglycemia (glycogen storage diseases and gluconeogenesis defects). As the majority of IEM can predominantly present with neurologic manifestations, three articles were designated to discuss IEM with neurologic involvement. IEM with cognitive impairment, including metabolism defects of phenylalanine, homocysteine and methionine, purine and pyrimidine, and creatine, is then discussed. The article in this issue by Almannai and El-Hattab presents IEM with seizures, including defects of glycine and serine metabolism and co-factor-related disorders. This is followed by an article by Parikh that summarizes IEM that can present with movement disorders, including defects in metal transport and neurotransmitter metabolism. Other common manifestations of IEM are myopathy and hepatopathy. IEM with myopathy (defects of fatty acid oxidation and carnitine transport) is then discussed and is followed by IEM with hepatopathy (metabolism defects of galactose, fructose, and tyrosine). After that, IEM involving complex molecules (lysosomal and peroxisomal storage diseases) is discussed, followed by IEM with complex phenotypes (mitochondrial disorders and congenital disorders of glycosylation). Finally, the last article, by Sutton and colleagues, discusses the history, current status, and future directions of newborn screening.

We thank the truly amazing group of authors, who have contributed articles that are both practical and on the cutting edge of their field of expertise. While reading and editing the articles, we found many clinical pearls that will make us better physicians and know that you will as well.

Ayman W. El-Hattab, MD, FAAP, FACMG
Division of Clinical Genetics and Metabolic Disorders
Pediatrics Department
Tawam Hospital
Al-Ain 15258, United Arab Emirates

V. Reid Sutton, MD, FACMG
Department of Molecular and Human Genetics
Baylor College of Medicine and
Texas Children's Hospital
6701 Fannin Street Suite 1560
Houston, TX 77030, USA

E-mail addresses:
elhattabaw@yahoo.com (A.W. El-Hattab)
vrsutton@texaschildrens.org (V.R. Sutton)

Inborn Errors of Metabolism Overview
Pathophysiology, Manifestations, Evaluation, and Management

Jean-Marie Saudubray, MD[a],*, Àngels Garcia-Cazorla, MD, PhD[b]

KEYWORDS

- Inborn errors of metabolism (IEM) • IEM diagnostic approach • IEM classification
- IEM in neonates • IEM acute presentations • Metabolic comas
- IEM with chronic encephalopathy • Treatable IEM

KEY POINTS

- More than 750 inborn errors of metabolism have been described so far.
- Many inborn errors of metabolism present in extremis and can be easily diagnosed based on plasma/urine metabolic tests performed in laboratories specialized in biochemical genetics.
- Some inborn errors of metabolism are treatable and require early and urgent intervention to prevent permanent sequelae.
- Most treatable inborn errors of metabolism can be identified by newborn screening.

INTRODUCTION

About 60 years after Garrod's premonitory dissertations on 4 inborn errors of metabolism (IEM), the first edition of the classic textbook *The Metabolic Basis of Inherited Disease* by Stanbury and colleagues was published in 1960, a time when IEM were being rediscovered and slowly redefined as molecular diseases. Since then, the study of IEM has made important progress and the 8th edition of the *Metabolic and Molecular Basis of Inherited Diseases* published in 2001 by Scriver and colleagues[1] encompassed 4 volumes, and the description of about one thousand

No commercial or financial conflicts of interest are declared. À. Garcia-Cazorla is supported by the "Plan Nacional de I+D+I and Instituto de Salud Carlos III- Subdireccion General de Evaluacion y Fomento de la Investigacion Sanitaria", project PI15/01082, and the European Regional Development Fund (FEDER [PI15/01082]).
a Department of Neurology, Neurometabolic Unit, Hopital Pitié Salpétrière, 47-83 Boulevard de l'Hopital, Paris 75013, France; b Neurology Department, Neurometabolic Unit, Hospital Sant Joan de Deu and CIBERER-ISCIII, Passeig Sant Joan de Deu 28950 Esplugues de Llobregat, Barcelona, Spain
* Corresponding author. 22 rue Juliette Lamber, Paris 75017, France.
E-mail address: jmsaudubray@orange.fr

Pediatr Clin N Am 65 (2018) 179–208
https://doi.org/10.1016/j.pcl.2017.11.002
0031-3955/18/© 2017 Elsevier Inc. All rights reserved.

pediatric.theclinics.com

rare, inherited metabolic disorders and mechanisms. The book is now being updated and is only available on-line. More recently, in the classic clinical textbook *Inborn Metabolic Diseases Diagnosis and Treatment*, more than 300 "new" disorders were described in the 5 years between the fifth (2011) and the sixth (2016) editions, 85% presenting with predominantly neurologic manifestations.[2] However, the specialized study of IEM remains underrepresented worldwide in the great majority of medical faculty teaching programs. This lack is partly due to the traditional classification of diseases based on organs and systems (cardiology, pulmonology, neurology, hematology, etc), whereas IEM may present with many symptoms and affect any organs at any age in any scenario, which means they do not all fall into any one of the traditional categories for diseases. This situation is made even less favorable by the very poor transfer of cell biology and biochemistry knowledge obtained from academic training to physicians' daily clinical practice. To successfully perceive and diagnose an IEM, it is crucial that metabolic physicians have sound clinical training in these elements. Given the increasing complexity of biochemical and molecular tests and the difficulty of keeping up with this evolving field for busy practicing physicians, these effective but complex, time-consuming, and expensive methods of testing are at risk of being used in an uncontrolled and uncritical way. Appropriate educational programs are of utmost importance as a strategy to create a critical and pathophysiology-based thinking in medical doctors.

For physicians on the front line not to miss a treatable disorder, the clinical diagnosis of IEM should rely on a small number of important principles[2,3] (**Box 1**). IEM are individually rare but collectively numerous. The application of tandem mass spectrometry to newborn screening and prenatal diagnosis has enabled presymptomatic diagnosis for some IEM (see Reid Sutton and colleagues' article, "Newborn Screening: History, Current Status, and Future Directions," in this issue). However, for most IEM, neonatal screening tests are either too slow, too expensive, or unreliable; consequently, clinical screening is mandatory before starting the sequence of sophisticated biochemical tests required to identify many IEM.

Box 1
Principles for clinical diagnosis of IEM: Do not miss a treatable disorder

- In the appropriate clinical context, consider an IEM in parallel with other more common conditions.

- Be aware that symptoms that persist and remain unexplained after the initial treatment and the usual tests for more common disorders have been performed and ruled out, may be owing to an IEM.

- Do not confuse a symptom or a syndrome with etiology—the underlying cause may be an IEM yet to be defined.

- Remember that an IEM can present at any age, from conception through old age.

- If you are looking for a family connection to an IEM remember that although most metabolic errors are hereditary, they are often transmitted as recessive disorders, making the majority of individual cases seem to be sporadic.

- Consider and try to diagnose IEMs that are amenable to treatment (mainly those that cause intoxication) first.

- In emergency situations, first provide care to the affected individual (emergency treatment) and then to the family (genetic advice).

Abbreviation: IEM, inborn error of metabolism.

PATHOPHYSIOLOGIC CLASSIFICATION OF INBORN ERRORS OF METABOLISM

The vast majority of IEM involve abnormalities in enzymes and transport proteins and can be divided into the following 2 large clinical categories.

Category 1 includes disorders that either involve only one functional system (such as the endocrine system, immune system, or coagulation factors) or affect only 1 organ or anatomic system (such as the intestine, renal tubules, erythrocytes, or connective tissue). Presenting symptoms are uniform (eg, a bleeding tendency in coagulation factor defects or hemolytic anemia in defects of glycolysis), and the correct diagnosis is usually easy to predict.

Category 2 includes diseases in which the basic biochemical lesion either affects 1 metabolic pathway common to a large number of cells or organs (eg, storage diseases owing to lysosomal catabolic disorders, energy deficiency in mitochondrial disorders) or is restricted to one organ but gives rise to humoral and systemic consequences (eg, hyperammonemia in urea cycle defects, hypoglycemia in hepatic glycogenosis). The diseases in this category have a great diversity of presenting symptoms but can be divided into 3 diagnostically useful groups: group 1 includes disorders of intermediary metabolism affecting small molecules, group 2 includes disorders involving primarily energy metabolism, and group 3 includes disorders involving complex molecules.

Group 1: Disorders of Intermediary Metabolism Affecting Small Molecules

Intermediary metabolism can be defined as an immense network of biochemical reactions of degradation (catabolism), synthesis (anabolism), and recycling that allows a cycle of continuous exchanges between cells and the nutrients brought on by alimentation (carbohydrates, lipids, proteins) and respiration (oxygen). It involves thousands proteins, mostly enzymes and transporters, the deficit of which cause IEM. Deficits can affect small or complex molecules.

This group 1 is very large and there are many different mechanisms involved. It includes IEM that lead to acute or progressive intoxication from the accumulation of normal or unusual compounds proximal to the metabolic block. They encompass classical inborn errors of amino acid catabolism (phenylketonuria, maple syrup urine disease, homocystinuria, tyrosinemia, etc), most organic acidurias (methylmalonic, propionic, isovaleric, biotin responsive multiple carboxylase deficiency; see Shawn E. McCandless and colleagues' article, "Inborn Errors of Metabolism with Acidosis: Organic Acidemias and Defects of Pyruvate and Ketone Body Metabolism," in this issue), urea cycle defects and related disorders (triple H syndrome, lysinuric protein intolerance; see David A. Weinstein and colleagues' article, "Inborn Errors of Metabolism with Hypoglycemia: Glycogen Storage Diseases and Inherited Disorders of Gluconeogenesis," in this issue), galactose (galactosemia), and fructose (hereditary fructose intolerance) metabolism defects (see Gerard T. Berry and colleagues' article, "Inborn Errors of Metabolism with Hepatopathy: Metabolism Defects of Galactose, Fructose, and Tyrosine," in this issue), and porphyrias.

Metal disorders can behave like intoxication in cases of accumulation (Wilson disease, hemochromatosis, neuroferritinopathies) and neurodegeneration with brain iron accumulation syndromes, cirrhosis dystonia syndrome (with hypermanganesemia, etc), but also like complex molecule disorders (disturbing glycosylation, trafficking, etc) in the case of metal deficiencies, like in the recently described inherited manganese deficiency linked to *SLC39A8* mutations[4] (see Sumit Parikh and colleagues' article, "Inborn Errors of Metabolism with Movement Disorders: Defects in Metal Transport and Neurotransmitter Metabolism," in this issue; **Box 2**).

> **Box 2**
> **Clinical similarities of classical intoxication disorders**
>
> - They do not interfere with embryo and fetal development.
> - They present with a symptom-free interval (days, months, or years).
> - Clinical signs of intoxication may be acute (vomiting, coma, liver failure, thrombosis, etc) or chronic (failure to thrive, developmental delay, ectopia lentis, cirrhosis, ichthyosis, cardiomyopathy, etc), even progressive (neurodegeneration).
> - They present with acute metabolic attacks provoked by fasting, catabolism, fever, intercurrent illness, and food intake.
> - Clinical expression is often both late in onset and intermittent.
> - The diagnosis is straightforward and most commonly relies on plasma and urine amino acid, organic acid, and acylcarnitine chromatography.
> - Most of these disorders are treatable and require the emergency removal of the toxin by special diets, extracorporeal procedures, vitamins or cleansing drugs (carnitine, sodium benzoate, penicillamine, etc).

Inborn errors of neurotransmitter synthesis, catabolism and transport (monoamines, gamma aminobutyric acid, and glycine) and inborn errors of brain amino acid synthesis (serine, glutamine, asparagine, and proline and ornithine) or transport (mostly branched chain amino acids)[5] display a somewhat different clinical presentation and pathophysiology: they can be present at birth and may interfere with embryo–fetal development; they do not have metabolic attacks, and they can be progressive. A new mechanism of neurotransmitters defect have been recently described that involved a co-chaperone of the HSP70 family encoded by *DNAJC12*, which interacts with phenylalanine, tyrosine, and tryptophan hydroxylase. All manifestations reversed on early treatment with tetrahydrobiopterin (BH4) and/or neurotransmitter precursors.[6]

Inborn errors of neurotransmitter and brain amino acid synthesis are also included in this group, because they share many biochemical characteristics: their diagnosis relies on plasma, urine, and cerebrospinal fluid investigations (amino acid, organic acid analyses, etc); and some are amenable to treatment even when the disorder is present in utero—for example, 3-phosphoglycerate-dehydrogenase deficiency[7] (see Ayman W. El-Hattab and Mohammed Almannai's article, "Inborn Errors of Metabolism with Seizures: Defects of Glycine and Serine Metabolism and Cofactor Related Disorders," and Sumit Parikh and colleagues' article, "Inborn Errors of Metabolism with Movement Disorders: Defects in Metal Transport and Neurotransmitter Metabolism;" in this issue).

Group 2: Disorders Involving Primarily Energy Metabolism

These disorders consist of IEM with symptoms due, at least in part, to a deficiency in energy production or use within the liver, myocardium, muscle, brain, or other tissues. Membrane carriers of energetic molecules (glucose, fatty acids, ketone bodies, and monocarboxylic acids) display many tissue specific isozymes as glucose transporter 1 (the glucose cerebral transporter), and glucose transporter 2 (the glucose hepatointestinal transporter), the deficiencies of which cause neurologic and hepatic signs, respectively.

Mitochondrial defects are the most severe and are generally untreatable. They encompass the aerobic glucose oxidation defects presenting with congenital lactic acidemias (pyruvate transporter, pyruvate carboxylase, pyruvate dehydrogenase system, and Krebs cycle defects), the mitochondrial respiratory chain disorders involving either the respiratory chain itself, the mitochondrial transporters of energetic molecules, amino acids, ions, metals and vitamins, or the biosynthesis of coenzyme Q (see Eva Morava and colleagues' article, "Complex Phenotypes in Inborn Errors of Metabolism: Overlapping Presentations in Congenital Disorders of Glycosylation and Mitochondrial Disorders," in this issue), and the fatty acid oxidation and ketone body defects (see Areeg El-Gharbawy and Jerry Vockley's article, "Inborn Errors of Metabolism with Myopathy: Defects of Fatty Acid Oxidation and the Carnitine Shuttle System," in this issue). Only the latter are even partially treatable.

Cytoplasmic energy defects are generally less severe. They include disorders of glycolysis, glycogen metabolism and gluconeogenesis, hyperinsulinism, and glucose transporter defects (all treatable disorders), the disorders of creatine metabolism (partially treatable), and the inborn errors of the pentose phosphate pathways (untreatable). Vesicular glycolysis was recently discovered to be capable of providing a constant intrinsic source of energy, independent of mitochondria, for the rapid axonal movement of vesicles over long distances[8] (**Box 3**).

Group 3: Disorders Involving Complex Molecules

This expanding group encompasses diseases that disturb the synthesis, processing, quality control, and catabolism of complex molecules. These complex processes take place in organelles (mitochondria, lysosomes, peroxisomes, endoplasmic reticulum, and the Golgi apparatus). Symptoms are permanent, very often progressive, and independent of intercurrent events, unrelated to food intake. Most patients do not present with crises. This group includes lysosomal storage disorders, peroxisomal disorders, carbohydrate-deficient glycoprotein (CDG) syndrome, inborn errors of purine and pyrimidine, inborn errors of cholesterol and bile acid synthesis, inborn errors of intracellular triglycerides, phospholipids and glycosphingolipids synthesis and remodeling, and many other defects affecting systems involved in intracellular vesiculation trafficking, processing of complex molecules, and quality control processes.

Lysosomal storage disorders (mostly defects of sphingolipids, mucopolysaccharides, and oligosaccharides catabolism) are responsible for intracellular accumulation of non/poor soluble material in reticuloendothelial cells (see Michael F. Wangler and colleagues' article, "Inborn Errors of Metabolism Involving Complex Molecules: lysosomal and Peroxisomal Storage Diseases," in this issue). Besides these well-known catabolic defects with visible storage material, a number of new disorders affecting the synthesis and recycling of sphingolipids, mucopolysaccharides, and oligosaccharides have been described recently (discussed elsewhere in this article).[9–11]

Box 3
Common symptoms of energetic disorders

- Hypoglycemia, hyperlactatemia, acidosis, and hyperketonemia or hypoketonemia.

- Hepatomegaly, severe generalized hypotonia, myopathy, cardiomyopathy, failure to thrive, cardiac failure, circulatory collapse, sudden unexpected death in infancy, eye (optic atrophy), and brain involvement.

- Recurrent crisis triggered by intercurrent events (catabolism).

- Some of the mitochondrial disorders and pentose phosphate pathway defects can interfere with embryo and fetal development, and can cause dysmorphism, dysplasia, and malformations.

- Diagnosis is difficult and relies on function tests measuring energetic molecules (glucose, lactate, ketones, etc) in cycles both in fed and fasted states, enzymatic analyses requiring biopsies or cell culture, and molecular analyses.

- Only a few are treatable (fatty acid oxidation defects, hepatic glycogenosis, coenzyme Q synthesis defects).

Peroxisomal disorders encompass a number of molecular defects affecting either the peroxisome biogenesis or a specific matrix enzyme (see Michael F. Wangler and colleagues' article, "Inborn Errors of Metabolism Involving Complex Molecules: Lysosomal and Peroxisomal Storage Diseases," in this issue). Nonmitochondrial fatty acid homeostasis defects share many similarities with peroxisomal disorders like Sjögren Larsson syndrome or Elongase 4 deficiency (ichthyosis, spastic paraplegia, and ocular findings).

CDG syndromes are an expanding group of disorders (>100 defects described so far) that display very diverse clinical presentations (see Eva Morava and colleagues' article, "Complex Phenotypes in Inborn Errors of Metabolism: Overlapping Presentations in Congenital Disorders of Glycosylation and Mitochondrial Disorders," in this issue).

Inborn errors of purine and pyrimidine disturb nucleic acid metabolism. Some defects are treatable like, uridine responsive epilepsy,[12] or uridine responsive congenital orotic aciduria with megaloblastic anemia (see Evgenia Sklirou and Uta Lichter-Konecki's article, "Inborn Errors of Metabolism with Cognitive Impairment: Metabolism Defects of Phenylalanine, Homocysteine and Methionine, Purine and pyrimidine, and Creatine," in this issue).

Inborn errors of cholesterol and bile acid synthesis present either with multiple malformation syndromes (like the Smith-Lemli-Opitz syndrome and about 6 other disorders), neonatal cholestasis (about 10 disorders), or with late onset neurodegenerative disorders (like the cerebrotendinous xanthomatosis, which is treatable by chenodeoxycholic acid).

Inborn errors of intracellular triglycerides, phospholipids, and glycosphingolipids synthesis and remodeling compose a rapidly expanding new group (>22 disorders described so far).[9,10] Intracellular triglycerides disorders display noncerebral presentations, mostly hepatic steatosis with hypertriglyceridemia, neutral lipid storage disorders (Chanarin Dorfman syndrome), congenital lipodystrophy with insulin resistance and diabetes, and recurrent myoglobinuria crisis (lipin 1 deficiency). Phospholipids and glycosphingolipid synthesis and remodeling defects display a variety of neurodegenerative symptoms (spastic paraplegia, spinocerebellar ataxia, polyneuropathy, infantile epilepsy, infantile neuroaxonal dystrophy, neurodegeneration with brain iron accumulation, etc) myopathy and cardiomyopathy (like in Barth or Sengers syndromes); orthopedic signs (bone and chondrodysplasia, malformation); syndromic ichthyosis; and retinal dystrophy. At present, few of these disorders can be screened for using lipidomics[13] and diagnosis depend on molecular techniques.

Many other defects affecting systems involved in intracellular vesiculation trafficking, processing of complex molecules, and quality control processes (like protein folding and autophagy) can be anticipated. This is illustrated, for example, by the CEDNIK neurocutaneous syndrome owing to mutation of SNAP29 implicated in intracellular vesiculation,[14] as well as by mutations in AP5Z1, the cellular phenotype of which bears striking resemblance to features described in a number of lysosomal storage disorders.[15] This is also the case of the synaptic vesicle cycle.[16] Congenital disorders of autophagy are another emerging class of IEM presenting as complex neurometabolic disorders like SENDA or Vici syndrome.[17] These new defects, all found by exome sequencing without obvious metabolic markers, raise the question of a broader definition of lysosomal storage disorders with the accumulation of indigestible material in the endosomal–lysosomal system.

This oversimplified classification does not take into account the diversity and risks of cellular biology. The newly described metabolic disorders affecting cytoplasmic and mitochondrial transfer RNA synthetases and other factors implicated in the logistics and regulation of the cell challenge our current classification based on organelles and form a bridge between "classic" metabolic diseases with metabolic markers and those caused by structural proteins mutations without such markers and which are most often diagnosed by molecular techniques.[18]

Disorders affecting catabolism and the synthesis and recycling of complex molecules are summarized in **Tables 1** and **2**.

There are many overlapping metabolic and genetic mechanisms that challenge this simplified classification:

1. Some mitochondrial enzymes such as those implicated in the urea synthesis (carbamyl phosphate-synthetase I, ornithine-transcarbamylase, glutamate dehydrogenase) are regulated by SIRTUINS (SIRT), proteins that are induced by nutritional state.[19]
2. Tissue-specific proteins and the forthcoming clinical consequences of their mutations remain largely impossible to foresee. For example, the deficiency of adenylate kinase 2, an enzyme that is expressed in many tissues, presents with reticular dysgenesia syndrome, which is associated with a sensory neural deafness.[20]
3. The clinical consequences of compounds accumulated proximal to an enzymatic block can be unexpected; for example, thymidine accumulation in thymidine phosphorylase deficiency results in impaired mitochondrial DNA maintenance responsible for MNGIE syndrome (mitochondrial neurogastrointestinal encephalopathy); abnormal accumulation of polyols in the fetus, osmolyte substances implicated in fetal water metabolism is responsible for hydrops fetalis with the oligohydramnios observed in transaldolase deficiency.[21]
4. Ubiquitous dominant activating mutations can lead to unexpected organ-specific manifestations, like hyperinsulisms associated with hyperammonemia, or those induced by exercise in glutamate dehydrogenase and monocarboxylate transporter 1 genes mutations, respectively.[22]

Table 1
Inborn errors of complex molecules: Catabolism defects with visible storage material: "Storage disorders"

Biochemical Compounds	Defect and Location	Inherited Disorders (n) Major Clinical Findings
SPL	SPL degradation (lysosome, Golgi)	Sphingolipidosis[10] HSM, neurodeterioration, bone and neurologic crisis
Lipopigments	Degradation (lysosome)	Ceroid lipofuscinoses[13] Epilepsy, mental regression, optic atrophy, retinitis (RP)
Glycosaminoglycans (GAG)	Degradation (lysosome)	Mucopolysaccharidosis[14] Dysostosis multiplex, HSM, neurologic, eye findings
Oligosaccharides Glycoproteins/sialic acid	Degradation (lysosome)	Oligosaccharidosis, glycoproteinosis, mucolipidosis, sialidosis[14] Dysostosis multiplex, HSM, cognitive impairment, angiokeratoma
Glycogen	Degradation (cytosol, lysosome)	Glycogenosis[21] Hepatomegaly, hypoglycemia, myopathy, cardiomyopathy (Pompe) Cerebral glycogenosis (Lafora disease, etc)
Neutral lipids	Degradation (cytosol, lysosome)	Neutral lipid storage diseases[2] Many IEM with secondary steatosis

Abbreviations: HSM, hepatosplenomegaly; IEM, inborn errors of metabolism; RP, retinitis pigmentosa; SPL, sphingolipids.

Table 2
Inborn errors of complex molecules: Defects of synthesis and recycling: No storage material

Biochemical Compound	Defect and Localization	Inherited Disorders (n) Major Clinical Findings
Liver and muscle glycogen	Synthesis (cytoplasm)	GSD 0a: Ketotic hypoglycemia GSD 0b, Glycogenin: Myopathy, cardiomyopathy
Long, very long, and ultralong chain fatty acids, fatty alcohol, eicosanoids (prostaglandins, leukotrienes)	Extra mitochondrial synthesis and degradation (ER, microsome, peroxisome)	Peroxisomal β/α-oxidation[21] Fatty acid elongation defects[5] Eicosanoids/other defects (>5) Nervous system, bone, eye, skin, liver, inflammasome
TG, neutral lipids	Synthesis and recycling (cytosol, ER, lipid droplets)	TG synthesis, lipolytic defects (7 + 2 neutral lipid storage) Liver, muscle, skin
SPL 1. Ceramide 2. Phosphosphingolipids containing phosphate (sphingomyelin) 3. Glycosphingolipids containing sugar residue (gangliosides, globosides, cerebrosides, sulfatides, etc)	Synthesis and recycling (ER, Golgi, membranes)	Ceramide and SPL synthesis recycling defects[9] Nervous system (central and peripheral), skin (ichthyosis), retina (dystrophy)
GAG	Synthesis and recycling (cytosol, ER, Golgi)	GAG synthesis and recycling defects[20] Connective tissues: bone, cartilage, ligaments, skin, sclerae
PL including plasmalogen, cardiolipin, and polyphosphoinositides	Synthesis and recycling (cytosol, ER, peroxisome, mitochondrial membrane)	PL synthesis defects[11] including 5 plasmalogen defects PL remodeling defects[21] Nervous system, muscle, skin, bone, eye, immune system
Glycosylated proteins and lipids	Synthesis, processing, recycling (cytosol, ER, Golgi)	N-linked CDG (>60) O-CDG (>10) GPI/glycolipid (>15) Glycanopathy (>25) Nervous system, muscle, skin, eye, liver, bone
Isoprenoids (>30)	Synthesis, recycling (microsomes, ER, mitochondria, peroxisome)	Cholesterol[8]: congenital morphogenic anomalies Bile acids[8]: cholestasis, neurodegeneration Steroids synthesis defects[5] Dolichol (>5): CDG Ubiquinone[5]: mitochondrial defects
Dyslipidemias (>20)	Synthesis, recycling, transport	Atherosclerosis, premature coronary artery disease

Abbreviations: CDG, congenital disorders of glycosylation; ER, endoplasmic reticulum; GAG, glycosaminoglycans; GPI, glycosylphosphatidylinositol; GSD, glycogen storage disease; PL, phospholipids; SPL, sphingolipids; TG, triglycerides.

CLINICAL PRESENTATIONS OF INBORN ERRORS OF METABOLISM

A few metabolic disorders are recognized through newborn screening of the general population (as for phenylketonuria) or of at-risk families. Apart from these few, metabolic disorders present in 6 major groups of clinical circumstances.

Antenatal Symptoms

These can be classified in 3 major clinical categories[23]:

1. True major malformations (such as skeletal malformations, congenital heart disease, visceral aplasias, and neural tube defects);
2. Dysplasias (like cortical heterotopias, cortical cysts, posterior fossa abnormalities, polycystic kidneys, liver cysts); and
3. Functional signs (such as intrauterine growth retardation, hydrops fetalis, hepatosplenomegaly, microcephaly, coarse facies or facial dysmorphism).

According to this classification, true irreversible major malformations are only observed in O-glycosylation disorders that are primary, or secondary to manganese transporter *SLC39A8* mutations[4]; in cholesterol synthesis defects; in amino acid synthesis disorders, as with glutamine and asparagine synthetase deficiency (lissencephaly), and rarely in severe energetic defects such as glutaric aciduria type II; some respiratory chain disorders; and in the mitochondrial thiamine pyrophosphate carrier defect (*SLC25A19*) responsible for the Amish lethal microcephaly. A recently described omega 3 fatty acid transporter defect (MFSD2A) produce major brain gyration abnormalities and early death.[24] The vast majority of "true intoxication" disorders (amino acids and organic acids catabolism disorders) do not interfere with the embryofetal development.

Neonatal and Early Infancy Period

Acute encephalopathy and metabolic crash

- The neonate has a limited repertoire of responses to severe illness. IEM may present with nonspecific symptoms such as respiratory distress, hypotonia, poor sucking reflex, vomiting, lethargy, and seizures—problems that can easily be attributed to sepsis or some other common cause.

The death of a sibling previously from a similar IEM may have been attributed to sepsis, cardiac failure, or intraventricular hemorrhage. Group 1 disorders (intoxication) are illustrated by an infant born at full term who, after a normal pregnancy and delivery and an initial symptom-free period, relentlessly deteriorates for no apparent reason and does not respond to symptomatic therapy. The interval between birth and clinical symptoms may range from hours to weeks. Tests routinely performed on sick neonates include a chest radiograph, cerebrospinal fluid examination, bacteriologic studies, and cerebral ultrasound examination; all yield normal results. This unexpected and "mysterious" deterioration after a normal initial period is the most important indicator for this group of IEM. Careful reevaluation of the child's condition is then warranted. Neurologic deterioration (coma, lethargy) is the most frequent presenting sign in "intoxication" disorders. Typically, the first reported sign is poor sucking and feeding, after which the child sinks into an unexplained coma despite supportive measures. At a more advanced state, neurovegetative problems with respiratory abnormalities, hiccups, apneas, bradycardia, and hypothermia can occur. In the comatose state, characteristic changes in muscle tone and involuntary movements occur. Generalized hypertonic episodes with opisthotonus, boxing, or pedaling movements and slow limb elevations are observed in maple syrup urine disease. Because most nonmetabolic causes of coma are associated with hypotonia, the presence of "normal" peripheral muscle tone in a comatose child reflects a relative hypertonia. In organic acidurias, axial hypotonia and limb hypertonia with fast, large-amplitude tremors and myoclonic jerks (often mistaken for convulsions) are usual. Abnormal urine and body odor is present in some diseases in which volatile metabolites accumulate; for example, a maple syrup odor in maple syrup urine disease and the sweaty feet odor in isovaleric acidemia and glutaric acidemia type II (see Shawn E. McCandless and colleagues' article, "Inborn Errors of Metabolism with Acidosis: Organic Acidemias and Defects of Pyruvate and Ketone Body Metabolism," in this issue).

In energy deficiencies, the clinical presentation is less obvious and displays a more variable severity. In many conditions, there is no symptom-free interval. The most frequent findings are a severe generalized hypotonia, rapidly progressive neurologic deterioration, and possible dysmorphism or malformations. In contrast with the intoxication group, lethargy and coma are rarely initial signs. Hyperlactatemia with or without metabolic acidosis is frequent. Cardiac and hepatic involvement are also commonly associated with energy deficiencies.

In the neonatal period, only a few lysosomal storage disorders present with neurologic deterioration. By contrast, many peroxisomal biogenesis defects present at birth with dysmorphism and severe neurologic dysfunction. Severe forms of CDG involving N- and O-glycosylation, glycosylphosphatidylinositol anchor, and dolichol phosphate biosynthesis may also present with acute congenital neurologic dysfunction although they more often present with hypotonia, seizures, dysmorphism, malformations, and diverse visceral involvement.

Seizures

- Always consider the possibility of an IEM in a neonate with unexplained and refractory epilepsy.

Neonatal metabolic seizures are often a mixture of partial, erratic myoclonus of the face and extremities, or tonic seizures. Classically, the term "early myoclonic encephalopathy" has been used if myoclonic seizures dominate the clinical pattern. The electroencephalogram often shows a burst–suppression pattern; however, myoclonic jerks may occur without electroencephalographic abnormalities (see Mohammed Almannai and Ayman W. El-Hattab's article, "Inborn Errors of Metabolism with Seizures: Defects of Glycine and Serine Metabolism and Cofactor Related Disorders," in this issue).

Five treatable disorders can present in the neonatal period, predominantly with intractable seizures: pyridoxine-responsive seizures, folinic acid–responsive epilepsy (both allelic to antiquitin deficiency), pyridox(am)ine-5'-phosphate oxidase deficiency, 3-phosphoglycerate dehydrogenase deficiency responsive to serine supplementation, and persistent hyperinsulinemic hypoglycemia. Also, biotin-responsive holocarboxylase synthetase deficiency may rarely present predominantly with neonatal seizures. Glucose transport 1 (brain glucose transporter) deficiency, which is responsive to a ketogenic diet, and biotin-responsive biotinidase deficiency can also present in the first months of life as epileptic encephalopathy, but in these 2 disorders the early neonatal period is normally free of symptoms.

There are other recently described disorders presenting with severe early seizures in which a potential treatment has been suggested. These disorders are (i) manganese deficiency owing to SLC39A8 mutations (potentially treated by galactose, uridine and manganese)[4] and (ii) CAD mutations encoding a multifunctional enzyme involved in de novo pyrimidine biosynthesis, and responsive to uridine.[12]

Many other untreatable inherited disorders can present in the neonatal period with severe epilepsy: nonketotic hyperglycinemia (that can be due to the well-known glycine cleavage system defects and to the new disease related to *SLC6A9* mutations encoding a glycine transporter), D-glyceric aciduria, and mitochondrial glutamate transporter defect (all 3 presenting with myoclonic epilepsy and a burst–suppression electroencephalographic pattern), peroxisomal biogenesis defects, respiratory chain disorders, sulfite oxidase deficiency, Menkes' disease, and the new forms of CDG syndromes, dolichol, and glycosylphosphatidylinositol anchor biosynthesis defects. In all these conditions, epilepsy is severe, has an early onset, and can present with spasms, myoclonus, and partial or generalized tonic–clonic crises.

Hypotonia
Severe hypotonia is a common symptom in sick neonates. It is more generally observed in nonmetabolic severe fetal neuromuscular disorders. Only a few IEM present with iso-lated hypotonia in the neonatal period, and very few are treatable. The most severe metabolic hypotonias are observed in the congenital hyperlactatemias, respiratory chain disorders, urea cycle defects, nonketotic hyperglycinemia, sulfite oxidase defi-ciency, peroxisomal disorders, Lowe syndrome, and trifunctional enzyme deficiency. Severe forms of Pompe disease (alpha-glucosidase deficiency) can initially mimic res-piratory chain disorders or trifunctional enzyme deficiency when generalized hypotonia is associated with cardiomyopathy. However, Pompe disease does not strictly start in the neonatal period. Prader-Willi syndrome, one of the most frequent causes of isolated neonatal hypotonia at birth, can mimic hypotonia–cystinuria syndrome. Severe global hypotonia and hypomotility mimicking neuromuscular diseases can occur in some treat-able IEM, such as biogenic amine defects, primary carnitine deficiency (not strictly in the neonatal period), fatty acid oxidation defects, genetic defects of riboflavin transport, pri-mary coenzyme Q10 defects. Pyridostigmine responsive congenital myasthenic syn-drome can be a presenting sign in ALG2, ALG14, DPAGT1, GFPT1, and GMPPB-CDGs.

Other severe motor dysfunctions
Neonatal hypertonia is very common in sulfite oxidase deficiency and in hyperplexia owing to abnormal glycinergic transmission (mutations in receptors and transporters). Severe pontocerebellar hypoplasias (regardless of the specific genetic cause), early neonatal forms of Krabbe disease, and gangliosidosis can also produce major hypertonia with hyperexcitability signs. Fluctuating muscle strength, switching rapidly from a normal state to hypertonus of the extremities and trunk, can be the equivalent of dystonic move-ments in the immature newborn brain. Oculogyric crisis and other dyskinetic movements (orofacial and distal) can be associated. In such a clinical scenario, disorders with prom-inent basal ganglia dysfunction should be considered (eg, mitochondrial disorders, neurotransmitter defects). These neurologic presentations are summarized in **Table 3**.

Hepatic and gastrointestinal presentations
Six main clinical groups can be identified.

- Hepatomegaly with hypoglycemia and seizures without liver failure suggest glyco-genosis type I or III (typically massive hepatomegaly), gluconeogenesis defects, or severe hyperinsulinism (both with moderate hepatomegaly (see David A. Weinstein and colleagues' article, "Inborn Errors of Metabolism with Hypoglycemia: Glycogen Storage Diseases and Inherited Disorders of Gluconeogenesis," in this issue).
- Liver failure (jaundice, coagulopathy, hepatocellular necrosis with elevated serum transaminases, and hypoglycemia with ascites and edema) suggests fructosemia (now rare because infant formulas are fructose free); galactosemia; tyrosinemia

Table 3
Neurologic presentations in neonate and in early infancy

Predominant Clinical Symptom	Main Clinical Signs	Biological Signs	Best Diagnoses (Disorder/Enzyme Deficiency)
Neurologic deterioration: mostly metabolic and treatable	Lethargy, coma, hiccups, poor sucking, hypothermia, hypotonia, hypertonia, abnormal movements, large amplitude tremor, myoclonic jerks, "burst suppression," abnormal odor	Ketosis, acidosis	MSUD (odor)
		Hyperlactacidemia	MMA, PA, IVA (odor)
		Hyperammonemia	MCD
		Bone marrow suppression	Urea cycle defects
		Characteristic changes of AAC or OAC	CAVA deficiency
			GA II (odor)
Seizures: sometimes metabolic, sometimes treatable	Isolated	Metabolic ketoacidosis	MCD
	Generalized	Typical OAC profile	
		None	Pyridoxine responsive, folinic acid responsive (antiquitin deficiency)
		Hypocalcemia with hypomagnesemia	Congenital magnesium malabsorption
	Generalized hypsarrhythmia	Severe hypoglycemia	PHHI
	Major microcephaly	Low serine (plasma/CSF)	PGD (serine)
		Low blood manganese and a CDG type II profile	SLC39A8 (manganese)
	Severe hypotonia	Low HVA, 5 HIAA in CSF, vanillactic acid (urine)	PNPO (pyridoxamine phosphate responsive)
	Myoclonic jerks	Hyperglycinemia	NKH
	Burst suppression	None	Glutamate transporter
		S-Sulphocysteine	Sulfite oxidase
	Facial dysmorphia Malformations Severe hypotonia	VLCFA, phytanic, plasmalogen	Peroxisomal defects
		Glycosylated transferrin	CDG syndrome
		Sterols in plasma	Cholesterol biosynthesis
	Global psychomotor delay	Dyserythropoietic anemia (seen on a blood smear)	CAD defect (uridine)

Severe hypotonia: rarely metabolic, many not treatable	Isolated	None	Prader-Willi syndrome Hypotonia cystinuria syndrome
	Predominant dysmorphia	Massive cystinuria VLCFA, phytanic, plasmalogen Sterols in plasma Glycosylated transferrin APO-B glycosylation	Peroxisomal defects Cholesterol defects Glycosylation defects Multiple malformation syndromes with muscular dystrophy (Walker-Warburg syndrome, with muscle, eye, brain, other anomalies)
	Malformations		
	Cataract	Hyperlactatemia	Lowe syndrome
	Tubulopathy	Enzyme/DNA analyses	Respiratory chain
	Cardiomyopathy	Vacuolated lymphocytes	Pompe disease
	Abnormal movements (dystonia-parkinsonism, oculogyric crises), feeding difficulties, temperature instability	Abnormal CSF biogenic amines/pterins, glycine	Neurotransmitter disorders
	Pyridostigmine responsive congenital myasthenic syndrome	Serum transferrin IEF type 1 pattern in some Normal CK	ALG2, ALG14, DPAGT1, GFPT1, and GMPPB-CDGs
	Macroglossia	Hyperlactatemia	Respiratory chain
	Hepatopathy	Acylcarnitine	Trifunctional enzyme (FAO) Carnitine transporter, Riboflavin transporter
		COQ10 fibroblasts, muscle	Primary COQ10 defects

Abbreviations: 3 PGD, 3-phosphoglycerate dehydrogenase; 5 HIAA, 5-hydroxy indole acetic acid; AAC, amino acid chromatography; APO-B, apolipoprotein B; CAD, gene that encodes a multifunctional enzyme complex (comprising glutamine amidotransferase, carbamoyl phosphate synthase, aspartate transcarbamylase, dihydroorotase); CAVA, carbonic anhydrase VA isoform; CDG, congenital disorders of glycosylation; CK, creatine kinase; CoQ10, coenzyme Q10; CSF, cerebrospinal fluid; FAO, fatty acid oxidation; GA II, glutaric aciduria type II; HVA, homovanillic acid; IEF, isoelectric focusing; IVA, isovaleric acidemia; MCD, multiple carboxylase deficiency; MMA, methylmalonic aciduria; MSUD, maple syrup urine disease; NKH, nonketotic hyperglycinemia; OAC, organic acid chromatography; PA, propionic acidemia; PHHI, primary hyperinsulinemic hypoglycemia of infancy; PNPO, pyridox(am)ine-5'-phosphate oxidase; VLCFA, very long chain fatty acids.

type I (after 3 weeks; see Gerard T. Berry and colleagues' article, "Inborn Errors of Metabolism with Hepatopathy: Metabolism Defects of Galactose, Fructose, and Tyrosine," in this issue); neonatal hemochromatosis; respiratory chain disorders (and notably mitochondrial DNA depletion syndromes); and transaldolase deficiency, a disorder of the pentose phosphate pathway that can present with hydrops fetalis and severe anemia.[21] Severe fetal growth retardation, lactic acidosis, failure to thrive, hyperaminoaciduria, very high serum ferritin concentrations, hemosiderosis of the liver, and early death suggest GRACILE syndrome (Finnish lethal neonatal metabolic syndrome). The recently described mutations in *IARS* and *LARS* (coding for cytoplasmic isoleucyl and leucyl-tRNA synthetase, respectively) present with hypoalbuminemia, recurrent acute infantile liver failure, anemia, seizures, and encephalopathic crises.[25] Recently, *NBAS* mutations were also identified as a new molecular cause of fever-dependent episodes of recurrent acute infantile liver failure with onset in infancy.[26] A recent case of cytosolic phosphoenolpyruvate carboxykinase deficiency in a young child with liver failure, accumulation of tricarboxylic acid cycle metabolites on urine organic acid analysis, and hyperammonaemia with an amino acid profile suggestive of a proximal urea cycle defect, has been described. This is a treatable disease, reversible with intravenous dextrose.[27] Investigating individuals with severe hepatic failure is difficult with many pitfalls. At an advanced state, nonspecific abnormalities secondary to liver damage can be present. Melituria (galactosuria, glycosuria, fructosuria), hyperammonemia, hyperlactatemia, hypoglycemia after a short fast, hypertyrosinemia (>200 μmol/L), and hypermethioninemia (sometimes higher than 500 μmol/L) are encountered in most cases of advanced hepatocellular disease.

- Cholestatic jaundice with failure to thrive is a predominant finding in alpha1-antitrypsin deficiency, Byler disease, inborn errors of bile acid metabolism, peroxisomal disorders, Niemann-Pick type C disease, CDG syndromes, citrin deficiency and hepatocerebral syndrome owing to mitochondrial DNA depletion. Long-chain 3-hydroxyacyl-CoA dehydrogenase deficiency can present early in infancy as cholestatic jaundice, liver failure, and hepatic fibrosis. Cerebrotendinous xanthomatosis, citrin deficiency, arginase deficiency, and Niemann-Pick type C disease can present as a transient asymptomatic jaundice before neurologic signs manifest later in life. Two complex lipid synthesis disorders may also present with transient cholestatic liver disease: the MEGDHEL syndrome (*SERAC* mutation), which can mimic Niemann-Pick type C disease with a positive filipin test and the spastic paraparesis type 5 owing to oxysterol 7-hydroxylase deficiency.[9,10]

- Liver steatosis: Hepatic presentations of fatty acid oxidation disorders and urea cycle disorders consist of acute steatosis or Reye's syndrome presenting with normal bilirubin rather than true liver failure. Long-chain 3-hydroxyacyl-CoA dehydrogenase deficiency is an exception, which may present early in infancy (but not strictly in the neonatal period) as cholestatic jaundice, liver failure, and hepatic fibrosis. Chanarin-Dorfman syndrome (*ABHD5* mutations) presents early in infancy with liver steatosis, cataract, deafness, congenital ichthyosis, and myopathy, whereas the newly described cytoplasmic glycerol-3-phosphate dehydrogenase 1 deficiency displays an asymptomatic early infantile hepatomegaly and steatosis with transient hypertriglyceridemia[9,10]

- Hepatosplenomegaly with other signs of storage disorders (coarse facies, macroglossia, hydrops fetalis, ascites, edema, dysostosis multiplex, vacuolated lymphocytes) are observed in lysosomal diseases. Hepatosplenomegaly with inflammatory syndrome, including hematologic or immunologic features, may be observed in lysinuric protein intolerance (a macrophage-activating syndrome and leukopenia), mevalonic aciduria, (inflammatory syndrome and recurrent severe anemia), and transaldolase deficiency (hydrops fetalis with severe anemia).

- Congenital diarrheal disorders may be caused by mutations in genes related to disaccharidase deficiency, ion or nutrient transport defect like *SLC26A3* mutations causing congenital secretory chloride diarrhea, pancreatic insufficiency, lipid trafficking, or *PMI-CDG(Ib)* and ALG8-CDG(Ih). A disorder presenting with congenital diarrheal disorders linked to *DGAT1* mutations involved in triglycerides synthesis has been described recently. Affected neonates present with vomiting, colicky pain, and nonbloody, watery diarrhea, protein-losing enteropathy, hypoalbuminemia, and hyperlipidemia.

Cardiac presentations

Some metabolic disorders can present predominantly with cardiac disease. Heart failure and a dilated hypertrophic cardiomyopathy, most often associated with hypotonia, muscle weakness, and failure to thrive, suggests fatty acid oxidation disorders, respiratory chain disorders, or Pompe disease. Consider the possibility of a carnitine-uptake defect (systemic carnitine defect), which responds dramatically to carnitine administration. CDG syndrome can sometimes present in infancy with cardiac failure owing to pericardial effusion, cardiac tamponade, and cardiomyopathy. Many defects of long-chain fatty acid oxidation can present with cardiomyopathy, arrhythmias, or conduction defects, which may lead to cardiac arrest.

Initial approach to investigation

If clinical assessment suggests IEM, general supportive measures and laboratory investigations should be undertaken concurrently (**Table 4**). Abnormal urine odor can be diagnostic. Acetonuria (2–3+) in a newborn is always abnormal and is an important sign of metabolic disease. The metabolic acidosis of organic acidurias is usually accompanied by an elevated anion gap. Hyperammonemia with ketoacidosis suggests an underlying organic acidemia. An elevated ammonia level alone can induce respiratory alkalosis. Propionic, methylmalonic, and isovaleric acidemias frequently present with granulocytopenia and thrombocytopenia, which may be mistaken for sepsis. Adequate amounts of plasma, urine, blood on filter paper, and cerebrospinal fluid should always be stored, because they may later be important in establishing a diagnosis. How to make use of these precious samples should be carefully planned after getting advice from specialists in IEM.

Approach to therapy

Immediate therapy of acute encephalopathy owing to any of the likely IEM involves measures to decrease the production of offending metabolites and to increase their excretion. Treatment should include the following steps.

1. Ensure adequate cardiorespiratory function to allow removal of any accumulating metabolites. Adequate hydration is essential to maintain good urine output, because many of the offending diffusible metabolites are freely filtered at the glomerulus.
2. Reverse the catabolic state and reduce exposure to the offending nutrients. Neonates with severe ketoacidosis present with intracellular dehydration that is often underestimated. In this situation, aggressive rehydration with hypotonic fluids and alkalization may cause or exacerbate preexisting cerebral edema. Acidosis can be partially corrected with bicarbonate via intravenous administration, especially if it does not improve with the first measures applied for toxin removal. However, aggressive therapy with repeated intravenous doses of bicarbonate may induce hypernatremia, cerebral edema, and even cerebral hemorrhage. In mildly affected individuals, hydration can be performed using a standard 5% to 10% glucose solution

Table 4
Protocol for emergency investigations (neonatal and late-onset situations)

	Immediate Investigations	Storage of Samples
Urine	Smell (special odor) Look (special color) Urine dipstick tests for acetone, reducing substances, pH, sulfites Electrolytes (Na, K), urea, creatinine Uric acid	Urine collection: collect fresh sample and put it in the refrigerator Freezing: freeze samples collected before and after treatment at −20°C, and collect an aliquot 24 h after treatment Metabolic investigation: OAC, AAC, orotic acid, porphyrins
Blood	Blood cell count Electrolytes (search for anion gap) Glucose, calcium Blood gases (pH, P_{CO_2}, HCO_3, H, P_{O_2}) Uric acid Prothrombin time Transaminases (and other liver tests) CK Ammonia Lactic 3-hydroxybutyrate Free fatty acids	Plasma (5 mL) heparinized at −20°C Blood on filter paper: 2 spots (as "Guthrie" test) Whole blood (10 mL) collected on EDTA and frozen (for molecular biology studies) Major metabolic investigations: Total homocysteine, AAC, acylcarnitine (tandem MS), OAC, porphyrins, neurotransmitters
Miscellaneous	Lumbar puncture Chest radiograph Cardiac ultrasound, ECG Cerebral ultrasound, EEG	Skin biopsy (fibroblast culture) CSF (1 mL), frozen (neurotransmitters, AA) Postmortem: liver, muscle biopsies

Abbreviations: AA, amino acid; AAC, amino acid chromatography; CK, creatine kinase; CSF, cerebrospinal fluid; DNPH, dinitrophenylhydrazine; ECG, electrocardiogram; EDTA, ethylenediaminetetraacetic acid; EEG, electroencephalogram; MS, mass spectrometry; OAC, organic acid chromatography.

containing 75 mmol/L of Na^+ (4.5 g/L of NaCl) and 20 mmol/L of K^+ (1.5 g/L of KCl). High-calorie, protein-free nutrition should be started in parallel, using carbohydrates and lipids to provide 100 kcal/kg/d. Initially, for the 24- to 36-hour period needed to test gastric tolerance, parenteral and enteral nutrition are used together.

3. After these measures have been instituted, and even before a precise biochemical diagnosis has been made, begin hemodialysis or hemofiltration to remove the offending small molecules as quickly as possible if the affected individual is comatose or semicomatose.

4. Provide therapy specific to the disease, for example,:
   A. Whatever the disease, nutrition is extremely important and both the method of administration and the appropriate diet and nutrition must be rapidly determined. Briefly, 4 types of diet can be considered: normal, low protein, carbohydrate restricted, and high glucose, with or without lipid restriction.
   B. Cofactor administration, which sometimes improves the function of a genetically defective enzyme (eg, vitamin B_6 in recurrent intractable seizures, vitamin B_{12} in some cases of methylmalonic aciduria because it is a cofactor for methylmalonyl-CoA mutase).
   C. Metabolic manipulation and cleansing drugs, such as administering sodium benzoate in hyperammonemias or carnitine in organic acidurias, to divert a toxic substrate to a benign excretable form.

Later Onset, Acute, and Recurrent Attacks (Late Infancy and Beyond)

In about 50% of individuals with IEM, onset of symptoms is delayed. The symptom-free period is often longer than 1 year and may extend into late childhood, adolescence, or even adulthood. Each attack can follow a rapid course ending either in spontaneous improvement or unexplained death despite supportive measures. Between attacks, the affected individual may seem to be normal. The onset of acute disease may occur without an overt cause, but may be precipitated by an intercurrent event related to excessive protein intake, prolonged fasting, prolonged exercise, or any condition that enhances protein catabolism.

- Recurrent crises in a context of chronic encephalopathy or neurologic deterioration is an important signal for an IEM.

Coma, strokes, and attacks of vomiting with lethargy

Acute encephalopathy is a common problem in children and adults with IEM. All types of coma may be indicative of an IEM, including those presenting with focal neurologic signs (**Table 5**). Neither the age at onset, the accompanying clinical signs (hepatic, gastrointestinal, neurologic, psychiatric, etc), the mode of evolution (improvement, sequela, death), nor the routine laboratory data allow an IEM to be ruled out a priori. These comas may present with or without focal neurologic signs. The main varieties of metabolic coma may be observed in these late-onset, acute diseases, such as predominant metabolic acidosis, hypoglycemia, hyperammonemia, hyperlactacidemia, or combinations of these abnormalities. Many late-onset ornithine transcarbamylase deficiencies are first diagnosed with viral encephalitis and treated with Zovirax. Our aphorism to our residents was, "Write on the Zovirax box: did you test for hyperammonemia?" A neurologic coma with focal signs, seizures, severe intracranial hypertension, strokes, or strokelike episodes may be also observed in some individuals with organic acidemias and urea cycle defects. Strokes and cerebrovascular accidents are frequently presenting signs of all homocystinurias. Major findings are summarized in **Table 5**.

In summary, all these disorders should be considered in the differential diagnosis of strokes or strokelike episodes. In fact, these apparent initial acute manifestations are frequently preceded by other premonitory symptoms, such as acute ataxia, persistent anorexia, chronic vomiting, failure to thrive, hypotonia, and progressive developmental delay.

- Vaguely defined or undocumented diagnoses, such as encephalitis, basilar migraine, intoxication, poisoning, or cerebral thrombophlebitis, should therefore be questioned, particularly when even moderate ketoacidosis, hyperlactatemia, or hyperammonemia is present.

Acute psychiatric symptoms

Late-onset forms of congenital hyperammonemia, mainly partial ornithine transcarbamylase deficiency, can present late in childhood or in adolescence with psychiatric symptoms. Because hyperammonemia and liver dysfunction can be mild even at the time of acute attacks, these intermittent late-onset forms of urea cycle disorders can easily be misdiagnosed as hysteria, schizophrenia, or alcohol or drug intoxication. Acute intermittent porphyria and hereditary coproporphyria present classically with recurrent attacks of vomiting, abdominal pain, neuropathy, and psychiatric symptoms. *ATP1A3* and *RYR* 1 mutations encoding the ryanodine receptor mutations may be also a cause of childhood-onset schizophrenia and other acute psychiatric manifestations. Individuals with homocysteine remethylation defects may present with schizophrenia-like episodes that are responsive to folate.

Table 5
Diagnostic approach to recurrent attacks of coma and vomiting with lethargy

Clinical Presentation	Laboratory Studies	Other Features	Most Frequent Diagnosis (Disorder/Enzyme Deficiency)	Differential Diagnosis
Metabolic coma (without focal neurologic signs)	Acidosis (metabolic; pH <7.20,[a] CO$_3$H <10 mmol, Pco$_2$ <25 mm)	With Ketosis +	Organic acidurias,[a] MSUD[a] MCD,[a] PC, RCD Ketolysis defects,[a] MCT1[a] Gluconeogenesis defects[a] CAVA defect[a] TANGO II[a]	Diabetes Intoxication Encephalitis
	with or without hyperammonemia (NH$_3$ >100 μmol/L)	Without Ketosis –	PDH,[a] ketogenesis defects[a] FAO,[a] FDP,[a] EPEMA Riboflavin transporter[a]	
	Hyperammonemia (NH$_3$ >100 μmol/L)	Normal glucose	Urea cycle defects[a] Triple H,[a] LPI[a] TANGO II[a]	Reye syndrome Encephalitis Intoxication
	Respiratory alkalosis (pH >7.45, Pco$_2$ <25)	Hypoglycemia	FAO (MCAD)[a] HMG-CoA lyase[a]	
	Hypoglycemia (<2 mmol/L)	Acidosis +	Gluconeogenesis defects[a] MSUD[a] (ketosis +) HMG-CoA lyase[a] FAO[a] (ketosis –)	Drugs and toxin Ketotic hypoglycemia Adrenal insufficiency GH deficiency Hypopituitarism
	Hyperlactatemia (>4 mmol/L)	Normal glucose	PC, MCD,[a] Krebs cycle Respiratory chain PDH[a] (without ketosis) EPEMA syndrome	
		Hypoglycemia	Gluconeogenesis defects[a] (ketosis variable) FAO[a] (moderate hyperlactatemia, no ketosis) TANGO II	

Category	Clinical feature	Metabolic disorders	Differential diagnosis
Neurologic coma (with focal signs, seizures, or intracranial hypertension)	Biological signs are very variable, can be absent or moderate; see "Metabolic coma"		
	Cerebral edema	MSUD,[a] OTC[a]	Cerebral tumor Migraine Encephalitis Moyamoya syndrome
	Hemiplegia (hemianopsia)	MSUD,[a] OTC,[a] MMA,[a] PA,[a] PGK	Vascular hemiplegia
	Extrapyramidal signs	MMA,[a] GA I,[a] Wilson's disease[a] Homocystinuria[a]	
	Basal ganglia necrosis	BBGD (caudate and putamen necrosis)[a] Leigh syndrome[a]	
	Stroke and Strokelike symptoms	UCD,[a] MMA,[a] PA,[a] IVA[a] Respiratory chain (MELAS) Homocystinurias[a] CDG syndrome Thiamine-responsive megaloblastic anemia[a] Fabry[a] (rarely presenting sign) Maltase acid (rare) GLUT 10 ATP1A3	Cerebral thrombophlebitis Infectious acute necrotizing encephalitis Cerebral tumor Reye's syndrome
	RECA (some of them develop generalized dystonia)		
Abnormal coagulation	Thromboembolic accidents	Homocystinurias (all kinds)[a]	
Hemolytic anemia		CDG, PGK	

(continued on next page)

Table 5
(continued)

Clinical Presentation	Laboratory Studies	Other Features	Most Frequent Diagnosis (Disorder/Enzyme Deficiency)	Differential Diagnosis
Hepatic coma (hepatomegaly cytolysis or liver failure)	Normal bilirubin; Slight elevation of transaminases	Steatosis and fibrosis	FAO,[a] UCD[a]	Hepatitis; Reye's syndrome
Reye syndrome	Hyperlactatemia; Hemolytic jaundice	Liver failure; Cirrhosis	Respiratory chain defects; Wilson's disease[a]; Manganese transporter deficiency[a]	
	Hypoglycemia	Exudative enteropathy	Hepatic fibrosis with enteropathy (CDG Ib)[a]	

Abbreviations: BBGD, biotin-responsive basal ganglia disease also known as biotin–thiamine-responsive basal ganglia disease; CDG, carbohydrate–deficient glycoprotein syndrome; EPEMA, encephalopathy, petechiae, ethylmalonic aciduria syndrome; FAO, fatty acid oxidation; FDP, fructose 1-6 diphosphatase; GA, glutaric aciduria; GH, growth hormone; GLUT 10, Glucose transporter 19; HMG-CoA, 3-hydroxy-3-methylglutaryl coenzyme A; IVA, isovaleric acidemia; LPI, lysinuric protein intolerance; MCD, multiple carboxylase deficiency; MCT, monocarboxylic acid transporter; MELAS, mitochondrial encephalopathy lactic acidosis stroke-like episodes; MMA, methylmalonic acidemia; MSUD, maple syrup urine disease; OTC, ornithine transcarbamylase; PA, propionic acidemia; PC, pyruvate carboxylase; PDH, pyruvate dehydrogenase; PGK, phosphoglycerate kinase; RCD, respiratory-chain defects; RECA, relapsing encephalopathy with cerebellar ataxia; TANGO II, transport and Golgi organization 2; UCD, urea cycle disorders.

[a] Treatable disorders.

- In view of these possible diagnoses, it is justified to systematically measure ammonia, porphyrins, and plasma homocysteine in every individual presenting with unexplained acute psychiatric symptoms.[28]

Reye's syndrome, sudden unexpected death in infancy, and near miss

There is now considerable evidence that many IEM responsible for Reye's syndrome (mostly fatty acid oxidation and urea cycle defects) were misdiagnosed in the past because of inadequate research into IEM. True sudden unexpected death in infancy owing to an IEM is a rare event despite the large number of publications on the topic and despite the fact that at least 30 metabolic defects are possible causes.[29] However, it is important to note that this assertion is not true in the first week of life.

- Fatty acid oxidation disorders are a major cause of sudden unexpected death in infancy or near-miss in the first weeks of life.

Exercise intolerance and recurrent myoglobinuria

In the glycolytic disorders mostly observed in late childhood, adolescence, or adulthood, exercising muscle is most vulnerable during the initial stages of exercise and during intense exercise. A "second-wind" phenomenon sometimes develops. The creatine kinase level remains elevated in most affected individuals. The most frequent and typical disorder in this group is McArdle's disease.

In the fatty acid oxidation disorders, attacks of myoglobinuria occur typically after mild to moderate prolonged exercise and are particularly likely when affected individuals are under additional stress during fasting, cold, or infection (see Jerry Vockley and Areeg El-Gharbawy's article, "Inborn Errors of Metabolism with Myopathy: Defects of Fatty Acid Oxidation and the Carnitine Shuttle System," in this issue).

Mutations in *TANGO2* encoding transport and Golgi organization 2 homolog have been described recently in infants and children with episodic rhabdomyolysis, hypoglycemia, hyperammonemia, and susceptibility to life-threatening cardiac tachyarrhythmias mimicking a fatty acid oxidation defect.[30] Mutations in *RYR 1* encoding the ryanodine receptor present with muscle rigidity and rhabdomyolysis when affected individuals are exposed to general anesthesia in infancy. *Lipin1* mutations have been found recently to be the second most frequent cause of unexplained recurrent myoglobinuria triggered by fever after exclusion of primary fatty acid oxidation disorder in infancy. Respiratory chain disorders can present with recurrent muscle pain and myoglobinuria from the neonatal period to adolescence.

Chronic Gastrointestinal Involvement, Failure to Thrive, Anemia, and Recurrent Infections

Gastrointestinal nonspecific findings (anorexia, failure to thrive, chronic vomiting) and osteoporosis occur in a wide variety of IEM. Unfortunately, their cause often remains unrecognized, further delaying diagnosis. Persistent anorexia, feeding difficulties, chronic vomiting, failure to thrive, frequent infections, osteopenia, generalized hypotonia in association with chronic diarrhea, anemia, and bone marrow suppression are frequent presenting symptoms and signs in IEM. They are easily misdiagnosed as cow's milk protein intolerance; celiac disease; chronic ear, nose, and throat infections; late-onset chronic pyloric stenosis; and so on. Congenital immunodeficiencies are also frequently considered, although only a few congenital immunodeficiencies present early in infancy with this clinical picture.

- When there is no definitive diagnosis despite extensive gastroenterological, hematologic, and immunologic testing, it is necessary to seriously consider

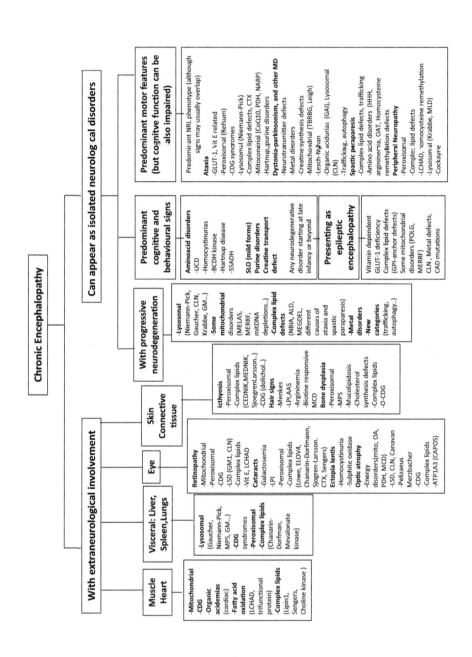

conditions such as organic aciduria-methylmalonic aciduria, propionic acidemia, isovaleric acidemia, urea cycle defects, lysinuric protein intolerance, and respiratory chain defects

Developmental Delay and Neurologic Syndromes

Neurologic symptoms are very frequent and encompass progressive psychomotor retardation, seizures, several neurologic abnormalities in both the central and peripheral nervous systems, sensorineural defects, and psychiatric symptoms.[31–33] In the 21st century, many new disorders involving the nervous system were revealed using a genome-wide next-generation sequencing approach, in an individual in whom clinical suspicion of an IEM was low before genetic testing. This finding is mostly true for the mitochondrial disorders (>300 new defects), congenital disorders of glycosylation (>100 new defects), and the new category of complex lipid and fatty acid synthesis and remodeling defects (>60 new disorders). A highly simplified general approach to identification of IEM associated with chronic encephalopathy is shown in **Fig. 1**. Some IEM start in early childhood with rather unspecific or insidious symptoms and become characteristic only in adulthood.[34]

- The clinical approach should be always based on searching for associated extraneurologic symptoms. These signs are sometimes obvious, like generalized ichthyosis, massive hepatosplenomegaly, bone dysplasia, or severe myocardiopathy, and so on, but may also be subtle and easily missed if not systematically investigated like isolated moderate splenomegaly, interstitial pneumonia, retinitis pigmentosa, macrocytic anemia, or poikilocytosis.

Table 6 presents laboratory tests for investigating neurologic syndromes and focuses on treatable IEM. Disorders requiring urgent attention (in hospital emergency facilities) are noted.

Specific Organ Signs and Symptoms

IEM can involve any organ or system in any scenarios at any age, the specific description of which is beyond the scope of this general article.

Fig. 1. Diagnostic approach to chronic encephalopathy. AAS, arginino succinic aciduria; ALD, adrenoleukodystrophy; BCDH, branched chain dehydrogenase; CAD, gene that encodes a multifunctional enzyme complex (comprising glutamine amidotransferase, carbamoyl phosphate synthase, aspartate transcarbamylase, dihydroorotase); CAPOS, episodic cerebellar ataxia, areflexia (peripheral neuropathy), optic atrophy, and sensorineural hearing loss; CDG, congenital disorders of glycosylation; CLN, ceroid neuronal lipofuscinosis; CoQ10, coenzyme Q10; CTX, cerebrotendinous xantomatosis; GAI, Glutaric aciduria type I; GLUT-1, glucose transporter deficiency type 1; GM, gangliosidosis; GPI, glycosidilphosphoinositol; HHH, hyperornithinemia, hyperammonaemia, homocitrullinuria; LCHAD, long-chain 3-hydroxyacyl-CoA dehydrogenase; LPI, lysinuric protein intolerance; LSD, lysosomal storage disorders; MCD, multiple carboxylase deficiency; MD, movement disorders; MEGDEL, 3-methylglutaconic aciduria, deafness, encephalopathy, Leigh-like disease; MELAS, mitochondrial encephalomyopathy, lactic acidosis, strokelike episodes; MERRF, myoclonic epilepsy, ragged-red fibers; MLD, metachormatic leukodystrophy; MPS, mucopolysaccharidoses; NARP, neuropathy, ataxia, retinopathy, peripheral neuropathy; NBIA, neurodegeneration with brain iron accumulation; OA, organic acidurias; OAT, ornithine aminotransferase; PDH, pyruvate dehydrogenase; POLG, polymerase gamma deficiency; SLO, Smith-Lemli-Opitz syndrome; SSADH, succinyl semialdehyde dehydrogenase; TBRBG, thiamine biotin responsive basal ganglia disease; UCD, urea cycle disorders.

Table 6
Recommended laboratory tests in neurologic syndromes focused on treatable inborn errors of metabolism[a]

Predominant Neurologic Syndrome	Laboratory Tests (Rational Approach Based on Associated Clinical Signs and Treatable Disorders)	Disorders
Isolated developmental delay/ID	• Basic laboratory tests[b]: blood glucose, acid–base status, blood counts, liver function, creatine kinase, uric acid, thyroid function, alkaline phosphatase • Plasma: lactate, ammonium, amino acids, total homocysteine, folate, biotinidase activity • Urine: creatine metabolites, organic acids (including 4-hydroxybutyric acid), amino acids, GAGs, purines, pyrimidines, • Consider maternal phenylalanine	PKU,[a] homocystinurias,[a] urea cycle defects,[a] amino acid synthesis defects, thyroid defects,[a] biotinidase deficiency,[a] Hartnup disease[a]
With dysmorphic features	• Consider also plasma sterols, peroxisomal studies (very long-chain fatty acids, phytanic acid, plasmalogens), transferrin isoelectric focusing for glycosylation studies (CDG), mucopolysaccharides and oligosaccharides in urine • For the study of ID with or without dysmorphic features, genetic tests (cytogenetic studies, microarrays, NGS, and targeted studies) have the highest diagnostic yield.	SLO syndrome, peroxisomal diseases (only partially by some supplements) mucopolyclysaccharidosis Oligosaccharidosis Sialidosis CDG Some PL synthesis
Behavioral and psychiatric manifestations including autistic signs	• Basic laboratory tests[b] • Plasma: ammonium, amino acids, total homocysteine, folate, sterols (including oxysterols), copper, ceruloplasmin • Urine: GAGs, organic acids (4-hydroxybutyric acid), amino acids, purines, creatine, creatinine, and guanidinoacetate • Depending on additional clinical signs and brain MRI pattern: peroxisomal studies, lysosomal studies	PKU,[a] urea cycle disorders,[a] homocystinurias,[a] folate metabolism[a] Wilson's disease,[a] BCKDH kinase deficiency, CTD, mild forms of SLO, Niemann-Pick type C disease, X-ADL (at some stages), Hartnup disease, MPS III

| Epilepsy | • Basic laboratory tests[b] adding calcium, magnesium and manganese
• Plasma: lactate, ammonium, amino acids, total homocysteine, folate, biotinidase activity, copper and ceruloplasmin, VLCFA
• Urine: organic acids, creatine, creatinine and guanidinoacetate, sulfite test, purines and pyrimidines, pipecolic acid and 5-AASA
• CSF: glucose, lactate, amino acids, 5-MTHF, pterins, biogenic amines, GABA
• Consider lysosomal studies and targeted tests if PME
• Consider genetic tests for GPI-anchor biosynthesis pathway defects and other defects of complex lipid synthesis (FA2H, ELOVL4, GM3 synthetase) | GLUT-1,[a] homocystinurias,[a] IEM of folate metabolism,[a] organic acidurias,[a] biotinidase deficiency,[a] creatine synthesis defects, serine biosynthesis defects, Menkes disease (only partially treatable), late-onset forms of pyridoxine-dependent epilepsy,[a] pterin defects (DHPR),[a] AADC deficiency,[a] MoCo deficiency (cyclic pyranopterin monophosphate: treatment recently introduced) |
| Ataxia | • Basic laboratory tests[b] adding albumin, cholesterol, triglycerides, and alpha-fetoprotein
• Plasma: lactate, pyruvate, ammonium, amino acids, biotinidase activity, vitamin E, sterols (including oxysterols), ceruloplasmin, peroxisomal studies (including phytanic acid), coenzyme Q10, transferrin electrophoresis
• Urine: organic acids (including 4-hydroxybutyric and mevalonic acids), amino acids, purines
• CSF: glucose, lactate, pyruvate
• Consider lysosomal/mitochondrial/NBIA studies depending on the clinical and brain MRI signs. Consider lipidome studies (plasma, CSF)
• Consider genetic panels of inherited ataxias | PDH deficiency (thiamine-responsive; ketogenic diet),[a] biotinidase deficiency,[a] GLUT-1,[a] abetalipoproteinemia, CTX,[a] Refsum disease, coenzyme Q10 deficiencies,[a] Harnup disease, Niemann-Pick type C disease
CDGs |

(continued on next page)

Table 6
(continued)

Predominant Neurologic Syndrome	Laboratory Tests (Rational Approach Based on Associated Clinical Signs and Treatable Disorders)	Disorders
Dystonia-Parkinsonism	• Basic laboratory tests[b] • Plasma: lactate, pyruvate, ammonium, amino acids, biotinidase activity, sterols (including oxysterols), copper, ceruloplasmin, uric acid, manganese • Urine: organic acids, uric acid, creatine, creatinine and guanidinoacetate, purines, GAGs, oligosaccharides • CSF: glucose, lactate, pyruvate, amino acids, 5-methyltetra-hydrofolate, pterins, biogenic amines, GABA • Consider lysosomal/mitochondrial/NBIA studies depending on the clinical and brain MRI signs • Consider genetic panels of inherited dystonias, parkinsonism, and other NGS techniques	Neurotransmitter defects,[a] GLUT-1 deficiency,[a] thiamine transport defects (TBBGD),[a] PDH defects,[a] organic acidurias,[a] homocystinurias,[a] IEM of folate metabolism,[a] defects of creatine biosynthesis, Wilson's disease,[a] biotinidase deficiency,[a] Niemann-Pick type C disease, CTX,[a] manganese defects[a]
Chorea	• Basic laboratory tests[b] • Plasma: lactate, pyruvate, ammonium, amino acids, total homocystinuria, folate, biotinidase activity, sterols (including oxysterols), copper, ceruloplasmin, uric acid, galactose 1 P, transferrin electrophoresis • Urine: organic acids, uric acid, creatine, creatinine and guanidinoacetate, purines, galactitol, sulfite test • CSF: glucose, lactate, pyruvate, amino acids, 5-methyltetra-hydrofolate, pterins, biogenic amines, GABA • Consider NCL studies and GPI-anchor synthesis defect genetic tests Consider genetic panels of inherited choreas, and other NGS techniques	Glutaric aciduria I and other classic organic acidurias (MMA, PA), GAMT, GLUT-1, homocystinurias, pterin and neurotransmitter defects, Niemann-Pick disease type C, Wilson's disease,[a] galactosemia, cerebral folate deficiency owing to FOLR mutations, MoCo deficiency, NKH

Spasticity	• Basic laboratory tests[b] • Plasma: lactate, pyruvate, ammonium, amino acids, total homocystinuria, folate, biotinidase activity, vitamin E, triglycerides, cholesterol, sterols, peroxisomal studies • Urine: organic acids, amino acids, GAGs, oligosaccharides, sialic acid, purines • CSF: biogenic amines, pterins and 5-MTHF • Consider lysosomal/mitochondrial/NBIA studies depending on clinical and MRI findings • Consider genes related to HSP and plasma, CSF lipidome	HHH, arginase deficiency, ornithine aminotransferase deficiency, homocysteine remethylation defects, biotinidase deficiency, cerebral folate deficiencies, dopamine synthesis defects (atypical TH), CTX, vitamin E deficiency
Peripheral neuropathy	• Basic laboratory tests[b] • Plasma: lactate, pyruvate, ammonium, amino acids, folate, vitamin E, triglycerides, cholesterol, acylcarnitines, sterols, peroxisomal studies, transferrin electrophoresis • Urine: amino acids, GAGs, oligosaccharides, thymidine, porphyrins • Consider lysosomal/mitochondrial/NBIA studies depending on clinical and MRI findings	Refsum disease, X-ADL (treatable at some stages), homocysteine remethylation defects, CTX, abetalipoproteinemia, LCHAD, trifunctional protein, PDH, vitamin E malabsorption, ornithine aminotransferase, serine deficiency

Abbreviations: 5-AASA, 5-aminoadipic semialdehyde; 5-MTHF, 5-methyltetrahydrofolate; AADC, amino acid decarboxylase; BCKDH, branched chain keto acid dehydrogenase; CDG, carbohydrate-deficient glycoprotein syndrome; CSF, cerebrospinal fluid; CTD, carnitine transport defect; CTX, cerebrotendinous xanthomatosis; DHPR, dihydropteridine reductase; FOLR, folate receptor; GABA, gamma aminobutyric acid; GAG, glycosamineglycan; GAMT, guanidinoacetate methyltransferase; GLUT-1, glucose transport I; GPI, glycosylphosphatidylinositol; HHH, hyperammonemia, hyperornithinemia, homocitrullinuria; HSP, hereditary spastic paraparesis; ID, intellectual disability; IEM, inborn errors of metabolism; LCHAD, long-chain 3-hydroxyacyl-CoA dehydrogenase; MMA, methylmalonic aciduria; MoCo, molybdenum cofactor deficiency; MPS, mucopolysaccharidoses; NBIA, neurodegeneration with brain iron accumulation; NCL, neuronal ceroid lipofuscinosis; NGS, next-generation sequencing; NKH, nonketotic hyperglycinemia; PA, propionic academia; PDH, pyruvate dehydrogenase deficiency; PKU, Phenylketonuria; PL, phospholipids; PME, progressive myoclonus epilepsy; SLO, Smith-Lemli-Optiz syndrome; TH, tyrosine hydroxylase; VLCFA, very long chain fatty acids; X-ADL, x-linked adrenoleukodystrophy.

[a] Treatable disorders.

[b] These basic laboratory tests should be considered as a routine screening in every neurologic syndrome.

Adapted from Saudubray JM, Baumgartner M, Walter J. Inborn metabolic diseases diagnosis and treatment, vol. 1. 6th edition. Heidelberg (Germany): Springer; 2016. p. 658.

WHEN AND HOW FAR TO INVESTIGATE A METABOLIC DISORDER

All organs being dependent on cellular metabolism, it could be anticipated that IEM can potentially disturb all organs and cellular systems in any scenario at any age and with any mode of heredity. But of course this does not mean that extensive metabolic investigations are required in all individuals with unexplained symptomatology.

Despite the massive progress accomplished in medical and scientific research that has to do with the brain, mainly in neurophysiology, brain imaging, classical and molecular karyotyping, and molecular testing, many individuals with an intellectual disability remain undiagnosed. Isolated developmental delay or intellectual disability of apparently unknown cause has become one of the most important concern in public health because it affects up to 3% of the pediatric population.[31]

The hope for a treatable, disorder-specific illness or at least a prognosis and genetic counseling motivates affected individuals and their families to pursue a specific diagnosis as early as possible. In this context, IEM are very attractive possibilities (as compared with other potential diagnoses), because many of them are easily identified using plasma or urine tests, have a well-understood pathophysiology, are amenable to treatment, and can be recognized early in pregnancy. However, even in countries where phenylketonuria is detected by newborn screening, IEM are rarely the cause of isolated intellectual disability. Furthermore, there is no international agreement about what type of metabolic tests should be performed on individuals with unspecific intellectual disability and there are 2 common extremes: physicians with no real knowledge of IEM who unintentionally miss a diagnosis and potentially life-saving treatment because they do not consider IEM at all, and inexperienced or overly systematic professionals performing time- and money-consuming metabolic investigations in situations that do not call for them because of the pressure for a diagnosis from affected individuals and their families.

In neurology, several review papers have been published recently describing clinical algorithms and metabolic protocols in the most frequent neurologic syndromes (mental retardation, epilepsy, leukodystrophy, abnormal movements, and peripheral neuropathy) in children[30–32] and in adults.[34] Per current research, metabolic investigations can be considered mandatory in 3 circumstances (**Box 4**).

Most disorders treatable by special diets, vitamins, or cleansing drugs belong to the intoxication group of intermediary metabolism. Metabolic disturbances can be transient and may only be present during the acute attack. Some affected individuals can die during an attack before any metabolic sampling has been performed. Some metabolic disorders with an acute crisis do not disturb the first-line metabolic profile.

Box 4
Circumstances for mandatory metabolic investigation

1. In urgent situations, owing to an acute decompensation or to a rapid actual or potential deterioration, it is important to rule out all treatable metabolic disorders. In such circumstances, sample first, treat, and then think.

2. In case of a new and unexpected pregnancy, appropriate metabolic investigations with regard to the clinical context of the index case are mandatory to give rapid and accurate genetic counseling and not to miss an antenatal diagnosis.

3. When symptoms (like intellectual disability and neurologic syndromes) are persistent, progressive, and remain unexplained after the usual investigations for more common disorders have been performed, a comprehensive metabolic investigation is also warranted. The other neurologic scenario where metabolic studies are greatly required is in early unexplained encephalopathies.

Some metabolic disturbances must be interpreted in the clinical context. A fasting hypoglycemia associated with permanent hepatomegaly, lactic acidosis, or without concomitant acetonuria is almost always related to an IEM. Conversely, a sporadic fasting ketotic hypoglycemia without acidosis and hepatomegaly is rarely, if ever, related to an IEM. That is also true for isolated periodic vomiting with no lethargy, no hepatomegaly, and no acidosis.

In these contexts, think first and then sample, and send to appropriate laboratories for specific targeted investigations rather than performing a systematic checklist, which is time consuming and has a low cost to benefit ratio (see **Table 6**). In all other circumstances, as soon as the basal metabolic tests for identifying treatable disorders have been performed, it is advisable to wait and see, and to repeat the clinical evaluation.

REFERENCES

1. Scriver CR, Beaudet AL, Valle D, et al. 8th edition. The metabolic and molecular basis of inherited diseases, vol. 4. New York: Mc Graw hill; 2001. p. 6338.
2. Saudubray JM, Baumgartner M, Walter J. 6th edition. Inborn metabolic diseases diagnosis and treatment, vol. 1. Heidelberg (Germany): Springer; 2016. p. 658.
3. Saudubray JM, Sedel F, Walter JH. Clinical approach to treatable inborn metabolic diseases: an introduction. J Inherit Metab Dis 2006;29:261–74.
4. Park JH, Hogrebe M, Grüneberg M, et al. SLC39A8 deficiency: a disorder of manganese transport and glycosylation. Am J Hum Genet 2015;97:894–903.
5. Tarlungeanu DC, Deliu E, Dotter CP, et al. Impaired amino acid transport at the blood brain barrier is a cause of autism spectrum disorder. Cell 2016;167:1481–94.
6. Anikster Y, Haack TB, Vilboux T, et al. Biallelic mutations in DNAJC12 cause hyperphenylalaninemia, dystonia, and intellectual disability. Am J Hum Genet 2017; 100:1–10.
7. De Koning TJ, Klomp LW, van Oppen AC, et al. Prenatal and early postnatal treatment in 3-phosphoglycerate-dehydrogenase deficiency. Lancet 2004;364:2221–2.
8. Zala D, Hinckelmann MV, Yu H, et al. Vesicular glycolysis provides on-board energy for fast axonal transport. Cell 2013;152:479–91.
9. Lamari F, Mochel F, Saudubray JM. An overview of inborn errors of complex lipid biosynthesis and remodeling. J Inherit Metab Dis 2015;38:3–18.
10. Garcia-Cazorla A, Mochel F, Lamari F, et al. The clinical spectrum of inherited diseases involved in the synthesis and remodeling of complex lipids. A tentative overview. J Inherit Metab Dis 2015;38:19–40.
11. Sasarman F, Maftei C, Campeau PM, et al. Biosynthesis of glycosaminoglycans: associated disorders and biochemical tests. J Inherit Metab Dis 2016;39:173–88 [review].
12. Koch J, Mayr JA, Alhaddad B, et al. CAD mutations and uridine-responsive epileptic encephalopathy. Brain 2017;140:279–86.
13. Vaz FM, Pras-Raves M, Bootsma AH, et al. Principles and practice of lipidomics. J Inherit Metab Dis 2015;38:41–52.
14. Sprecher ED, Ischida-Yamamoto A, Mizrahi-Koren M, et al. A mutation in SNAP29,-coding for a SNARE protein involved in intracellular trafficking, causes a novel neurocutaneous syndrome characterized by cerebral dysgenesis, neuropathy, ichthyosis, and palmoplantar keratoderma. Am J Hum Genet 2005;77:242–51.
15. Hirst J, Edgar JR, Esteves T, et al. Loss of AP-5 results in accumulation of aberrant endolysosomes: defining a new type of lysosomal storage disease. Hum Mol Genet 2015;24:4984–96.

16. Cortès-Saladelafont E, Tristán-Noguero A, Artuch R, et al. Diseases of the synaptic vesicle: a potential new group of neurometabolic disorders affecting neurotransmission. Semin Pediatr Neurol 2016;23(4):306–20.
17. Ebrahimi-Fakhari D, Saffari A, Wahlster L, et al. Congenital disorders of autophagy: an emerging novel class of inborn errors of neuro-metabolism. Brain 2016;139:317–37.
18. Morava E, Rahman S, Peters V, et al. Quo vadis: the redefinition of inborn metabolic diseases. J Inherit Metab Dis 2015;38:1003–6.
19. Nakagawa T, Lomb DJ, Haigis MC, et al. SIRT5 Deacetylates carbamoyl phosphate synthetase 1 and regulates the urea cycle. Cell 2009;137:560–70.
20. Lagresle-Peyrou C, Six EM, Picard C, et al. Human adenylate kinase 2 deficiency causes a profound hematopoietic defect associated with sensorineural deafness. Nat Genet 2009;41:106 11.
21. Valayannopoulos V, Verhoeven NM, Mention K, et al. Transaldolase deficiency: a new cause of hydrops fetalis and neonatal multi-organ disease. J Pediatr 2006; 149:713–7.
22. Arnoux JB, Saint-Martin C, Montravers F, et al. An update on congenital hyperinsulinism: advances in diagnosis and management. Expert Opin Orphan Drugs 2014;2:779–95.
23. Collardeau-Frachon S, Cordier MP, Rossi M, et al. Antenatal manifestations of inborn errors of metabolism: autopsy findings suggestive of a metabolic disorder. J Inherit Metab Dis 2016;39:597–610.
24. Guemez-Gamboa A, Nguyen LN, Yang H, et al. Inactivating mutations in MFSD2A, required for omega-3 fatty acid transport in brain, cause a lethal microcephaly syndrome. Nat Genet 2015;47:809–13.
25. Casey JP, Slattery S, Cotter M, et al. Clinical and genetic characterization of infantile liver failure syndrome type I, due to recessive mutations in LARS. J Inherit Metab Dis 2015;38:1085–93.
26. Staufner C, Haack TB, Köpke MG, et al. Recurrent acute liver failure due to NBAS deficiency: phenotypic spectrum, disease mechanisms, and therapeutic concepts. J Inherit Metab Dis 2016;39:13–6.
27. Santra S, Cameron JM, Shyr C, et al. Cytosolic phosphoenolpyruvate carboxykinase deficiency presenting with acute liver failure following gastroenteritis. Mol Genet Metab 2016;118:21–7.
28. Walterfang M, Bonnot O, Mocellin R, et al. The neuropsychiatry of inborn errors of metabolism. J Inherit Metab Dis 2013;36:687–702.
29. van Rijt WJ, Koolhaas GD, Bekhof J, et al. Inborn errors of metabolism that cause sudden infant death: a systematic review with implications for population neonatal screening programmes. Neonatology 2016;109:297–302.
30. Lalani SR, Liu P, Rosenfeld JA, et al. Recurrent muscle weakness with rhabdomyolysis, metabolic crises, and cardiac arrhythmia due to Bi-allelic TANGO2 mutations. Am J Hum Genet 2016;98:347–57.
31. García-Cazorla A, Wolf NI, Serrano M, et al. Mental retardation and inborn errors of metabolism. J Inherit Metab Dis 2009;31:597–608.
32. García-Cazorla A, Wolf NI, Serrano M, et al. Inborn errors of metabolism and motor disturbances in children. J Inherit Metab Dis 2009;31:618–29.
33. Wolf NI, García-Cazorla A, Hoffmann GF. Epilepsy and inborn errors of metabolism in children. J Inherit Metab Dis 2009;31:609–17.
34. Hollak C, Lachmann RH. Inherited metabolic diseases in adults. A clinical guide, vol. 1. Oxford: Oxford University Press; 2016. p. 626.

Inborn Errors of Metabolism with Acidosis

Organic Acidemias and Defects of Pyruvate and Ketone Body Metabolism

Lori-Anne P. Schillaci, MD, Suzanne D. DeBrosse, MD,
Shawn E. McCandless, MD*

KEYWORDS

- Organic acidemia • Ketone utilization • Pyruvate metabolism • Metabolic acidosis
- Ketoacidosis • Inborn error of metabolism

KEY POINTS

- Early identification and treatment of inborn errors of metabolism can prevent irreversible damage.
- A normal newborn screen does not rule out an inborn error of metabolism.
- Acute treatment to reverse catabolism does not require precise diagnosis.
- Collect and freeze extra serum and urine samples during the acute presentation.

Pediatricians know that inborn errors of metabolism (IEM) require early diagnosis and early treatment to prevent permanent neurologic damage.[1] Most patients present acutely in the neonatal period with nonspecific symptoms, but they can appear later with a few common presentations, including hypoglycemia; hyperammonemia; neurologic abnormalities; and, the focus of this article, increased anion gap metabolic acidosis. This article intends to help the practicing provider use basic laboratory findings to identify those children at highest risk for an IEM and initiate life-saving and brain-sparing treatments.

Metabolic acidosis is the accumulation of excess hydrogen ions in the blood. Lower pH reflects a higher concentration of unbuffered (free) hydrogen ions. Although this is the physiologically significant issue in most cases of acidosis, accurate diagnosis and

Disclosure Statement: The authors have nothing to disclose related to the subject matter of this article.
Department of Genetics and Genome Sciences, Case Western Reserve University, Center for Human Genetics, University Hospitals Cleveland Medical Center, 11100 Euclid Avenue, Suite 1500 Lakeside Building, Cleveland, OH 44106, USA
* Corresponding author. Center for Human Genetics, 11100 Euclid Avenue, Suite 1500 Lakeside Building, Cleveland, OH 44106.
E-mail address: Shawn.McCandless@case.edu

management is more concerned with the anions accumulating in association with the hydrogen ion and, in the IEM, these anions may cause toxicity. Metabolic acidosis can be readily demonstrated through blood gas and electrolyte measurements and is characterized by decreased blood pH, decreased bicarbonate (HCO_3^-), and decreased Pco_2. Specifically, metabolic acidosis is defined as pH less than 7.30, Pco_2 less than 30, and serum HCO_3^- less than 15.[2] The reduced Pco_2 reflects the respiratory response to compensate, confirming that the acidosis is not secondary to respiratory insufficiency, thus it is a metabolic acidosis.

Basic blood chemistries measure the most common cations and anions in the serum, sodium (Na^+) being the major cation, and chloride (Cl^-) and HCO_3^- representing the major anions. Potassium does not contribute much to the total cation load in the serum because it is primarily intracellular, and it tends to vary because of physiologic variation and artifacts due to hemolysis of blood samples. For the purpose of this discussion, the anion gap (normal = 7–16) is defined as the difference between the serum Na^+ and the sum of the serum Cl^- plus HCO_3^-.

These are not all of the ions present in the serum; there is a gap between the measured cations and anions. The physiologic requirement for electroneutrality does not allow a true gap between the concentration of cations and anions in the serum, thus a difference represents the sum of all of the unmeasured ions. An increase in the anion gap can result from either a decrease in unmeasured cations (eg, hypokalemia, hypocalcemia, hypomagnesemia) or an increase in unmeasured anions (additional organic compounds circulating).[3]

Metabolic acidosis can be classified into 2 categories: high anion gap or normal anion gap acidosis. A reduction in unmeasured cations or an increase in negatively charged plasma proteins may not be associated with acidosis, thus the anion gap in the absence of acidosis reflects other types of physiologic disruption that are not discussed in this article.

Metabolic acidosis with an anion gap greater than 16, reflecting an increase in an unmeasured anion, is one of the most specific laboratory findings suggestive of an IEM causing acidosis. **Box 1** shows the commonly used mnemonic to remember the differential diagnosis of high anion gap metabolic acidosis. Initial history and laboratory results should reveal most of these etiologic factors, leaving only unexplained anions from IEM or significant poisonings in the differential.[3] In normal anion gap metabolic acidosis the decrease in serum HCO_3^- is matched by an equivalent increase in serum Cl^-, resulting from direct loss of HCO_3^- from the gastrointestinal tract

---

Box 1
Differential diagnosis of high anion gap metabolic acidosis

MUDPILES

Methanol

Uremia

Diabetic ketoacidosis (ketones)

Propylene glycol ingestion

IEM, infection, isoniazid intoxication, or iron intoxication

Lactic acid (ischemia or hypotension)

Ethylene glycol ingestion

Salicylates

(diarrhea), the kidney from renal tubular injury or defect, or from administration of Cl⁻ rich solutions during hospitalization.

Once metabolic acidosis is classified as high anion gap acidosis, other basic laboratory tests can be helpful in narrowing down the differential. These tests can be readily performed in most laboratories and results are available quickly:

- Glucose
- Electrolytes
- Liver function tests
- Lactate
- Ammonia
- Serum (or urine) ketones.

A diagnostic approach is outlined in **Fig. 1**. Hypoglycemia, in the presence of significant acidosis, is highly suggestive of an IEM. Evidence of liver or kidney dysfunction may be an indicator of severe hypoxia or organ hypoperfusion; either complicates the interpretation of IEM.

The metabolism of both lactic acid and ammonia can be altered in defects of mitochondrial intermediate metabolism, thus their presence in the setting of acute acidosis may suggest an IEM. The diagnostic approach to a pure lactic acidosis is shown in **Fig. 2**.

The absence of ketones is a major clinical clue. Ketosis is a physiologic response to fasting, catabolic state, or ketogenic diet. Lack of ketones with hypoglycemia or a fasting state can indicate a disorder of fatty acid oxidation or a disorder in ketone synthesis. (See Areeg El-Gharbawy and Jerry Vockley's article, "Inborn Errors of Metabolism with Myopathy: Defects of Fatty Acid Oxidation and the Carnitine Shuttle System," in this issue.) When unanticipated ketosis is present (eg, ketones without fasting and normoglycemia), an IEM should be suspected.[3]

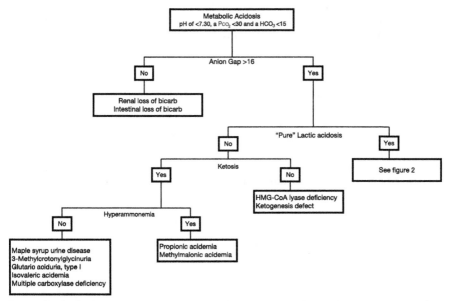

Fig. 1. The likely diagnostic outcome in a child presenting with metabolic acidosis based on simple screening laboratory results that are available within hours of admission in most health care facilities. HCO_3^-, bicarbonate; HMG-CoA, 3-hydroxymethylglutaryl–coenzyme A.

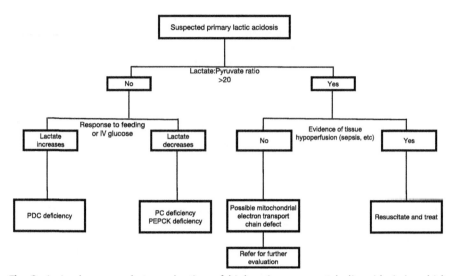

Fig. 2. A simple approach to evaluation of high anion gap metabolic acidosis in which lactate elevation accounts for the entire increase in anion gap, thus a pure lactic acidosis. IV, intravenous; PC, pyruvate carboxylase; PDC, pyruvate dehydrogenase complex; PEPCK, phosphoenolpyruvate carboxykinase.

Once these basic laboratory tests have been reviewed, other, more specific biochemical testing should be performed. Samples of serum, plasma, and urine should be collected during the acute episode and frozen to be sent later for more specific testing; these critical tests[3] are shown in **Box 2**.

It is important to briefly discuss the limitations of newborn screening (NBS). (See discussion of detailed NBS in Ayman W. El-Hattab and colleagues' article, "Newborn Screening: History, Current Status, and Future Directions," in this issue.) Many, but not all, of the IEM that present with acidosis can be identified before, or around the time of, becoming symptomatic. **Box 3** shows those commonly identified by NBS. Unfortunately, a low risk NBS may cause some providers to forget to include IEM in their differential. Not all IEM are identified by the acylcarnitine profile, which is the assay used in NBS for organic acidurias and defects of fatty acid oxidation. Also, NBS is a screening test and, although highly sensitive, it can be falsely negative in some (eg, low excretors with glutaric aciduria type I [GA-I][4] or variant maple syrup urine disease [MSUD][5]).

The underlying biochemical defects in these conditions are permanent, but increased concentrations of the poorly metabolized compounds are consistently present in blood and urine. Physiologic mechanisms to maintain homeostasis and acid-base balance during metabolic stress allow the affected individual to live in a compensated state with normal pH and normal serum HCO_3^-. Normal individuals have a large

---

Box 2
Critical samples to be collected at the time of acute presentation acidosis

- Plasma amino acids
- Plasma carnitine and acylcarnitine analysis
- Urine organic acids
- Urine acylglycines

Box 3
Inborn errors of metabolisms typically identified by newborn screening

- Maple syrup urine disease
- Glutaric aciduria, type I
- Propionic acidemia
- Methylmalonic acidemias
- Isovaleric acidemia
- Beta-ketothiolase deficiency
- Biotinidase deficiency
- Holocarboxylase deficiency
- 3-Hydroxymethylglutaryl–coenzyme A lyase deficiency
- 2-Methyl-3-hydroxybutyric acidemia
- 3-Methylglutaconic aciduria
- 3-Methylcrotonyl–coenzyme A carboxylase deficiency

---

capacity to buffer the increased production of organic acids produced during stress; however, the individual with an IEM producing excess acid has markedly diminished reserve capacity. During periods of increased catabolism of proteins due to intercurrent illness, prolonged fasting, surgery, or intense physical or emotional stress, these compensatory mechanisms are rapidly overwhelmed, resulting in acute, and often severe, acidosis.

This acute metabolic decompensation is a true medical emergency and, like most medical emergencies, is best managed by anticipation and avoidance rather than by correction after it has occurred. For this reason, families are instructed to contact their metabolic provider during episodes of illness, particularly with fever, vomiting, or anorexia due to illness; or before fasting for medical or social reasons. Prophylactic hospital admission is often necessary to provide aggressive nutritional and fluid support and is, in fact, the standard of care if appropriate support cannot be safely and reliably provided at home.

Questions have been raised in the popular press regarding the safety of vaccines in individuals with IEM. Few studies directly address this issue, but the safety of routine immunizations in individuals with IEM is accepted.[6,7] In a study of metabolically fragile children with urea cycle disorders, there was no increase in frequency of metabolic decompensation in the 21 days after vaccine administration than in the 7 days before, suggesting that vaccines, and the inflammatory response they produce, are not a significant cause of metabolic decompensation.[6] In a survey of metabolic specialists, 78% reported never having had a child have an adverse outcome related to a vaccine, and another 21% reported only seldom or once, with more than 90% agreeing that "the benefits outweigh the risks" for routine administration of recommended vaccines for children with IEM.[7] In sum, lacking significant evidence to the contrary, and consistent with widely held expert opinion, children with IEM associated with acute acidosis should receive all immunizations according to the current recommendations.

Details of acute support during metabolic decompensation are shown in **Fig. 3**. Scrupulous attention to maintenance of electrolytes, minerals, and appropriate free water is critical; and, in the face of significant acidosis (pH <7.2), is best accomplished in an intensive care setting. Appropriate fluid resuscitation is critical because individuals

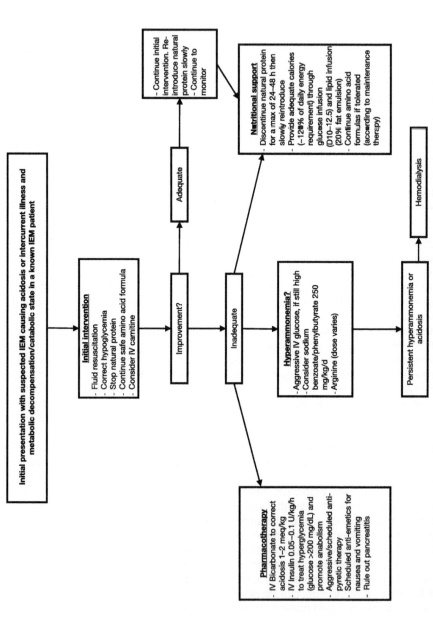

Fig. 3. The general approach to treatment of metabolic acidosis due to IEM. See the article for specific examples of situations in which modification of this standard approach is needed.

are often dehydrated at the time of presentation, but close monitoring is needed because of the risk of cerebral edema in the acutely decompensated, acidotic child.

A not uncommon complication of systemic acidosis in most or all of these conditions is acute pancreatitis.[8,9] The specific mechanism is not known, although it has been speculated that the systemic acidosis leads to activation of trypsin and other proteases inside the pancreas, whereas typically these proteases are maintained in a proform until exposed to acid in the duodenum. Because the symptoms of acute pancreatitis may be overlooked in the acutely ill child with vomiting for other reasons, it is prudent to order biochemical testing early in the evaluation (amylase and lipase are generally reasonable markers) and whenever there is an unexpected deterioration in clinical status.

Management of acute pancreatitis is not significantly different in children with IEM than those with other causes. Intravenous (IV) lipid infusion has been found to be generally safe and well tolerated during treatment of acute pancreatitis,[10] thus this mainstay of metabolic support in treatment of acute metabolic acidosis does not need to be stopped if pancreatitis is diagnosed as a complication of the acidosis. Avoidance of hypertriglyceridemia, whether due to IV lipid emulsions or high glucose-infusion rates, is important, because it may be an independent risk factor for the development of pancreatitis.

Chronic pancreatitis has also been described in association with IEM associated with recurrent acidosis. Both acute and chronic pancreatitis can cause mortality in these conditions.[11]

The use of IV HCO_3^- in the treatment of acute metabolic acidosis has been somewhat controversial.[12,13] In young children with diabetic ketoacidosis, there is a suggestion that HCO_3^- infusion increases the risk of cerebral edema.[14] The argument against HCO_3^- infusion is that it is rapidly converted into carbon dioxide (CO_2) in the plasma, which unlike HCO_3^- easily moves into the intracellular environment, potentially worsening intracellular acidosis. Absent a definitive study, clinical experience suggests that in some cases, particularly in the ketone utilization defects, infusion of HCO_3^- may speed recovery, thus the practitioner is left to use her or his own judgment. Consideration should be given to using IV HCO_3^- therapy only in moderately severe acidosis (pH <7.2) or worse, in the setting of renal insufficiency or renal tubular acidosis (eg, methylmalonic acidemia [MMA]), when the pH is not improving despite adequate fluid resuscitation and treatment to enhance anabolism, or in the setting of altered mental status that is worsening (with care taken regarding the possibility of cerebral edema).

The rest of this article focuses on the finding of metabolic acidosis as the presenting sign of an IEM.

DEFECTS OF ORGANIC ACID METABOLISM

Organic acids occur as intermediates in several intracellular metabolic pathways, most typically amino acid degradation.[3] In contrast to amino acidopathies, for example, phenylketonuria, organic acidemias frequently disturb mitochondrial energy metabolism, at least in part by sequestration of free coenzyme A (CoA), leading to acute metabolic decompensation and acidosis. Some metabolites, including methylmalonic and propionic acid metabolites, are able to inhibit other enzyme systems, particularly those involved in oxidative phosphorylation,[15,16] the glycine cleavage system,[17,18] and the urea cycle.[19] This can lead to multiorgan complications, including neurologic distress, cardiomyopathy, or renal disease.

Table 1 shows clinical findings and details regarding the most common organic acidemias. See later discussion of examples of several of the more common types of organic acidemias, with focus on the acute treatment, chronic management, and prognosis of each.

Table 1
Typical laboratory and clinical findings with some more common organic acidemias

Organic Acidemia	Ketones[a]	Lactic Acidosis[a]	NH4[+a]	Typical Urine Organic Acids	Typical Plasma Acyl-Carnitines	Sources	Clinical Notes
PA	+++	++	++	↑ 3-OH-propionic ↑ propionylglycine ↑ methylcitric	↓ free or total ↑ propionyl-	Propiogenic precursors: Isoleucine Threonine Methionine Valine Odd-chained fatty acids Cholesterol side chain	Cardiomyopathy
MMA	+++	++	++	↑ methylmalonic ↑ 3-OH-propionic ↑ propionylglycine ↑ methylcitric	↓ free or total ↑ propionylcarnitine ↑ methylmalonylcarnitine	See PA (propiogenic precursors)	Multiple causes, including B12 deficiency or metabolic defect; B12 defects can also have ↑ plasma homocysteine
MSUD[b]	+++ (alpha ketones)	+	+	↑ alpha-ketoacids: ↑ 2-oxoisocaproate ↑ 2-oxo-3-methylvalerate ↑ 2-oxoisovalerate ↑ 2-OH-isovalerate ↑ 2-OH-isocaproate ↑ 2-OH-3-methylvalerate	N/A	Branched-chain amino acids: Isoleucine Valine Leucine	Urine, sweat, and earwax have maple syrup odor; a common spice, fenugreek, can cause a similar odor in urine
IVA	+++	++	+	↑ isovalerylglycine ↑ 3-OH-isovaleric	↓ free or total ↑ isovalerylcarnitine	Leucine	Odor of sweaty socks
3-MCG	+++	−	−	↑ 3-OH-isovaleric ↑ 3-methylcrotonylglycine	↓ free or total ↑ 3-OH-isovalerylcarnitine	Leucine	Part of multiple carboxylase deficiency; NBS suggests that most cases are relatively mild, raising questions about clinical significance of the biochemical finding

			Urine organic acids	Plasma acylcarnitine	Amino acids/precursors	Comments
GA-I	+++	+	+	↑ glutaric acid ↑ 3-OH-glutaric acid	↓ free or total ↑ glutarylcarnitine	Tryptophan Lysine Hydroxylysine	Urinary glutarylcarnitine may be helpful to diagnose in low excretors of urine glutaric acid
BTND	+++	+++	+	↑ 3-OH-isovaleric ↑ 3-OH-propionic ↑ propionylglycine ↑ methylcitric ↑ 3-methylcrotonylglycine	↓ free or total ↑ 3-OH-isovalerylcarnitine ↑ propionylcarnitine	Propiogenic precursors Fatty acids Leucine Glucose or pyruvate	Required cofactor for holocarboxylase synthesis; causes multiple carboxylase deficiency
HCSD	+++	+++	+	↑ 3-OH-isovaleric ↑ 3-OH-propionic ↑ propionylglycine ↑ methylcitric ↑ 3-methylcrotonylglycine	↓ free or total ↑ 3-OH-isovalerylcarnitine ↑ propionylcarnitine	See BTND	Multiple carboxylase deficiency, includes: 3-methylcrotonyl-CoA, propionyl-CoA, pyruvate, and acetoacetyl-CoA carboxylases
3-HMG-CoA lyase	−	+	+	↑ 3-OH-methylglutaric ↑ 3-OH-isovaleric ↑ 3-methylglutaconic ↑ 3-methylglutaric	↑ 3-methylglutarylcarnitine	N/A	Also needed for ketone synthesis

−, never; +, occasionally; ++, most of the time; +++, always.

Abbreviations: 3-HMG-CoA lyase, 3-hydroxymethylglutaryl-CoA lyase; 3-MCG, 3-methylcrotonylglycinuria; 3-OH-, 3-hydroxy-; BTND, biotinidase deficiency; HCSD, holocarboxylase synthetase deficiency; IVA, isovaleric acidemia; N/A, not applicable; NH_4^+, ammonia; PA, propionic acidemia.

[a] During acute presentation and episodes of metabolic decompensation.

[b] Branched-chain ketoacid dehydrogenase deficiency.

After establishing a diagnosis in a symptomatic individual, **Fig. 3** describes a reasonable general treatment plan. Acute treatment of organic acidemias involves maintaining normal protein synthesis and avoiding catabolism, preventing imbalances or deficiencies of amino acids and metabolic intermediates, restoring energy homeostasis, and promoting anabolism. Treatment then shifts to long-term or chronic treatment, which is usually focused on a low-protein diet supplemented with special amino acid formulas that do not contain specific precursor amino acids. The following few paragraphs discuss common treatment issues, with special conditions (see later discussion of the detailed discussions of specific disorders).

Feeding difficulties are relatively common in children with severe organic acidemias[20]; some may require gastrostomy or nasogastric tube feeding. Poor weight gain is also relatively common and has been attributed to a variety of potential mechanisms, including inadequate dietary protein or energy intake.[21]

It is often the practice to provide IV L-carnitine during acute treatment and to provide oral supplementation chronically.[21,22] One hypothetical argument for this use is shown in **Fig. 4**. Unfortunately, this hypothesis has not been rigorously tested. It is difficult to rapidly achieve marked increases in cytoplasmic carnitine concentrations because of the kinetics of the transporters involved; thus most L-carnitine delivered by IV is rapidly filtered by the glomerulus and excreted in the urine. That said, plasma carnitine, which reflects intracellular carnitine stores, is often low in individuals with organic acidemias who do not use regular carnitine supplementation when stable. Therefore, in the absence of compelling data for or against acute administration, many experts choose to give it. Doses vary but most often 50 to 100 mg/kg/d divided into 2 to 4 doses is used. Although there is no specific maximum dose, individual doses greater than 1 g are unusual.

Chronic L-carnitine supplementation is often used and is clearly effective at preventing secondary carnitine deficiency. Other potential benefits include enhanced excretion of potentially toxic organic acids in the less toxic form of acylcarnitines. Experience[23,24] suggests that carnitine therapy is possibly effective and reasonably safe, although the latter issue has been questioned by recent work suggesting the possibility that long-term supplementation with carnitine may increase risk of coronary artery disease later in life because of the metabolites of carnitine produced by gut flora.[25,26] Another potential benefit of carnitine supplementation is suggested by data showing in-vitro antioxidant capacity similar to vitamin E (α-tocopherol).[27] In a survey of European metabolic treatment centers, most recommend carnitine for individuals with MMA, and presumably other organic acidemias.[22]

The use of HCO_3^- infusion, previously discussed, is often not needed after attending to fluid deficits and providing adequate calories. If these steps do not lead to correction of the acidosis, searches for other contributing factors, including unsuspected infection or pancreatitis, should be considered.

MAPLE SYRUP URINE DISEASE

MSUD is caused by a deficiency of the branched-chain alpha-ketoacid dehydrogenase complex enzyme, the second step of branched-chain amino acid metabolism (leucine, isoleucine, and valine). Although all 3 branched-chain amino acid concentrations are found to be elevated in the blood, elevated leucine and its metabolite 2-ketoisocaproic acid are thought to be the most toxic.[28]

Clinical Manifestations

MSUD has both severe and milder presentations depending on the residual enzyme activity. Classic MSUD (75% of cases) usually presents within the first weeks after

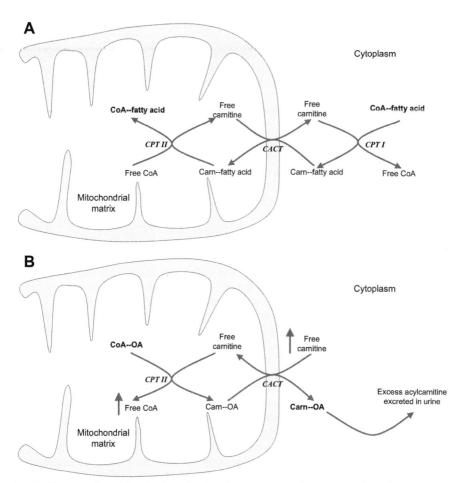

Fig. 4. The use of carnitine is primarily aimed at optimizing free CoA pools in the mitochondria by delivering high concentrations of carnitine that will drive the exchange of free carnitine into the mitochondria in exchange for organic acid bound to carnitine coming out. (*A*) The usual physiologic role for the carnitine pathway involves formation of acylcarnitine (with a long-chain fat as the acylcarnitine group) by carnitine palmitoyltransferase (CPT) I, which is transported into the mitochondria in exchange for a free carnitine coming out via the carnitine acylcarnitine translocase (CACT). Inside the mitochondrion CPT II reverses the reaction and reforms the long-chain fatty acyl-CoA that then enters the beta-oxidation pathway. (*B*) CoA cannot cross the mitochondrial membrane, and it cannot be rapidly generated inside the mitochondria in response to sequestration by an accumulating organic acid-CoA (CoA-OA) due to a metabolic block. Because CoA is an essential cofactor for a large number of mitochondrial reactions, the accumulation of a specific acid bound to CoA that cannot be furthered metabolized leads to acute free CoA deficiency and, ultimately, mitochondrial energy failure. The 3 enzyme process (CPT I, CACT, CPT II) is reversible, thus an excess of free carnitine in the cytoplasm should drive the removal of the excessive organic acid, in the form of acylcarnitines (Carn-OA), from the mitochondria, thus freeing up CoA.

birth with maple syrup odor, feeding problems, lethargy, and acute metabolic acidosis. Without treatment, MSUD progresses to coma with involuntary movements and central respiratory failure.[29] In older individuals, acute increases in plasma leucine lead to intoxication symptoms, including ataxia, slurred speech, lethargy, vomiting, and progressive alteration in mental status. If untreated, cerebral edema and death follow.

With careful management, affected individuals can have normal psychomotor and neurologic development. Early diagnosis by NBS has decreased the number of days with toxic leucine levels and improved neurologic outcomes in these individuals.[29]

Treatment

As in **Fig. 3**, with the following exceptions, reintroduce isoleucine and valine supplementation when blood levels decrease below 400 to 600 µmol/L to maximize the rate of reduction of plasma leucine concentrations. Remember that the only mechanism for reducing high plasma amino acid values is to increase incorporation into protein, and isoleucine and valine are critical to achieve this goal. Dietary management guidelines have been published.[10]

PROPIONIC ACIDEMIA AND METHYLMALONIC ACIDEMIA

Both propionic acidemia (PA) and MMA are defects in the propionate catabolism pathway involving isoleucine, valine, threonine, and methionine, as well as odd-chain fatty acids, cholesterol, and propionic acid produced by gut bacteria.

Excess propionyl-CoA is used for fatty acid synthesis in these individuals, so that as much one-third of their adipose tissue may be composed of odd-chain length fats.[30] Therefore, suppression of lipolysis of endogenous fat during acute illness is particularly important to prevent release of propionic acid during oxidation of these odd-chain length fats (beta-oxidation ends with the 3-carbon propionyl-CoA instead of the 2-carbon acetyl-CoA).

PA is caused by a deficiency of propionyl-CoA carboxylase (PCC), a biotin-dependent enzyme composed of PCCA and PCCB subunits; mutations in either gene (*PCCA* or *PCCB*) can cause PA.[31]

Vitamin B12 is a cofactor for the methylmalonyl-CoA mutase. The MMAs are a genetically heterogeneous group of disorders of methylmalonate or cobalamin (vitamin B12) metabolism leading to deficient activity of methylmalonyl-CoA mutase. Mutations in *MUT* (the gene coding the methylmalonyl-CoA mutase) causing no residual mutase enzyme activity (MUT^0) are associated with a more severe phenotype than in individuals with *MUT* mutations causing some residual enzyme activity (MUT$^-$) or cobalamin defects.

Clinical Manifestations

These conditions classically present within the first few days of life with hypotonia, poor feeding, vomiting, metabolic acidosis, and hyperammonemia. Children become progressively encephalopathic and without treatment ultimately progress to coma and death. Individuals with milder variants can present at any age with a more variable clinical picture.

Neurologic symptoms can include hypotonia, developmental delay, progressive psychomotor delay, seizures, and movement disorders. Neurologic complications can present as an acute or progressive extrapyramidal syndrome associated with changes in the basal ganglia. Stroke-like episodes may occur at any age and are more frequent in MMA.[31] Hematologic findings include neutropenia, thrombocytopenia, and pancytopenia. In the acute setting, these can be confused with sepsis.

Cardiomyopathy (acute or chronic) is a major complication in PA (less commonly in MMA) and can be responsible for rapid deterioration. Both dilated and hypertrophic cardiomyopathies have been reported and can occur in metabolically stable individuals. Individuals with PA can also develop life-threatening cardiac arrhythmias, specifically, long QT interval. Cardiac manifestations can occur with or without carnitine deficiency.[32]

Chronic kidney disease is a common and severe long-term complication of MMA[33] but not PA, eventually requiring hemodialysis or kidney transplant. Optic neuropathy has also been increasingly recognized as a complication.[34]

Early detection (NBS) and treatment of MMA and PA, has significantly improved long-term survival. Unfortunately, recent work has shown that, despite early diagnosis and treatment, these conditions continue to be associated with long-term intellectual disability.[9] In both MMA and PA, movement disorders are frequent and metabolic stroke-like events can occur during, or just after, metabolic decompensation (even in individuals stable before the crisis).[31]

Treatment

The mainstay of long-term management in PA and MMA is dietary therapy. This includes a low-protein diet, limiting the propionic acid precursor amino acids while ensuring essential requirements are met. Natural protein tolerance should be individualized. In addition, diets are usually supplemented with additional precursor-free formula (amino acids) to supplement natural protein intake to achieve the recommended protein requirements.

Intermittent courses of antibiotics (metronidazole or neomycin) reduce the production of propionyl-CoA from anaerobic bacterial fermentation of carbohydrates in the gut.[31]

Vitamin B12 responsiveness should be assessed in every individual with MMA. Hydroxocobalamin can be compounded to concentrations as high as 25 mg/mL for subcutaneous injection and daily doses titrated to effect.[35]

Liver transplantation can be considered in children with frequent metabolic decompensation poorly controlled with dietary and pharmacologic treatment. Several reports of successful liver transplants suggest a decrease in hospital admissions and improvement in quality of life.[36] Neurologic complications have still been found to occur even after liver transplantation.[37]

GLUTARIC ACIDURIA TYPE I

GA-I is caused by a deficiency of glutaryl-CoA dehydrogenase in the catabolic pathway of the amino acids tryptophan, lysine, and hydroxylysine. The clinical symptoms of GA-I seem to result from glutaric acid and 3-hydroxyglutaric acid accumulating in the brain, causing neurotoxicity.[38]

Clinical Manifestations

About half of affected individuals initially present with nonspecific neurologic symptoms, such as hypotonia and motor delays. Macrocephaly is commonly found at birth or shortly after. Untreated, 80% to 90% of affected infants will suffer from an acute encephalopathic crisis during the first 6 years of life (most commonly between 3 and 36 months of age). These crises result in characteristic neurologic sequelae, specifically, bilateral striatal injury and subsequent development of a dystonic movement disorder. Crises are often triggered by infections, fever, or surgical intervention. There have also been reports of individuals experiencing striatal injury in the absence of a specific encephalopathic crisis. Early clinical diagnosis is difficult because there are no characteristic or pathognomonic clinical signs or symptoms that occur before encephalopathic crisis. Fortunately, GA-I is now included in NBS making early, pre-symptomatic diagnosis possible.[39]

A subgroup of affected infants has only minimally elevated urinary glutarate excretion. They have a similar clinical course and are at high risk for neurologic complications.[4] It seems that urine glutarylcarnitine measured by liquid chromatography-mass spectroscopy (LC-MS) is more sensitive than urine glutaric acid in identifying these children.[40]

It is important for pediatricians to note that children with GA-I are at increased risk for subdural hematomas (SDHs), even in the absence of significant trauma. This is due to abnormal brain growth resulting in widening of the subarachnoid space, leading to increased tension on bridging veins, making them more susceptible to rupture even with minor trauma.[39] SDH is estimated to occur in up to 20% to 30% of children with GA I.[41] This has led to concern that children with isolated SDH being investigated for nonaccidental injury may actually have GA-I. SDH in GA-I always occurs in combination with other characteristic neuroradiologic abnormalities, including enlargement of the frontoparietotemporal space, or insular region, around the brain; therefore, isolated SDH without other abnormalities is not suggestive of GA-I.[41] GA-I can be readily ruled out by the combination of normal plasma and urine acylcarnitine profiles, urine organic acid analysis, and other brain MRI findings, with DNA testing rarely needed.

Of infants identified with GA-I by NBS and starting treatment before neurologic injury, 80% to 90% remain asymptomatic.[39,42] Unfortunately, NBS may not reliably identify all children with GA-I (especially low excretors).[4,39] After diagnosis by NBS, individuals generally have average intelligence and normal executive function, attention, gross motor skills, and visual memory, although, fine motor skills and speech may be impaired, despite early and appropriate treatment.[38] Outcomes are poor when diagnosis is made after irreversible neurologic injury has occurred, although treatment may help prevent further neurologic deterioration.

Treatment

Chronic management of GA-I includes a low-lysine diet, carnitine supplementation, and aggressive treatment during episodes of intercurrent illness. Treating with supraphysiologic doses of arginine has also been proposed.[43] Because arginine competes with lysine for uptake via a specific transporter at the blood–brain barrier, arginine supplementation may decrease cerebral concentrations of the neurotoxic metabolites, although more clinical evidence to support high-dose arginine supplementation is needed.[39]

L-Carnitine is often used. Anecdotal reports suggest biochemical improvement following riboflavin supplementation, although there is no standardized protocol for assessing riboflavin responsiveness and no clear objective evidence that riboflavin improves clinical outcomes.

MULTIPLE CARBOXYLASE DEFICIENCY (BIOTINIDASE DEFICIENCY AND HOLOCARBOXYLASE SYNTHETASE DEFICIENCY)

Biotin is a cofactor for 4 important carboxylases in different metabolic pathways. Biotinidase is responsible for biotin regeneration and liberating protein-bound biotin. Holocarboxylase synthase binds biotin to form the active carboxylases. Defects in either of these enzymes results in characteristic biochemical patterns because of deficiencies of PC (involved in gluconeogenesis), PCC (involved in branched-chain amino acid metabolism), 3-methylcrotonyl-CoA carboxylase (involved in leucine metabolism), and acetyl-CoA carboxylase (involved in fatty acid synthesis).

Clinical Manifestations

The clinical findings of biotinidase deficiency (BTND) and holocarboxylase synthetase deficiency are similar but are readily distinguished by enzyme testing (widely available for biotinidase) or DNA sequencing.

The typical presentation with holocarboxylase synthetase deficiency is in early infancy with emesis, lethargy, hypotonia, seizures, metabolic acidosis, skin rash, and alopecia. In untreated individuals, sensorineural hearing loss and vision loss have also been described.[44] BTND typically presents with these symptoms; however, children are usually older with symptoms appearing after the age of 3 months.[45] There are exceptions for both disorders.

Prognosis for these conditions is directly related to timing of initiation of treatment. Individuals diagnosed by NBS (or before the development of symptoms) seem to have normal development with no neurologic sequelae. Individuals symptomatic before biotin therapy may have residual neurologic problems. Although seizures, skin, and biochemical abnormalities resolve with biotin treatment, developmental delay, optic nerve atrophy, and hearing loss are usually irreversible.[45]

Treatment

It is critical that biotin supplementation be started immediately when these conditions are suspected, before confirmatory testing is back. Treatment is life-long oral biotin supplementation at a dose of 5 to 10 mg per day. Suspensions of the medicine are not recommended because of loss of activity and difficulty maintaining sterility. Capsules can be opened or tablets crushed to deliver the dose with food or drink if the child is too young to swallow the dosage intact.

Protein-restricted diets are not necessary in these conditions. However, raw eggs should be avoided because they contain avidin, an egg-white protein that binds biotin, decreasing the vitamin's availability. Cooking inactivates avidin in eggs, rendering it incapable of binding biotin.[45]

DEFECTS OF PYRUVATE METABOLISM

Persistent lactic acidosis without marked abnormalities in other organic acids points the clinician toward primary defects of pyruvate metabolism. Pyruvate is an intermediary in the metabolism of glucose, with the pyruvate dehydrogenase complex (PDC) being required for the complete oxidation of glucose, and pyruvate carboxylase (PC) as the first committed step in gluconeogenesis from amino acid carbon backbones via the tricarboxylic acid cycle. This presents an interesting clinical dichotomy in which IV dextrose therapy is a required in the treatment of gluconeogenic defects causing lactic acidosis (PC and phosphoenolpyruvate carboxykinase [PEPCK] deficiencies) but is contraindicated in PDC deficiency. A diagnostic approach is shown in **Fig. 2**. PC and cytosolic PEPCK deficiencies can present with acidosis but more typically present with hypoglycemia. (See discussion of these deficiencies in David A. Weinstein and colleagues' article, "Inborn Errors of Metabolism with Hypoglycemia: Glycogen Storage Diseases and Inherited Disorders of Gluconeogenesis," in this issue.)

Pyruvate and lactate are interconverted in the cytoplasm depending on the relative concentrations of oxidized and reduced nicotinamide adenine dinucleotide (NAD^+ and NADH, respectively) to drive the lactate dehydrogenase (LDH) reaction (lactic acid + NAD^+ ↔ pyruvic acid + NADH). Defects of the mitochondrial electron transport chain lead to accumulation of NADH in the cytoplasm and push the LDH reaction toward accumulation of lactate more than pyruvate. Thus, a normal ratio of lactate to pyruvate (<20) in the setting of increased lactate suggests that lactic acidosis is likely due to a primary defect of pyruvate metabolism. A lactate-to-pyruvate ratio greater than 20 suggests a primary defect of the mitochondrial electron transport chain or tissue hypoperfusion or hypoxia. (See discussion in Thatjana Gardeitchik and colleagues' article, "Complex Phenotypes in Inborn Errors of Metabolism: Overlapping Presentations in Congenital Disorders of Glycosylation and Mitochondrial Disorders," in this issue.)

High suspicion of a primary defect in pyruvate metabolism can be reached in the acute presentation when the increase in the anion gap can be entirely explained by the concentration of lactate in the blood (eg, an anion gap of 19, which is 4–6 points higher than normal, is entirely explained by a lactate of 6 mmol/L). In the acute setting, it is often not clear whether the lactate increase is secondary to an organic acidemia, in which high concentrations of dextrose are indicated, or a defect in PDC, in which dextrose may make things worse. In practice, if in doubt, it is prudent to start IV dextrose at the higher rate and remeasure lactate in 2 hours. If the repeat lactate is significantly increased and the clinical findings suggest possible PDC deficiency or a defect in the electron transport chain, reducing IV dextrose and consideration of adding other sources of energy, such as IV lipids, is indicated.

PYRUVATE DEHYDROGENASE COMPLEX DEFICIENCY

PDC, located in the mitochondrial matrix, converts pyruvate formed by the breakdown of glucose to CO_2 and acetyl-CoA, which can be further metabolized in the tricarboxylic acid cycle. The complex contains 6 proteins (3 catalytic, 2 regulatory, and a binding protein) and 3 cofactors (thiamine pyrophosphate, lipoic acid, and flavin adenine dinucleotide). Defects in any of these, as well as a variety of other interacting and regulatory factors, can lead to PDC insufficiency. The most common, however, is a defect in the X-linked *PDHA1* gene that codes for a critical catalytic enzyme.[46,47]

Clinical Manifestations

PDC deficiency presents with a range of neurologic symptoms and varying degrees of lactic acidosis.[46,48–50] Neonatal forms often include profound lactic acidosis, coma, and neonatal death. Older infants and toddlers may present with developmental delay, encephalopathy, hypotonia, and/or seizures. These children may have abnormalities on brain imaging, including agenesis or dysgenesis of the corpus callosum, ventriculomegaly, gray matter heterotopia or cystic changes, and Leigh syndrome. Older children may present with ataxia or neuropathy mimicking Guillain-Barre syndrome. Mortality is high and survivors often have varying degrees of intellectual disability.[46,47]

Treatment

There is no proven effective treatment of PDC deficiency. Use of a ketogenic diet that results in generation of acetyl-CoA from ketone bodies rather than from glucose to bypass the metabolic block has been reported to provide some benefit,[51] although concerns have been raised about long-term use.[52] A recent report suggests reasonable long-term efficacy and safety.[53] The ketogenic diet should only be used when the cause of the PDC deficiency is known because it can be dangerous in some secondary causes of PDC inhibition, PC, or PEPCK deficiencies, or mitochondrial respiratory chain defects. Dichloroacetate and phenylbutyrate[54] both inhibit pyruvate dehydrogenase kinase, thus activating the PDC,[55] and may have potential as therapy.[54,56] Some affected individuals may be responsive to thiamine, which is incorporated into the cofactor thiamine pyrophosphate.

DEFECTS OF KETONE METABOLISM

The formation of the ketone bodies (acetoacetate and 3-hydroxybutyrate) is an endpoint of fatty acid oxidation because these substrates can be used for energy in tissues, particularly the brain, that do not use fatty acid oxidation. **Fig. 5** shows the process of ketone synthesis in the hepatocytes and utilization in brain and other tissues.

KETONE UTILIZATION DEFECTS

A rare, and often difficult to diagnose, group of disorders that present with recurrent episodes of ketoacidosis with either low or normal serum glucose are defects of utilizing ketones (an excellent review is available[57]). Episodes are usually related to intercurrent viral illnesses and typically present with vomiting. Often, even modest dextrose infusions given as maintenance fluid can lead to slow resolution of the illness, which is often ascribed to dehydration. This can occur multiple times until recognition of excessive ketosis out of proportion to the fasting. Occasionally, the presentation with ketoacidosis is quite severe.

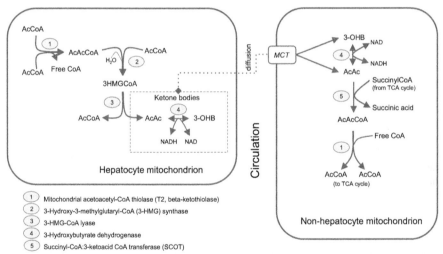

Fig. 5. Ketone body synthesis and utilization. In the hepatocyte ketone synthesis begins with condensation of 2 acetyl-CoA (AcCoA) molecules by (1) mitochondrial acetoacetyl-CoA thiolase (T2) or uses acetoacetyl-CoA (AcAcCoA) from the last steps of fat oxidation or oxidation of isoleucine. An AcAcCoA molecule is combined with a molecule of AcCoA by (2) 3-hydroxy-3-methylglutaryl-CoA (3-HMG) synthase. This redundant approach is necessary because the enzyme that directly releases CoA from AcAcCoA (see 5) is not expressed in the liver (thus, hepatocytes can make ketones but cannot use them). The 3-HMG produced is then used by (3) 3-HMG-CoA lyase, to release acetoacetate (AcAc) and AcCoA. Defects in all 3 enzymes are described (Fukao and colleagues[61]) associated with hypoketotic hypoglycemia. The ketone bodies, AcAc and its redox partner, 3-hydroxybutyrate (3-OHB), are kept in equilibrium based on the ratio of NAD to NADH in the mitochondrion using the enzyme (4) 3-OHB dehydrogenase. Ketone bodies leave the cell by diffusion and circulate to nonhepatic tissues via the bloodstream. They are taken up by the monocarboxylate transporter (MCT) on the membrane of ketone-utilizing cells, especially the brain. After diffusion into the mitochondrion, AcAcCoA is reformed from AcAc by (5) succinyl-CoA:3-ketoacid CoA transferase (SCOT), and 2 molecules of AcCoA are released by the mitochondrial acetoacetyl-CoA thiolase (T2). TCA, tricarboxylic acid.

There are 2 classic defects: succinyl-CoA:3-ketoacid CoA transferase (SCOT) deficiency and the mitochondrial acetoacetyl-CoA thiolase (T2) deficiency (the gene is *ACAT1* and the enzyme is confusingly also referred to as 2-methylacetoacetyl-CoA thiolase, and commonly known as beta-ketothiolase). Recently, a third defect, the monocarboxylate transporter (MCT) deficiency, responsible for cellular uptake of circulating ketone bodies, has been identified in several individuals with recurrent ketoacidosis.[58]

Clinical Manifestations

The clinical presentation of each of these is similar with ketosis out of proportion to fasting during periods of illness, often magnified by fever or vomiting. Symptoms include vomiting and lethargy, sometimes exacerbated by hypoglycemia because the gluconeogenic pathway is either overstretched by increased brain demand due to inability to use ketones or by relative sequestration of mitochondrial CoA pools by the accumulating ketones. The ketone bodies themselves are weak acids; therefore, as they accumulate in the circulation, acidosis becomes apparent.

Diagnosis requires the clinician to maintain a high level of clinical suspicion when evaluating a child with prominent acidosis and symptoms out of proportion to the degree of dehydration in the setting of gastroenteritis or intercurrent illness. SCOT deficiency may be associated with persistent mild ketosis, even when well, but this is not universal, thus the absence of persistent ketosis does not rule out SCOT deficiency.[59]

T2 deficiency does not typically have ketosis between exacerbations because the overlapping activity of the medium-chain CoA T2 that is part of the fatty acid oxidation pathway can metabolize modest amounts of acetoacetyl-CoA; however, it is not capable of handling the high demand during stress. On the other hand, in the isoleucine degradation pathway, T2 is needed to metabolize the 2-methyl-3-hydroxybutyryl-CoA (2MHB) intermediate, thus 2MHB and an unusual metabolite, tiglylglycine, are usually present in the urine. Carnitine esters of these acids may be found in plasma, even between acute episodes. This condition can be but is not always identified by NBS.[60] Importantly, laboratories using tandem mass spectroscopy (including NBS laboratory tests) to evaluate acylcarnitines cannot distinguish 2MHB-carnitine and tiglylcarnitine from other 5 carbon isomers, thus liquid chromatography-mass spectrometry is required. Gas chromatography-mass spectrometry used for urine organic acid analysis is able to distinguish the compounds.

The MCT does not have a unique profile of metabolites, either during acute decompensation nor when well.[58] Thus, for all of the defects of ketolysis, enzymatic or molecular diagnosis is required. Molecular diagnosis (DNA) can never rule out a disease because of the uncertainty of whether the disease-causing variant was detected in the assay chosen. Unfortunately, there are few remaining clinical laboratories offering testing for SCOT and T2 enzymatic activities, and none, to the authors' knowledge, measuring MCT activity. This creates a growing diagnostic challenge for clinicians, which is likely to become more critical in the future.

Treatment

The outcome of each of these defects of ketone utilization can be good if they are promptly identified and if severe and prolonged episodes of acidosis are avoided by routine admission for therapy with fluids and IV dextrose during intercurrent illnesses or periods of required fasting (eg, perioperatively). Generally, no treatment is required between episodes, except to avoid prolonged fasts beyond the time that glycogen stores can be relied on to maintain blood glucose as the primary source of energy for brain and kidney. If plasma carnitine deficiency develops in T2 deficiency, supplemental L-carnitine may be useful.

SUMMARY

1. Early identification and treatment can prevent irreversible neurologic damage in IEM.
2. A normal NBS does not rule out an IEM.
3. Any neonate or child presenting with a metabolic acidosis should prompt the following work-up:
   o Blood gas and finger stick blood sugar
   o Chemistry to calculate anion gap
   o Lactate level
   o Ammonia level
   o Ketone measurement in blood or urine.
4. Acute treatment includes
   o Treating the precipitating illness (eg, infection)
   o Reversing catabolism (high dextrose IV fluids and IV lipids)
   o Enhancing renal clearance of the accumulating compounds (carnitine administration)
   o Ensuring a high-energy intake as a calculated glucose infusion rate.
5. Collect and freeze extra plasma, serum, and urine samples during the acute presentation for future, more specific biochemical testing. These samples are precious.
6. Do not hesitate to call the nearest metabolic center for help.

REFERENCES

1. Burton BK. Inborn errors of metabolism in infancy: a guide to diagnosis. Pediatrics 1998;102(6):E69.
2. Ogier de Bauiny H, Dionisi-Vici C, Wendel U. Branched-chain organic acidurias/acidemias. In: Saudubray JM, Van den Berghe G, Walter JH, editors. Inborn metabolic diseases. 5th edition. New York: Springer; 2012. p. 277–93.
3. Hoffmann GF, Schulze A. Organic acidurias. In: Sarafoglou K, editor. Pediatric endocrinology and inborn errors of metabolism. 1st edition. New York: McGraw-Hill; 2009. p. 83–118.
4. Schillaci LA, Greene CL, Strovel E, et al. The M405V allele of the glutaryl-CoA dehydrogenase gene is an important marker for glutaric aciduria type I (GA-I) low excretors. Mol Genet Metab 2016;119(1–2):50–6.
5. Puckett RL, Lorey F, Rinaldo P, et al. Maple syrup urine disease: further evidence that newborn screening may fail to identify variant forms. Mol Genet Metab 2010; 100(2):136–42.
6. Morgan TM, Schlegel C, Edwards KM, et al. Vaccines are not associated with metabolic events in children with urea cycle disorders. Pediatrics 2011;127(5): e1147–53.
7. Barshop BA, Summar ML. Attitudes regarding vaccination among practitioners of clinical biochemical genetics. Mol Genet Metab 2008;95(1–2):1–2.
8. Kahler SG, Sherwood WG, Woolf D, et al. Pancreatitis in patients with organic acidemias. J Pediatr 1994;124(2):239–43.
9. Grunert SC, Mullerleile S, de Silva L, et al. Propionic acidemia: neonatal versus selective metabolic screening. J Inherit Metab Dis 2012;35(1):41–9.
10. Frazier DM, Allgeier C, Homer C, et al. Nutrition management guideline for maple syrup urine disease: an evidence- and consensus-based approach. Mol Genet Metab 2014;112(3):210–7.

11. Marquard J, El Scheich T, Klee D, et al. Chronic pancreatitis in branched-chain organic acidurias–a case of methylmalonic aciduria and an overview of the literature. Eur J Pediatr 2011;170(2):241–5.
12. Kraut JA, Madias NE. Lactic acidosis: current treatments and future directions. Am J Kidney Dis 2016;68(3):473–82.
13. Kamel KS, Schreiber M, Carlotti AP, et al. Approach to the treatment of diabetic ketoacidosis. Am J Kidney Dis 2016;68(6):967–72.
14. Glaser N, Barnett P, McCaslin I, et al. Risk factors for cerebral edema in children with diabetic ketoacidosis. The Pediatric Emergency Medicine Collaborative Research Committee of the American Academy of Pediatrics. N Engl J Med 2001;344(4):264–9.
15. Chandler RJ, Zerfas PM, Shanske S, et al. Mitochondrial dysfunction in mut methylmalonic acidemia. FASEB J 2009;23(4):1252–61.
16. Wajner M, Goodman SI. Disruption of mitochondrial homeostasis in organic acidurias: insights from human and animal studies. J Bioenerg Biomembr 2011;43(1):31–8.
17. Childs B, Nyhan WL, Borden M, et al. Idiopathic hyperglycinemia and hyperglycinuria: a new disorder of amino acid metabolism. I. Pediatrics 1961;27:522–38.
18. Corbeel L, Tada K, Colombo JP, et al. Methylmalonic acidaemia and nonketotic hyperglycinaemia. Clinical and biochemical aspects. Arch Dis Child 1975; 50(2):103–9.
19. Coude FX, Sweetman L, Nyhan WL. Inhibition by propionyl-coenzyme A of N-acetylglutamate synthetase in rat liver mitochondria. A possible explanation for hyperammonemia in propionic and methylmalonic acidemia. J Clin Invest 1979; 64(6):1544–51.
20. Grunert SC, Mullerleile S, De Silva L, et al. Propionic acidemia: clinical course and outcome in 55 pediatric and adolescent patients. Orphanet J Rare Dis 2013;8:6.
21. Knerr I, Weinhold N, Vockley J, et al. Advances and challenges in the treatment of branched-chain amino/keto acid metabolic defects. J Inherit Metab Dis 2012; 35(1):29–40.
22. Zwickler T, Lindner M, Aydin HI, et al. Diagnostic work-up and management of patients with isolated methylmalonic acidurias in European metabolic centres. J Inherit Metab Dis 2008;31(3):361–7.
23. Fries MH, Rinaldo P, Schmidt-Sommerfeld E, et al. Isovaleric acidemia: response to a leucine load after three weeks of supplementation with glycine, L-carnitine, and combined glycine-carnitine therapy. J Pediatr 1996;129(3):449–52.
24. de Sousa C, Chalmers RA, Stacey TE, et al. The response to L-carnitine and glycine therapy in isovaleric acidaemia. Eur J Pediatr 1986;144(5):451–6.
25. Koeth RA, Wang Z, Levison BS, et al. Intestinal microbiota metabolism of L-carnitine, a nutrient in red meat, promotes atherosclerosis. Nat Med 2013;19(5): 576–85.
26. Miller MJ, Bostwick BL, Kennedy AD, et al. Chronic oral L-carnitine supplementation drives marked plasma TMAO elevations in patients with organic acidemias despite dietary meat restrictions. JIMD Rep 2016;30:39–44.
27. Gulcin I. Antioxidant and antiradical activities of L-carnitine. Life Sci 2006;78(8): 803–11.
28. Wappner R, Gibson KM. Disorders of leucine metabolism. In: Blau N, Hoffmann GF, Leonard JV, et al, editors. Physician's guide to the treatment and follow-up of metabolic disease. Germany: Springer-Verlag Berlin Heidelberg; 2006. p. 59–79.

29. Couce ML, Ramos F, Bueno MA, et al. Evolution of maple syrup urine disease in patients diagnosed by newborn screening versus late diagnosis. Eur J Paediatr Neurol 2015;19(6).652–9.

30. Wendel U, Baumgartner R, van der Meer SB, et al. Accumulation of odd-numbered long-chain fatty acids in fetuses and neonates with inherited disorders of propionate metabolism. Pediatr Res 1991;29(4 Pt 1):403–5.

31. Baumgartner MR, Horster F, Dionisi-Vici C, et al. Proposed guidelines for the diagnosis and management of methylmalonic and propionic acidemia. Orphanet J Rare Dis 2014;9:130.

32. Fraser JL, Venditti CP. Methylmalonic and propionic acidemias: clinical management update. Curr Opin Pediatr 2016;28(6):682–93.

33. Horster F, Baumgartner MR, Viardot C, et al. Long-term outcome in methylmalonic acidurias is influenced by the underlying defect (mut0, mut-, cblA, cblB). Pediatr Res 2007;62(2):225–30.

34. Martinez Alvarez L, Jameson E, Parry NR, et al. Optic neuropathy in methylmalonic acidemia and propionic acidemia. Br J Ophthalmol 2016;100(1):98–104.

35. Carrillo-Carrasco N, Sloan J, Valle D, et al. Hydroxocobalamin dose escalation improves metabolic control in cblC. J Inherit Metab Dis 2009;32(6):728–31.

36. Niemi AK, Kim IK, Krueger CE, et al. Treatment of methylmalonic acidemia by liver or combined liver-kidney transplantation. J Pediatr 2015;166(6):1455–61.e1.

37. Kaplan P, Ficicioglu C, Mazur AT, et al. Liver transplantation is not curative for methylmalonic acidopathy caused by methylmalonyl-CoA mutase deficiency. Mol Genet Metab 2006;88(4):322–6.

38. Brown A, Crowe L, Beauchamp MH, et al. Neurodevelopmental profiles of children with glutaric aciduria type I diagnosed by newborn screening: a follow-up case series. JIMD Rep 2015;18:125–34.

39. Boy N, Muhlhausen C, Maier EM, et al. Proposed recommendations for diagnosing and managing individuals with glutaric aciduria type I: second revision. J Inherit Metab Dis 2017;40(1):75–101.

40. Moore T, Le A, Cowan TM. An improved LC-MS/MS method for the detection of classic and low excretor glutaric acidemia type 1. J Inherit Metab Dis 2012; 35(3):431–5.

41. Vester ME, Bilo RA, Karst WA, et al. Subdural hematomas: glutaric aciduria type 1 or abusive head trauma? A systematic review. Forensic Sci Med Pathol 2015; 11(3):405–15.

42. Strauss KA, Puffenberger EG, Robinson DL, et al. Type I glutaric aciduria, part 1: natural history of 77 patients. Am J Med Genet C Semin Med Genet 2003; 121C(1):38–52.

43. Strauss KA, Brumbaugh J, Duffy A, et al. Safety, efficacy and physiological actions of a lysine-free, arginine-rich formula to treat glutaryl-CoA dehydrogenase deficiency: focus on cerebral amino acid influx. Mol Genet Metab 2011; 104(1–2):93–106.

44. Donti TR, Blackburn PR, Atwal PS. Holocarboxylase synthetase deficiency pre and post newborn screening. Mol Genet Metab Rep 2016;7:40–4.

45. Wolf B. Biotinidase deficiency: "if you have to have an inherited metabolic disease, this is the one to have". Genet Med 2012;14(6):565–75.

46. DeBrosse SD, Okajima K, Zhang S, et al. Spectrum of neurological and survival outcomes in pyruvate dehydrogenase complex (PDC) deficiency: lack of correlation with genotype. Mol Genet Metab 2012;107(3):394–402.

47. Patel KP, O'Brien TW, Subramony SH, et al. The spectrum of pyruvate dehydrogenase complex deficiency: clinical, biochemical and genetic features in 371 patients. Mol Genet Metab 2012;106(3):385–94.

48. Imbard A, Boutron A, Vequaud C, et al. Molecular characterization of 82 patients with pyruvate dehydrogenase complex deficiency. Structural implications of novel amino acid substitutions in E1 protein. Mol Genet Metab 2011;104(4): 507–16.

49. Quintana E, Gort L, Busquets C, et al. Mutational study in the PDHA1 gene of 40 patients suspected of pyruvate dehydrogenase complex deficiency. Clin Genet 2010;77(5):474–82.

50. Barnerias C, Saudubray JM, Touati G, et al. Pyruvate dehydrogenase complex deficiency: four neurological phenotypes with differing pathogenesis. Dev Med Child Nourol 2010;52(2):e1–9.

51. Wexler ID, Hemalatha SG, McConnell J, et al. Outcome of pyruvate dehydrogenase deficiency treated with ketogenic diets. Studies in patients with identical mutations. Neurology 1997;49(6):1655–61.

52. Weber TA, Antognetti MR, Stacpoole PW. Caveats when considering ketogenic diets for the treatment of pyruvate dehydrogenase complex deficiency. J Pediatr 2001;138(3):390–5.

53. Sofou K, Dahlin M, Hallbook T, et al. Ketogenic diet in pyruvate dehydrogenase complex deficiency: short- and long-term outcomes. J Inherit Metab Dis 2017; 40(2):237–45.

54. Ferriero R, Iannuzzi C, Manco G, et al. Differential inhibition of PDKs by phenylbutyrate and enhancement of pyruvate dehydrogenase complex activity by combination with dichloroacetate. J Inherit Metab Dis 2015;38(5):895–904.

55. Whitehouse S, Randle PJ. Activation of pyruvate dehydrogenase in perfused rat heart by dichloroacetate (short communication). Biochem J 1973;134(2):651–3.

56. Stacpoole PW, Nagaraja NV, Hutson AD. Efficacy of dichloroacetate as a lactate-lowering drug. J Clin Pharmacol 2003;43(7):683–91.

57. Fukao T. Beta ketiothiolase deficiency. Orphanet encyclopedia. 2001. Available at: https://www.orpha.net/data/patho/GB/uk-T2.pdf. Accessed March 12, 2017.

58. van Hasselt PM, Ferdinandusse S, Monroe GR, et al. Monocarboxylate transporter 1 deficiency and ketone utilization. N Engl J Med 2014;371(20):1900–7.

59. Fukao T, Shintaku H, Kusubae R, et al. Patients homozygous for the T435N mutation of succinyl-CoA:3-ketoacid CoA Transferase (SCOT) do not show permanent ketosis. Pediatr Res 2004;56(6):858–63.

60. Sarafoglou K, Matern D, Redlinger-Grosse K, et al. Siblings with mitochondrial acetoacetyl-CoA thiolase deficiency not identified by newborn screening. Pediatrics 2011;128(1):e246–50.

61. Fukao T, Mitchell G, Sass JO, et al. Ketone body metabolism and its defects. J Inherit Metab Dis 2014;37(4):541–51.

Inborn Errors of Metabolism with Hyperammonemia
Urea Cycle Defects and Related Disorders

Marshall L. Summar, MD*, Nicholas Ah Mew, MD

KEYWORDS

- Hyperammonemia • Ammonia • Arginine • Citrulline • Liver • Urea cycle • Ornithine

KEY POINTS

- Symptoms of hyperammonemia include cerebral edema, lethargy, anorexia, hyperventilation or hypoventilation, hypothermia, seizures, neurologic posturing, and coma.
- Clinical awareness and suspicion of hyperammonemia is the most important component in the diagnosis and treatment of inborn errors of metabolism associated with elevated ammonia levels.
- For the pediatrician, recognition, stabilization, and rapid transport to a center with a metabolic specialist is the surest way to achieve an optimal outcome.
- Emergency management of hyperammonemia is based on 3 interdependent principles: physical removal of the ammonia by renal replacement therapy, reversal of the catabolic state, and pharmacologic scavenging of excess nitrogen.

INTRODUCTION

The urea cycle, first described by Krebs and Henseleit,[1] converts into urea the extra nitrogen produced by the breakdown of protein and other nitrogen-containing molecules (**Fig. 1**). A congenital or secondary deficiency of the urea cycle may, thus, result in the accumulation of ammonia and other precursor metabolites. Through a variety of mechanisms, hyperammonemia can cause cerebral edema, lethargy, anorexia, hyperventilation or hypoventilation, hypothermia, seizures, neurologic posturing, and coma.

The urea cycle as a nitrogen clearance system is limited primarily to the human liver and intestine with carbamyl phosphate synthetase (CPS1) and ornithine transcarbamylase (OTC) limited exclusively to those tissues. The enzymes downstream that process citrulline into arginine are ubiquitous in their distribution, because these enzymes participate in the production of nitric oxide (NO).

The authors have no commercial or financial interests. Both Drs M.L. Summar and N.A. Mew have and do receive funding from the NIH.

Rare Disease Institute, Children's National Medical Center, 111 Michigan Avenue Northwest, Washington, DC 20010, USA

* Corresponding author.

E-mail address: msummar@cnmc.org

Pediatr Clin N Am 65 (2018) 231–246
https://doi.org/10.1016/j.pcl.2017.11.004
0031-3955/18/© 2017 Elsevier Inc. All rights reserved.

pediatric.theclinics.com

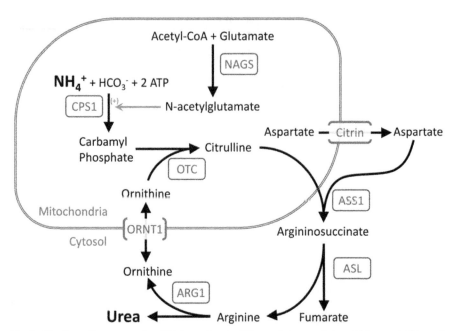

Fig. 1. The hepatic urea cycle. ARG1, arginase; ASL, argininosuccinic acid lyase; ASS1, argininosuccinic acid synthase; ATP, adenosine triphosphate; CoA, coenzyme A; CPS1, carbamyl phosphate synthetase 1; NAGS, *N*-acetylglutamate synthase; ORNT1, mitochondrial ornithine transporter 1; OTC, ornithine transcarbamylase.

A primary urea cycle disorder (UCD) results from an inherited defect in one of the 6 enzymes or 2 transporters of the urea cycle (see **Fig. 1**). Infants with near or total absence of activity of any of these proteins, in particular the first 4 urea cycle enzymes (CPS1, OTC, argininosuccinate synthase [ASS1], and argininosuccinate lyase [ASL]) or the cofactor producer (*N*-acetyl glutamate synthetase [NAGS]), often initially seem to be normal, but within days develop signs and symptoms of hyperammonemia. With partial urea cycle enzyme deficiencies, individuals may go decades before encountering an environmental stress that overwhelms their marginal ureagenesis capacity, resulting in a hyperammonemic episode. Commonly distributed, functional polymorphisms in the urea cycle may not result in hyperammonemia, but instead affect the production of downstream metabolic intermediates (such as arginine) during key periods of need. These variations in intermediate molecule supply can affect other metabolic pathways such as the production of NO from citrulline and arginine, and potentially the tricarboxylic acid cycle through aspartate and fumarate.

A secondary defect in the urea cycle may occur if there is a functional deficiency of substrates of one of the urea cycle enzymes. Examples include low intramitochondrial bicarbonate in carbonic anhydrase 5A deficiency, or low ornithine in lysinuric protein intolerance and neonatal ornithine aminotransferase deficiency. Additionally, inhibition of the cofactor producer, NAGS, is a proposed mechanism of urea cycle dysfunction in several conditions, including the organic acidemias, valproate toxicity, and chemotherapy-induced hyperammonemia. Furthermore, generalized liver dysfunction caused by toxin, infection, poor perfusion, or other inborn errors of metabolism, may impair urea cycle function and result in hyperammonemia (**Box 1**).

Box 1
Causes of hyperammonemia

Factors that diminish urea cycle function or augment demands on the urea cycle:
- Genetic defect in an enzyme
- Damage to the liver (both chronic and acutely)
- Chemical toxins (ethyl alcohol, industrial, etc)
- Infectious processes

Drug effects on the cycle
- Direct interference with enzymes
  ○ Valproic acid
  ○ Chemotherapy (particularly cyclophosphamide)
- Damage or general disruption of hepatic function
  ○ Systemic antifungals
  ○ Chemotherapy from hepatotoxic effects
  ○ Acetaminophen

Other metabolic diseases
- Organic acidemias (in particular, propionic and methylmalonic acidemias)
- Carbonic anhydrase 5A deficiency
- Lysinuric protein intolerance
- Ornithine aminotransferase deficiency (in neonates)
- Pyruvate carboxylase deficiency
- Fatty acid oxidation defects
- Galactosemia
- Tyrosinemia type I
- Glycogen storage disease

Portosystemic shunt

Nitrogen overload
- Massive hemolysis (such as large bone fracture or trauma)
- Total parenteral nutrition
- Protein catabolism from starvation or bariatric surgery
- Postpartum stress
- Heart lung transplant
- Renal disease
- Gastrointestinal bleeding
- Catabolic stimuli
  ○ Corticosteroids
  ○ Gastric bypass
  ○ Prolonged fast or excessive protein restriction

EFFECT OF AMMONIA ON BRAIN

Ammonia toxicity is thought to cause brain edema, induce neuronal and glial cell death, and alter synaptic growth.[2] The developing brain is much more susceptible to the deleterious effects of ammonia than the adult brain,[3] although the adult brain inside closed cranial sutures is more susceptible to the effects of cerebral edema.

Ammonia diffuses freely from the blood stream across the blood–brain barrier and is rapidly condensed with glutamate to form glutamine by astrocytic glutamine synthetase. Glutamine is osmotically active. In addition, ammonia itself may perturb potassium homeostasis and alter water transport through aquaporin. Therefore, through a variety of mechanisms, acute hyperammonemia results in astrocyte swelling and cytotoxic brain edema.[4] Astrocyte swelling can precipitate pH and Ca^{2+}-dependent glutamate release from astrocytes as well as inhibit GLAST (glutamate-aspartate) transporter reuptake of glutamate, leading to an overabundance of glutamate in the synaptic space. This results in excess depolarization of glutamatergic neurons through the N-methyl-D-aspartate glutamate receptor, thereby inducing alterations in NO metabolism and the Na^+/K^+-ATPase. This process precipitates a shortage of adenosine triphosphate, mitochondrial dysfunction, and oxidative stress, which ultimately promote neuronal apoptosis.[2] Acute hyperammonemia may exert effects through metabotropic and alpha-amino-3-hydroxy-5-methyl-4-isoxazolepropionic acid glutamate receptors[5] and also alters cholinergic and serotoninergic systems.[2]

Chronic hyperammonemia may induce adaptive changes in N-methyl-D-aspartate receptor-mediated transmission and induction of astrocytosis. In the developing rat, ammonia inhibits axonal and dendritic growth, and disturbs signal transduction pathways.[6] These potential mechanisms may explain the cognitive impairment, behavioral difficulties, and epilepsy observed in older individuals with UCDs, even in the absence of acute hyperammonemia.

Symptoms and Signs of Urea Cycle Disorders

Acute symptoms from hyperammonemia progress from somnolence to lethargy and coma. Abnormal posturing and encephalopathy are often related to the degree of central nervous system swelling and pressure on the brain stem.[7–9] A significant portion of neonates with severe hyperammonemia have seizures, which may be subclinical and nonconvulsive. Hyperventilation, secondary to cerebral edema, is a common early finding in a hyperammonemic attack, which causes a respiratory alkalosis. Hypoventilation and respiratory arrest follow as pressure increases on the brain stem[8–11] (**Box 2**).

In milder (or partial) urea cycle enzyme deficiencies, ammonia accumulation may be triggered by illness or stress at almost any time of life, resulting in multiple mild increases in plasma ammonia concentration.[12] The hyperammonemia is less severe and the symptoms more subtle. In individuals with partial enzyme deficiencies, the first recognized clinical episode may be delayed for months or years. Although the clinical abnormalities vary somewhat with the specific UCD, in most, the hyperammonemic episode is marked by loss of appetite, cyclical vomiting, lethargy, and behavioral abnormalities. Sleep disorders, delusions, hallucinations, and psychosis may occur. An encephalopathic (slow wave) pattern on electroencephalography may be observed during hyperammonemia and nonspecific brain atrophy may be seen subsequently on MRI[8,10,12–14] (**Box 3**). The symptoms at first presentation are summarized in **Box 4**.

CAUSES OF UREA CYCLE DISORDERS

A brief review of disorder of the of the urea cycle follows. **Table 1** lists the enzymes and genes of the cycle associated with disease.

Box 2
Symptoms of newborns with urea cycle defects

- Normal appearance at birth
- Somnolence progressing to lethargy then coma
- Loss of thermoregulation (hypothermia)
- Feeding disruption (increases catabolism)
- Neurologic posturing (from cerebral edema)
- Seizures
- Hyperventilation and then hypoventilation

Box 3
Common clinical features for late onset urea cycle disorders

- Dramatic and rapid increase in nitrogen load from
  ○ Trauma
  ○ Rapid weight loss and autocatabolism
  ○ Increase in protein turnover from intravenous steroids
- Avoidance of dietary protein
- History of behavioral or psychiatric illnesses
- Rapid deterioration of neurologic status
- Severe encephalopathy inconsistent with medical condition
- Evidence for cerebral edema by clinical examination or radiograph
- Seizures in most cases
- Decrease in oral intake in leading up to decompensation

Carbamylphosphate Synthetase 1 Deficiency

Carbamylphosphate synthetase 1 (CPS1) is the first enzyme in the urea cycle and is found primarily in the liver. It condenses ammonia, bicarbonate, and adenosine triphosphate into carbamyl phosphate. CPS1 requires its cofactor *N*-acetylglutamate (NAG; see **Fig. 1**). Individuals with complete CPS1 deficiency rapidly develop hyperammonemia in the newborn period. Affected children who are successfully rescued from crisis are chronically at risk for repeated bouts of hyperammonemia. Individuals with partial CPS1 deficiency can present at almost any time of life with a stressful triggering event. Biochemical analyses may be highly suggestive of CPS1 deficiency, however, molecular testing is often required to make this diagnosis.

N-Acetylglutamate Synthetase Deficiency

NAGS catalyzes the conversion of glutamate and acetyl-CoA to NAG, the required cofactor of CPS1 (see **Fig. 1**). Without NAG, CPS1 cannot convert ammonia into carbamyl phosphate; thus, NAGS deficiency results in a functional deficiency of CPS1. Individuals with complete NAGS deficiency rapidly develop hyperammonemia in the

---

Box 4
Presenting symptoms in 260 affected individuals at first presentation of hyperammonemia

- Neurologic symptoms (100%)
- Decreased level of consciousness (63%)
- Abnormal motor function or tone (30%)
- Seizures (10%)
- Vomiting (19%)
- Infection (30%)
- Subjective: decreased appetite, fussy
- Physiologic: respiratory alkalosis (secondary to cerebral edema) followed by apnea

From Summar ML, Dobbelaere D, Brusilow S, et al. Diagnosis, symptoms, frequency and mortality of 260 patients with urea cycle disorders from a 21-year, multicentre study of acute hyperammonaemic episodes. Acta Paediatr 2008;97(10):1420–5; with permission.

Table 1
Enzymes and genes of urea cycle associated with disease: CPS1 deficiency

Gene Name	Gene Symbol	Location	Protein Name
Carbamyl phosphate synthetase 1	CPS1	2q35	Carbamyl phosphate synthase 1
Ornithine transcarbamylase	OTC	Xp21.1	Ornithine transcarbamylase
Argininosuccinate synthetase 1	ASS1	9q34	Argininosuccinate synthetase 1
Argininosuccinate lyase	ASL	7cen-q11.2	Argininosuccinate lyase
Arginase 1	ARG1	6q23	Arginase 1
N-acetyl glutamate synthetase	NAGS	17q21.3	N-acetyl glutamate synthetase
Solute carrier family 25 member 15	SLC25A15	13q14	Mitochondrial ornithine transporter 1 (ORNT1)
Solute carrier family 25 member 13	SLC25A13	7q21.3	Mitochondrial aspartate glutamate transporter (Citrin)

newborn period. Affected children who are successfully rescued from crisis are chronically at risk for repeated bouts of hyperammonemia. Individuals with partial NAGS deficiency can present at almost any time of life with a stressful triggering event. The use of an analog of NAG, carbamyl glutamate, has proven effective in the treatment of this condition.

Ornithine Transcarbamylase Deficiency

OTC combines carbamyl phosphate with ornithine to make citrulline (see **Fig. 1**). Like with CPS1 deficiency, children with complete OTC deficiency rapidly develop hyperammonemia in the newborn period and thereafter are at risk for repeated bouts of hyperammonemia. OTC is located on the X chromosome; therefore, the majority of severely affected individuals are male. Carrier females may rarely also be affected, owing to skewed lyonization. OTC deficiency is the most common UCD. Individuals with partial OTC deficiency can present at almost any time with a stressful triggering event.

Argininosuccinate Synthetase Deficiency (Citrullinemia I)

ASS1 conjugates citrulline and aspartate to form argininosuccinate (see **Fig. 1**). Individuals with complete ASS1 deficiency present with severe hyperammonemia in the newborn period. Citrulline levels in these individuals can be hundreds of times the normal values. Unlike CPS1, NAGS, and OTC, this enzyme is distributed throughout the body. ASS1 has also been shown to be involved in the production of NO.

Citrin Deficiency (Citrullinemia II)

Citrullinemia II results from a deficiency of the mitochondrial membrane glutamate-aspartate transporter, SLC25A15 (see **Fig. 1**). The reduced availability of aspartate for the enzyme argininosuccinic acid synthase results in a functional deficiency of the urea cycle. This disorder presents in adolescence or adulthood with recurrent hyperammonemia and neuropsychiatric symptoms. However, biallelic mutations in SLC25A15 more commonly present in newborns as neonatal intrahepatic cholestasis or in older children as failure to thrive and dyslipidemia. The majority of reported affected individuals have been Asian, owing to a common mutation.

Argininosuccinate Lyase Deficiency (Argininosuccinic Aciduria)

The products of ASL are arginine and fumarate. This enzymatic step is past the point in the urea cycle at which all the waste nitrogen from 1 revolution through the cycle has been incorporated (see **Fig. 1**). Because argininosuccinate is freely excreted in the urine, thereby disposing of 4 nitrogens, hyperammonemia is typically less severe and less frequent than the disorders proximal to this step in the urea cycle. This disorder is often marked by chronic hepatic enlargement and elevation of transaminases. Biopsy of the liver shows enlarged hepatocytes, which may over time progress to fibrosis, the etiology of which is unclear. These children can also develop trichorrhexis nodosa, a nodelike appearance of fragile hair, which usually responds to arginine supplementation.[8,10] Reports exist of affected individuals who have never had prolonged coma, but nevertheless have significant developmental disabilities, possibly owing to impairment of NO synthesis or the deleterious effects of argininosuccinic acid.

Arginase Deficiency (Hyperargininemia)

Arginase is the final step in urea synthesis. It cleaves arginine into ornithine and urea (see **Fig. 1**). Arginase deficiency is not typically characterized by rapid-onset hyperammonemia. Instead, affected individuals often present with developmental delay and progressive spasticity, in particular of the lower limbs. They also may develop seizures and gradually lose intellectual attainments. Growth is usually slow and without therapy they do not reach normal adult height. Other symptoms that may present early in life include episodes of irritability, anorexia, and vomiting.

Ornithine Translocase Deficiency (Hyperornithinemia, Hyperammonemia, Homocitrullinuria Syndrome)

The hyperornithinemia, hyperammonemia, homocitrullinuria syndrome is described in more than 50 individuals. The defect in ornithine translocase results in diminished ornithine transport into the mitochondria with ornithine accumulation in the cytoplasm and reduced intramitochondrial ornithine causing impaired ureagenesis, hyperammonemia, and orotic aciduria (see **Fig. 1**). Plasma ornithine concentrations are extremely high. Homocitrulline is thought to originate from carbamylation of lysine. Most affected individuals have intermittent hyperammonemia accompanied by vomiting, lethargy, and coma (in extreme cases). Growth is abnormal and intellectual development is affected. Spasticity is common, as are seizures.

DIAGNOSIS OF UREA CYCLE DISORDERS

The most important step in diagnosing UCDs is clinical suspicion of hyperammonemia. Time is not on the side of the clinician or the affected individual. Particular care should be taken in drawing blood ammonia, because there is significant variability depending on proper technique and handling, frequently resulting in false-positive results. The clinician should remember that treatment should not be delayed in efforts to reach a final diagnosis, and that later stages of treatment should be tailored to the specific disorder. In addition to plasma ammonia, helpful laboratory data include, pH, CO_2, anion gap, blood lactate, plasma acylcarnitine profile, plasma amino acids, and urine organic acids, including the specific determination of orotic acid.[15] Individuals with UCDs will typically have normal glucose and electrolyte levels. The pH and CO_2 can vary with the degree of cerebral edema and hyperventilation or hypoventilation; however, hyperammonemia in the context of a respiratory alkalosis is highly suggestive of a UCD. In neonates, it should be remembered that the basal ammonia level is elevated over that of adults, which typically is less than 35 μmol/L (less than

110 µmol/L in neonates). An elevated plasma ammonia level of 150 µmol/L (>260 µg/dL) or higher in neonates and greater than 100 µmol/L (175 µg/dL) in older children and adults, associated with a normal anion gap and a normal blood glucose level, is a strong indication for the presence of a UCD. Quantitative amino acid analysis can be used to evaluate these individuals and arrive at a tentative diagnosis. Elevations or depressions of the intermediate amino-containing molecules arginine, citrulline, ornithine, and argininosuccinate (see **Fig. 1**) will give clues to the point of defect in the cycle (**Fig. 2**). The levels of the nitrogen-buffering amino acid glutamine will also be quite high and can serve as confirmation of true hyperammonemia. If a defect in NAGS, CPS1, or OTC is suspected, the presence of elevated orotic acid in the urine

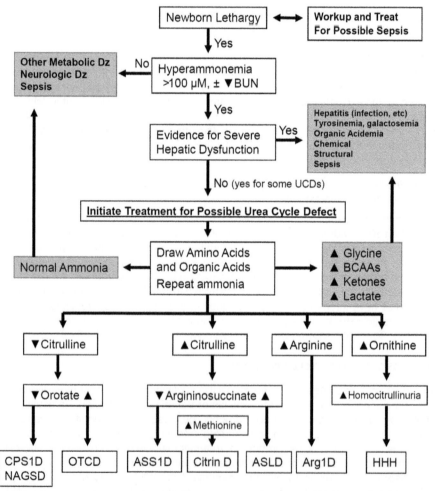

Fig. 2. Diagnostic algorithm for acute hyperammonemia. Arg1D, arginase deficiency; ASLD, argininosuccinic acid lyase deficiency; ASS1D, argininosuccinic acid synthase deficiency; BCAAs, branched chain amino acids; BUN, blood urea nitrogen; citrin D, citrin deficiency (citrullinemia type II); CPS1D, carbamyl phosphate synthetase 1 deficiency; Dz, disease; HHH, homocitrullinuria, hyperornithinemia, hyperammonemia; NAGSD, *N*-acetylglutamate synthase deficiency; OTCD, ornithine transcarbamylase deficiency; UCDs, urea cycle disorders; ▼, decreased; ▲, increased.

is highly suggestive of OTC deficiency. Orotic acid is produced when there is an over-abundance of carbamyl phosphate that spills into the pyrimidine biosynthetic system. The determination of urine organic acids and plasma acylcarnitines will also herald the presence of an organic aciduria.

DNA sequence analysis is available for all of these disorders and the clinician should consider a panel approach rather than a gene-by-gene approach. Enzymatic and genetic diagnosis is available for all of these disorders. For CPS1, OTC, and NAGS, enzymatic diagnosis is made on a liver biopsy specimen freshly frozen in liquid nitrogen. Enzymatic testing for ASS1 and ASL can be done on fibroblast samples and arginase activity can be tested in red blood cells.

TREATMENT OF UREA CYCLE DISORDERS

Disclaimer: The treatment of these disorders is complex and best conducted by a specialist in inborn errors of metabolism at a center equipped to do so. For the pediatrician, recognition, stabilization, and rapid transport are the surest way to achieve optimal outcome. Delays in treatment and failure to maximize appropriate treatment will have permanent and damaging effects on the affected individual.

This section provides an overview of UCDs management.[9,16,17] The treatment of these individuals requires a highly coordinated team of specialists trained in caring for individuals with inborn errors of metabolism (**Box 5**). The emergency management of affected individuals in hyperammonemic coma resulting from a UCD is based on 3 interdependent principles: first, physical removal of the ammonia by dialysis or some form of hemofiltration; second, reversal of the catabolic state through caloric supplementation and, in extreme cases, hormonal suppression (glucose/insulin drip); and third, pharmacologic scavenging of excess nitrogen (**Box 6**). These measures should be pursued in parallel as quickly as possible.

The extracorporeal clearance of ammonia should be considered regardless of ammonia level if the affected individual is grossly encephalopathic, or the increase in ammonia is rapid or refractory to medical therapy. Central venous access should be established at once and dialysis or rapid hemofiltration begun immediately at the highest available flow rate. Dialysis is very effective for the removal of ammonia and the clearance depends on the flow through the dialysis circuit.[18,19] Given the risk of dialysis in a newborn, consideration should be given to arteriovenous or venovenous hemofiltration with a variable speed bypass pump in the circuit. If possible, access to hemofiltration should be maintained until the child is stabilized and the catabolic state is reversed. Some individuals may experience a rebound in plasma ammonia levels and may require additional rounds of dialysis. This effect may be attenuated by converting the affected individual to continuous renal replacement therapy after the initial period of intermittent dialysis. Most affected individuals will have a slight increase in ammonia after dialysis, because removal by scavengers and the liver will not be as effective. This slight increase usually does not necessitate repeat dialysis. With more aggressive reintroduction of protein, the author has seen a reduction in this rebound effect.

The importance of the management of the catabolic state cannot be overstressed. Because the catabolism of protein stores is often the triggering event for hyperammonemia, the affected child will continue to produce ammonia and will not stabilize until the catabolic state is reversed. Fluids, dextrose, and intravenous lipid emulsion should be given to blunt the catabolic process. Most affected individuals are dehydrated at initial presentation owing to poor fluid intake. The affected individuals should be assessed for dehydration and fluids replaced. Because these individuals suffer from

---

Box 5
Treatment team and organization

- Metabolic specialist
  - Coordinate treatment and management
- Intensive care team
  - Assist with physiologic support
  - Ventilator management
  - Sedation and pain management
- Nephrologist or dialysis team
  - Manage dialysis
  - Manage renal complications
- Surgical team
  - Large-bore catheter placement
  - Liver biopsy as necessary
  - Gastrostomy tube placement (if indicated)
- Pharmacy staff
  - Formulate nitrogen scavenging drugs
  - Cross-check dosing orders in complex management
- Laboratory staff
  - Analyze large volume of ammonia samples in acute phase
  - Analyze amino acids and other specialty laboratory tests
- Nursing staff
  - Execute complex and rapidly changing management plan
  - Closely monitor for signs of deterioration or change
- Nutritionist
  - Maximize caloric intake with neutral nitrogen balance
  - Educate family in management of complex very low-protein diet
- Social work
  - Rapidly identify resources for complex outpatient treatment regimen
  - Work with families in highly stressful clinical situation
- Genetic counselor
  - Educate family in genetics of rare metabolic disease
  - Identify other family members at potential risk (ornithine transcarbamylase particularly)
  - Ensure proper samples are obtained for future prenatal testing
  - Contact research and diagnostic centers for genetic testing

---

Box 6
Emergency management at first symptoms

- Fluids, dextrose, and intralipid to mitigate catabolism and typical dehydration (attempt 80 cal/kg/d).
- Antibiotics and septic workup to treat potential triggering events or primary sepsis (continue through treatment course). A spinal tap should probably be avoided pending imaging.
- Contact and possible transport to treatment-capable institute as soon as possible.
- Remove protein from intake (by mouth or total parenteral nutrition).
- Establish central venous access.
- Provide physiologic support (pressors, buffering agents, etc). (Renal output is critical to long-term success).
- Stabilize airway; cerebral edema may result in sudden respiratory arrest.

cerebral edema, care should be taken to avoid fluid overload. The nitrogen scavenging drugs are usually administered in a large volume of fluid, which should be taken into consideration. A regimen of 80 to 120 kcal/kg/d is a reasonable goal. The administration of insulin is useful, but also requires experience, and should be reserved for the sickest individuals. At the same time, protein must be temporarily removed from intake (by mouth or total parenteral nutrition), for no longer than 12 to 24 hours. Refeeding the affected individuals as soon as practicable is useful, because more calories can be administered this way. The use of essential amino acid formulations in feeding can reduce the amount of protein necessary to meet basic needs, and should be strongly considered within the first 24 hours of admission. In lieu of introducing food into the gut, parenteral nutrition containing only essential amino acids as a nitrogen source can be used. Delivery through the gastrointestinal tract is the preferred method. These individuals have not shown themselves to be more prone to necrotizing enterocolitis.

Emergency pharmacologic management with intravenous ammonia scavengers is initiated as soon as possible using the drug combination sodium phenylacetate and sodium benzoate, ideally while the dialysis is being arranged and the diagnostic workup is under way. These 2 agents are used in combination to trap nitrogen in excretable forms. Sodium benzoate combines with glycine to make hippurate, and sodium phenylacetate combines with glutamine to make phenacetylglutamine, which are excreted by the kidneys (or removed in the dialysate).[20,21] The body replaces these amino acids using excess nitrogen. It is suspected that the removal of glutamine by phenylacetate has the additional benefit of removing a compound suspected of having a major role in the neurotoxicity of these disorders.[2,4,22,23] Currently, administering a second loading dose to the affected individual after the initial phase is not recommended, because there is toxicity associated with overdose.

Arginine must also be administered continuously intravenously in the acute phase of treatment of UCDs. Supplementation of arginine serves to replace arginine not produced by the urea cycle (in addition to the partial cycle function it can stimulate) and prevents its deficiency from causing additional protein catabolism. Because arginine is the precursor for NO production, it is worth considering reducing the arginine dose if the affected individual develops vasodilation and hypotension. Before diagnostic confirmation, affected individuals should be also started on the NAG analog carbamyl glutamate, because this agent may be effective in NAGS deficiency, some cases of CPS1 deficiency, and in the organic acidemias.

Table 2 lists doses for the acute management of these individuals according to the diagnosis at the time of treatment (information extracted from the US Food and Drug Administration package insert). Owing to the potential for toxicity (lethal in extreme cases) of these drugs, consultation with an experienced metabolic physician is recommended before initiating treatment.[24] A resource for finding these physicians and other treatment suggestions is found in the home page for this web site at: http://www.rarediseasesnetwork.org/ucdc.

After the initial loading phase and dialysis, the dose should be converted to the maintenance doses of the ammonia scavengers listed in the manufacturer's packaging insert (see **Table 2**). If the exact enzyme defect is known, the amount of arginine administered can be adjusted downward. If chronic therapy is warranted, the affected individual can then be switched to the oral prodrug of phenylacetate, sodium phenylbutyrate, or the pre-prodrug glycerol phenylbutyrate, which has a slower release and no taste. The drug insert packaging should be consulted for proper dosing. The usual total daily dose of phenylbutyrate tablets or powder for individuals with UCDs is 450 to 600 mg/kg/d in individuals weighing less than 20 kg, or 9.9 to 13.0 g/m^2/d in larger individuals. The tablets or powder are to be taken in equally divided amounts with each meal or

Table 2
Sodium phenylacetate and sodium benzoate dosage and administration

Affected Individual Population	Components of Infusion Solution			Dosage Provided		
	Sodium Phenylacetate and Sodium Benzoate	Arginine HCl Injection, 10%	Dextrose Injection, 10%	Sodium Phenylacetate	Sodium Benzoate	Arginine HCl
Neonates to young children						
NAGS, CPS and OTC Deficiency						
Loading dose (90 min)	2.5 (mL/kg)	2.0 mL/kg	≥25 mL/kg	250 mg/kg	250 mg/kg	200 mg/kg
Maintenance dose	2.5 mL/kg/24 h	2.0 mL/kg/24 h	≥ 25 mL/kg	250 mg/kg/24 h	250 mg/kg/24 h	200 mg/kg/24 h
Unknown, ASD and ASL deficiency						
Loading dose (90 min)	2.5 mL/kg	6.0 mL/kg	≥25 mL/kg	250 mg/kg	250 mg/kg	600 mg/kg
Maintenance dose	2.5 mL/kg/24 h	6.0 mL/kg/24 h	≥25 mL/kg	250 mg/kg/24 h	250 mg/kg/24 h	600 mg/kg/24 h
Older children and adults						
NAGS, CPS, and OTC deficiency						
Loading dose (90 min)	55 mL/m^2	2.0 mL/kg	≥25 mL/kg	5.5 g/m^2	5.5 g/m^2	200 mg/kg
Maintenance Dose	55 mL/m^2/24 h	2.0 mL/kg/24 h	≥25 mL/kg	5.5 g/m^2/24 h	5.5 g/m^2/24 h	200 mg/kg/24 h
Unknown, ASD and ASL deficiency						
Loading dose (90 min)	55 mL/m^2	6.0 mL/kg	≥25 mL/kg	5.5 g/m^2	5.5 g/m^2	600 mg/kg
Maintenance dose	55 mL/m^2/24 h	6.0 mL/kg/24 h	≥25 mL/kg	5.5 g/m^2/24 h	5.5 g/m^2/24 h	600 mg/kg/24 h

Abbreviations: ASL, argininosuccinate lyase; CPS, carbamyl phosphate synthetase; NAGS, N-acetyl glutamate synthetase; OTC, ornithine transcarbamylase.

feeding (ie, 3 to 6 times per day). Citrulline supplementation is recommended for individuals diagnosed with deficiency of NAGS, CPS1, or OTC. The daily recommended dose is 0.17 g/kg/d or 3.8 g/m^2/d. Arginine supplementation is needed for individuals diagnosed with deficiency of ASS1; arginine (free base) daily intake is recommended at 0.25 to 0.3 g/kg/d. In individuals with NAGS, the use of carbamyl glutamate has been demonstrated to be very effective,[25] and is approved by the US Food and Drug Administration for this disorder. The package insert should be consulted for dosing.

In all instances, intensive care treatment has to be meticulous. Ventilator or circulatory support may be required, in addition to anticonvulsive medications to control seizures. Sedation or head cooling to reduce cerebral activity could be of benefit to these individuals, but has not been fully clinically evaluated for efficacy. Antibiotic therapy and evaluation for sepsis is recommended because sepsis is an important consideration in the primary presentation and, if present, may lead to further catabolism. Electrolytes and acid–base balance are to be checked every 6 hours during the initial phase of treatment. The use of osmotic agents such as mannitol is not felt to be effective in treating the cerebral edema from hyperammonemia, because this condition is not thought to be osmotic in nature. In canines, opening the blood–brain barrier with mannitol resulted in cerebral edema by promoting the entry of ammonia into the brain fluid compartment.[26,27] Other measures include physiologic support (pressors, buffering agents to maintain pH and buffer arginine HCl, etc) and maintenance of renal output, particularly if ammonia scavengers are being used. Finally, it is imperative to reassess continuation of care after the initial phase of treatment.

Intravenous steroids should be avoided, because they promote catabolism. Valproic acid is also contraindicated because it may impair urea cycle function.

A rapid response to the hyperammonemia is indispensable for a good outcome.[28] Acute symptomatology centers around cerebral edema, disruptions in neurochemistry, and pressure on the brainstem. The resulting decrease in cerebral blood flow plus prolonged seizures, when they occur, are poor prognostic factors. In adults, because the sutures of the skull are fused, sensitivity to hyperammonemia seems to be considerably greater than in children.[29] Thus, treatment should be aggressive and intensified at a lower ammonia concentration than in children.

Cerebral studies should be conducted to determine the efficacy of treatment and whether continuation is warranted. Electroencephalography should be performed to assess both cerebral function and evidence of seizure activity, which may be nonconvulsive. If available, cerebral blood flow as determined by MRI can be used to establish if venous stasis has occurred from cerebral edema. Magnetic resonance spectroscopy may also be useful during the diagnostic stage. Evaluation of brain stem function and higher cortical function are useful to assess outcome. In the authors' experience, the appearance of the MRI in the postacute phase may be worse than what is seen in the long-term clinical outcome. Finally, the decision for continuation is based on baseline neurologic status, duration of coma, and potential for recovery, as well as whether the affected individual is a candidate for transplantation. In severe UCDs, early liver transplantation has become routine. Criteria for transplantation are, of course, linked back to neurologic status, duration of coma, and availability of donor organs. Diagnostic samples of DNA, liver, and skin should be obtained because they can be central in family counseling and future treatment issues.

LONG-TERM MANAGEMENT

Every effort should be made to avoid triggering events. It is imperative to prevent or quickly interrupt a catabolic state at an early stage of impending decompensation during subsequent illnesses or surgeries, as well as during any event resulting in significant bleeding or tissue damage. Because this conditions usually happens at home, it is essential to educate the family about how to react adequately. All affected individuals should carry an emergency card or bracelet containing essential information and phone numbers, as well as instructions on emergency measures. Every affected person should relate to physicians and a hospital with a dedicated team of metabolic specialists who can be reached at any time. For vacations, it is usually prudent to enquire about metabolic services in the respective destination.

Long-term diet modification with nutritional oversight is often necessary in individuals with chronic episodes of hyperammonemia, and should be done only in collaboration with a metabolic dietitian. Individuals with urea cycle defects should also avoid dehydration, an especially common occurrence among adults in connection with alcohol intake, hiking, and airline flights. Not all affected adults who recover from a hyperammonemic episode require chronic nitrogen scavengers, but they ought to be considered because many of these individuals can become more brittle as time goes on. Recommended evaluations for individuals with UCDs are listed in **Box 7**.

Should psychiatric problems occur over the long term, caregivers should be alert to the possibility of hyperammonemia. In addition, many individuals with UCDs, in particular OTC deficiency and citrullinemia type 2, have presented with mental disturbance.[30–34]

Clinical observations of individuals with ASL deficiency demonstrate a high incidence of chronic progressive cirrhosis with eventual fibrosis of the liver. This finding is not commonly seen in the other UCDs and studies are underway to better determine the exact pathophysiology. It is important to provide genetic counseling in order to assess risk to other family members.

Box 7
Recommended evaluations for individuals with UCD

During initial presentation:

Head ultrasound

Brain MRI (upon stabilization of acute hyperammonemia)

Hearing screen at discharge

Vision screen at discharge

Long term management:

Developmental testing

Echocardiogram every 2 years to evaluate for pulmonary hypertension (for argininosuccinate synthase and argininosuccinate lyase deficiencies)

Annual abdominal ultrasound and alpha-fetoprotein after age 20

Dual energy x-ray absorptiometry scan (every 5 years, starting at age 10)

Routine clinic visits

- Nutrition evaluation to include
  Growth parameters
  Dietary history

- Biochemical analysis
  Ammonia
  Amino acid profile
  Pre-albumin
  Vitamin D (yearly)

SUMMARY

UCDs present the physician with one of the most emergent and intellectually challenging scenarios they are likely to encounter. With optimized teamwork, rapid response, and early diagnosis, affected individuals can have a good outcome. The experts in the Urea Cycle Disorders Consortium, which is sponsored by the National Institutes of Health, are an excellent resource when confronting a newly affected individual, and the UCDC web site is an excellent place to start.

REFERENCES

1. Krebs H, Henseleit K. Untersuchungen uber die harnstoffbildung im tierkorper. Hoppe-Seyler's Z Physiol Chem 1932;210:325–32.
2. Braissant O, Mclin VA, Cudalbu C. Ammonia toxicity to the brain. J Inherit Metab Dis 2013;36(4):595–612.
3. Cagnon L, Braissant O. Hyperammonemia-induced toxicity for the developing central nervous system. Brain Res Rev 2007;56(1):183–97.
4. Gropman AL, Summar M, Leonard JV. Neurological implications of urea cycle disorders. J Inherit Metab Dis 2007;30(6):865–79.
5. Butterworth RF. Glutamate transporter and receptor function in disorders of ammonia metabolism. Ment Retard Dev Disabil Res Rev 2001;7(4):276–9.
6. Braissant O, Henry H, Villard AM, et al. Ammonium-induced impairment of axonal growth is prevented through glial creatine. J Neurosci 2002;22(22):9810–20.
7. Batshaw ML, Berry GT. Use of citrulline as a diagnostic marker in the prospective treatment of urea cycle disorders. J Pediatr 1991;118(6):914–7.
8. Brusilow SW. Disorders of the urea cycle. Hosp Pract (Off Ed) 1985;20(10):65–72.
9. Summar M. Current strategies for the management of neonatal urea cycle disorders. J Pediatr 2001;138(1 Suppl):S30–9.
10. Batshaw ML. Hyperammonemia. Curr Probl Pediatr 1984;14(11):1–69.
11. Summar M, Tuchman M. Proceedings of a consensus conference for the management of patients with urea cycle disorders. J Pediatr 2001;138(1 Suppl): S6–10.
12. Bourrier P, Varache N, Alquier P, et al. [Cerebral edema with hyperammonemia in valpromide poisoning. Manifestation in an adult, of a partial deficit in type I carbamylphosphate synthetase]. Presse Med 1988;17(39):2063–6 [in French].
13. Brunquell P, Tezcan K, Dimario FJ Jr. Electroencephalographic findings in ornithine transcarbamylase deficiency. J Child Neurol 1999;14(8):533–6.
14. Clancy RR, Chung HJ. EEG changes during recovery from acute severe neonatal citrullinemia. Electroencephalography Clin Neurophysiol 1991;78(3):222–7.
15. Steiner RD, Cederbaum SD. Laboratory evaluation of urea cycle disorders. J Pediatr 2001;138(1 Suppl):S21–9.
16. Brusilow SW, Maestri NE. Urea cycle disorders: diagnosis, pathophysiology, and therapy. Adv Pediatr 1996;43:127–70.
17. Haberle J, Boddaert N, Burlina A, et al. Suggested guidelines for the diagnosis and management of urea cycle disorders. Orphanet J Rare Dis 2012;7:32.
18. Summar M, Pietsch J, Deshpande J, et al. Effective hemodialysis and hemofiltration driven by an extracorporeal membrane oxygenation pump in infants with hyperammonemia. J Pediatr 1996;128(3):379–82.
19. Gupta S, Fenves AZ, Hootkins R. The role of RRT in hyperammonemic patients. Clin J Am Soc Nephrol 2016;11(10):1872–8.

20. Batshaw ML, Brusilow S, Waber L, et al. Treatment of inborn errors of urea synthesis: activation of alternative pathways of waste nitrogen synthesis and excretion. N Engl J Med 1982;306(23):1387–92.

21. Batshaw ML, Macarthur RB, Tuchman M. Alternative pathway therapy for urea cycle disorders: twenty years later. J Pediatr 2001;138(1 Suppl):S46–54 [discussion: S54–5].

22. Butterworth RF. Pathophysiology of hepatic encephalopathy: a new look at ammonia. Metab Brain Dis 2002;17(4):221–7.

23. Lichter-Konecki U. Profiling of astrocyte properties in the hyperammonaemic brain: shedding new light on the pathophysiology of the brain damage in hyperammonaemia. J Inherit Metab Dis 2008;31(4):492–502.

24. Praphanphoj V, Boyadjiev SA, Waber LJ, et al. Three cases of intravenous sodium benzoate and sodium phenylacetate toxicity occurring in the treatment of acute hyperammonaemia. J Inherit Metab Dis 2000;23(2):129–36.

25. Tuchman M, Caldovic L, Daikhin Y, et al. N-carbamylglutamate markedly enhances ureagenesis in N-acetylglutamate deficiency and propionic acidemia as measured by isotopic incorporation and blood biomarkers. Pediatr Res 2008;64(2):213–7.

26. Fujiwara M, Watanabe A, Shiota T, et al. Hyperammonemia-induced cytotoxic brain edema under osmotic opening of blood-brain barrier in dogs. Res Exp Med (Berl) 1985;185(6):425–7.

27. Fujiwara M. Role of ammonia in the pathogenesis of brain edema. Acta Med Okayama 1986;40(6):313–20.

28. Msall M, Batshaw ML, Suss R, et al. Neurologic outcome in children with inborn errors of urea synthesis. Outcome of urea-cycle enzymopathies. N Engl J Med 1984;310(23):1500–5.

29. Summar ML, Barr F, Dawling S, et al. Unmasked adult-onset urea cycle disorders in the critical care setting. Crit Care Clin 2005;21(4 Suppl):S1–8.

30. Kolker S, Garcia-Cazorla A, Valayannopoulos V, et al. The phenotypic spectrum of organic acidurias and urea cycle disorders. Part 1: the initial presentation. J Inherit Metab Dis 2015;38(6):1041–57.

31. Belanger-Quintana A, Martinez-Pardo M, Garcia MJ, et al. Hyperammonaemia as a cause of psychosis in an adolescent. Eur J Pediatr 2003;162(11):773–5.

32. Thurlow VR, Asafu-Adjaye M, Agalou S, et al. Fatal ammonia toxicity in an adult due to an undiagnosed urea cycle defect: under-recognition of ornithine transcarbamylase deficiency. Ann Clin Biochem 2010;47(Pt 3):279–81.

33. Sloas HA 3rd, Ence TC, Mendez DR, et al. At the intersection of toxicology, psychiatry, and genetics: a diagnosis of ornithine transcarbamylase deficiency. Am J Emerg Med 2013;31(9):1420.e5-6.

34. Kim SH, Lee JS, Lim BC, et al. A female carrier of ornithine carbamoyltransferase deficiency masquerading as attention deficit-hyperactivity disorder. Brain Development 2014;36(8):734–7.

Inborn Errors of Metabolism with Hypoglycemia

Glycogen Storage Diseases and Inherited Disorders of Gluconeogenesis

David A. Weinstein, MD, MMSc[a,b,*], Ulrike Steuerwald, MD[c],
Carolina F.M. De Souza, MD, PhD[d], Terry G.J. Derks, MD, PhD[e]

KEYWORDS

- Glycogen storage disease • Hypoglycemia • Ketosis • Lactate
- Disorders of gluconeogenesis • Ketotic hypoglycemia

KEY POINTS

- The mechanisms that maintain blood glucose are complex and controlled by hormones, glycogenolysis, gluconeogenesis, mitochondrial fatty acid oxidation, and ketogenesis.
- Glycogen storage diseases (GSDs) comprise several inherited diseases caused by abnormalities of the enzymes and transporters in glycogen synthesis and degradation.
- Hypoglycemia is the primary manifestation of the hepatic GSDs (types 0, I, III, VI, IX, and XI).
- Complications in the hepatic GSDs can be prevented or delayed if near optimal metabolic control is attained.
- Disorders of gluconeogenesis are typically characterized by fasting intolerance with associated recurrent hypoglycemia with lactic acidosis with or without ketosis.

The brain depends on a continuous supply of glucose because it can neither synthesize glucose nor store more than a few minutes supply as glycogen. Although delivery of glucose to the brain is critical for survival, the total amount of glucose in the blood

Disclosures: D.A. Weinstein and T.G.J. Derks collaborate in the Glyde trial (ClinicalTrials.gov identifier: NCT02318966), sponsored by Vitaflo International, Ltd. D.A. Weinstein, T.G.J. Derks, and C.F.M. De Souza serve on the Clinical Advisory Board for the DTX-401 gene therapy trial for GSD IA being planned with Ultragenyx Gene Therapy (Cambridge, MA). In addition, D. A. Weinstien has grant support from Ultragenyx Gene Therapy.
[a] University of Connecticut School of Medicine, Farmington, CT, USA; [b] Glycogen Storage Disease Program, Connecticut Children's Medical Center, 282 Washington Street, Hartford, CT 06106, USA; [c] Medical Center, National Hospital System, Torshavn, Faroe Islands; [d] Medical Genetics Service, Hospital de Clínicas de Porto Alegre, Porto Alegre, Rio Grande do Sul, Brazil; [e] Section of Metabolic Diseases, University of Groningen, University Medical Center Groningen, Beatrix Children's Hospital, Groningen, The Netherlands
* Corresponding author. Glycogen Storage Disease Program, Connecticut Children's Medical Center, 282 Washington Street, Hartford, CT 06106.
E-mail address: Weinstein@uchc.edu

stream can provide energy for the brain for less than 1 hour.[1] Regulation of blood glucose concentrations is, therefore, critical for survival. The body has multiple metabolic pathways (glycogenolysis, gluconeogenesis [GNG], mitochondrial fatty acid oxidation [mFAO], and ketogenesis) controlled by multiple hormones (glucagon, epinephrine, cortisol, and growth hormone), all of which combine to protect against hypoglycemia.[2] The differential diagnosis for hypoglycemia is fairly large, but the primary manifestations are divided into hormonal and metabolic etiologic factors (**Table 1**). A generalized approach to the evaluation of hypoglycemia is summarized in **Box 1** and **Fig. 1**. This article focuses on the inherited metabolic defects commonly associated with low glucose concentrations: glycogen storage diseases (GSDs) and inherited disorders of GNG.

PHYSIOLOGY OF FASTING

The liver plays a central role in maintaining normoglycemia during feeding-fasting transitions. During periods of fasting, the liver changes from synthesizing glycogen to endogenous glucose production by glycogenolysis and GNG. During more prolonged fasting, the origin of endogenous glucose production shifts from mainly glycogenolysis to GNG and the kidney's contribution increases (**Fig. 2**).[3]

Following a meal, glucose is predominantly stored as glycogen, a complex, highly branched spherical structure, which allows efficient storage and release of glucose. The liver is freely permeable to glucose, which is rapidly phosphorylated by glucokinase to form glucose-6-phosphate. Following conversion to glucose-1-phosphate, glycogen synthase catalyzes the formation of α-1,4-linkages that elongate into chains of glucose molecules. A branching enzyme leads to formation of α-1,6-linkages at approximately every 10 glucose units along the chain. This structure allows for compact storage of glucose and its slow release during periods of fasting. In between meals, a cascade of enzymatic reactions activates hepatic glycogen phosphorylase, the rate-limiting enzyme in glycogenolysis, which removes glucose from the outer branches of glycogen, and leads to formation of glucose-6-phosphate. Hydrolysis

---

Table 1
Metabolic and endocrine causes of hypoglycemia

Metabolic Causes	Hormonal Causes
Disorders of hepatic glucose release:	Hyperinsulinism:
• Glycogen storage disease types 0, I, III, VI, IX, XI	• Congenital hyperinsulinism
• Hereditary fructose intolerance	• Exogenous insulin
• Galactosemia	• Medications
Disorders of mFAO:	• Insulinomas
• Carnitine cycle	• Beckwith-Wiedemann syndrome
• Beta oxidation	Counter-regulatory hormone deficiency:
• Ketogenesis	• Growth hormone deficiency
Disorders of GNG:	• Corticotropin or cortisol deficiency
• Fructose-1,6-bisphosphatase deficiency	• Panhypopituitarism
• Pyruvate carboxylase deficiency	• Glucagon deficiency
• Phosphoenolpyruvate carboxykinase deficiency	IGF-II production:
Other metabolic defects:	• Cervical cancer
• Maple syrup urine disease	• Hepatoblastoma
• Glycerol kinase deficiency	• Wilms tumor
• Mitochondrial respiratory chain defects	• Hodgkin lymphoma
	• Other large mesenchymal tumors
	Glucagon-like peptide secretion:
	Dumping syndrome

Box 1

Approach for hypoglycemia

Depending on local situation, resources available, and collaborations, the following steps can be followed. It is important that diagnostics and management go in parallel and to emphasize laboratory studies in stress plasma and urine samples:

1. Before referral to center of expertise:
   a. Confirm hypoglycemia
   b. Analysis of stress samples of blood (lactate, ammonia, blood gas analysis, anion gap, insulin, and cortisol; store a spare plasma sample for later studies) and urine (ketones, store a spare urine sample for later studies), and regular blood samples of transaminases, uric acid, and lipids
   c. Assess:
      i. Family history: including consanguinity, sudden infant death syndrome, growth, hypoglycemias
      ii. Personal history: including detailed feeding history (timing and restrictions, of fruits or protein) and timing of hypoglycemia in relation to feeding moments and intercurrent infections, sleep, seizures, psychomotor development, and newborn screening results
      iii. Physical examination: including dysmorphic features, growth (height, weight, and head circumference) according to target range, liver size
   d. Request additional metabolite studies according to the phenotype in plasma (liver function tests, acylcarnitines, amino acids, asialotransferrins, biotinidase activity) and urine (organic acids, oligosaccharides)
   e. Consider dietary interventions and an emergency regimen based on the phenotype
   f. Controlled fasting studies are not recommended in this phase

2. In center of expertise:
   a. If laboratory studies in stress samples are not available, based on the history, the previously mentioned studies can be requested during an out-patient clinic visit after an overnight fast
   b. Objectify 24-hour glucose concentrations: by 8-point glucose measurements and/or the combination of continuous glucose monitoring plus ketone measurements
   c. Consider dietary interventions and an emergency regimen based on the phenotype
   d. Clear hypothesis for diagnosis?
      i. Yes: targeted enzymatic and/or DNA studies
      ii. No and if there are clinical arguments against idiopathic ketotic hypoglycemia: next-generation sequencing

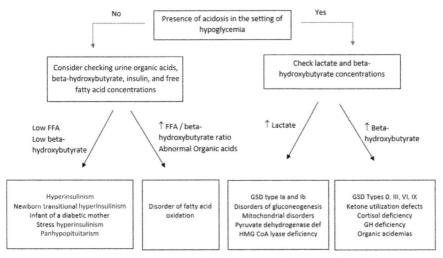

Fig. 1. Evaluation of hypoglycemia. FFA, free fatty acids; GH, growth hormone; HMG CoA, 3-hydroxy-3-methylglutaryl-CoA.

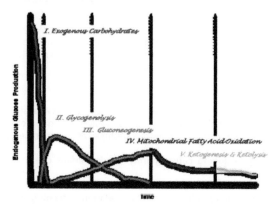

Fig. 2. Endogenous glucose production with fasting The major metabolic pathways responsible for glucose homeostasis. The time on the x-axis depends on age and is more compact with younger patients. Specific enzyme or transporter defects in these pathways are associated with fasting intolerance and (recurrent) hypoglycemia. Endocrine disorders are associated with abnormal exogenous carbohydrate (*blue*) requirements, such as congenital hyperinsulinism, hypocortisolism, and so forth. Other associations include glycogenolysis (*green*). GNG (*red*), defects of mFAO (*purple*), and defects in ketogenesis and ketolysis (*yellow*).

by glucose-6-phosphatase allows glucose to be released from the liver into the systemic circulation. Debranching enzyme is required for hydrolysis of α-1,6-linkages at branch points.[4]

Although glucose generated from glycogenolysis primarily is used to maintain normoglycemia early in fasting, endogenous glucose production from the gluconeogenic pathways also is important. In GNG, precursors are generated from 4 sources: lactate, pyruvate, glycerol, and alanine. These substrates are converted to glucose through pathways that depend on several key enzymes: pyruvate carboxylase (PC), phosphoenolpyruvate carboxylase, and fructose-1,6-bisphosphatase (FBPase).[5] GNG can occur in both the liver and kidney, and renal-derived glucose can account for up to 20% of endogenous glucose production, especially when systemic acidosis is present.[6] The percentage of glucose generated from GNG increases with the duration of fasting.

Prolonged fasting increases mFAO flux. With beta-oxidation, fatty acids are metabolized to acetyl coenzyme A (CoA) which can provide energy through the Krebs cycle. Formation of ketones from acetyl CoA by the liver also occurs, and ketones serve as an alternative energy source for the heart, muscles, and brain, thereby decreasing glucose utilization by these tissues.[7] The inherited disorders of mFAO will be reviewed in Areeg El-Gharbawy and Jerry Vockley's article, "Inborn Errors of Metabolism with Myopathy: Defects of Fatty Acid Oxidation and the Carnitine Shuttle System," in this issue.

HEPATIC GLYCOGEN STORAGE DISEASES

The GSDs comprise several inherited diseases caused by abnormalities of the enzymes and transporters that regulate glycogen synthesis and degradation. Glycogen is stored principally in the liver, muscle, and kidneys. Muscle, however, lacks glucose-6-phosphatase, and is consequently unable to generate glucose for systemic use. Hypoglycemia is the primary manifestation of the hepatic GSDs (types 0, I, III, VI, IX, and

XI), whereas weakness and/or muscle cramps are the primary features of the muscle GSDs (types II, III, IV, V, VII, X). Type GSD III is the only type of GSD with concomitant liver and muscle disease.[8] Type IV GSD (branching enzyme deficiency) results in scarring of the liver and cirrhosis in the classic form of the disease. Because hypoglycemia is not a manifestation of GSD IV until liver failure occurs, it is not discussed in this article (**Table 2**).

Glycogen Storage Disease Type I (von Gierke Disease)

Type I GSD is the classic form of the condition due to decreased glucose-6-phosphatase (G-6-Pase) function. There are 2 forms of GSD type I: type Ia and Ib. Type Ia is due to defects in the *G6PC* gene, which encodes for the enzyme and accounts for approximately 80% of the type I cases. Type Ib GSD results from mutations in the *SLC37A4* gene encoding the glucose-6-phosphate (G6P) transporter.[9] Because the G-6-Pase enzyme is located on the inner membrane of the endoplasmic reticulum, the transporter is required for G6P to reach the enzyme. The conversion of G6P to glucose is the final common pathway of all endogenous glucose production; hence, GSD I is associated with the most severe fasting intolerance of the GSDs.

The G-6-Pase enzyme complex is located in the liver, kidney, and intestine. Accumulation of glycogen results in hepatomegaly and nephromegaly, and shunting of G6P into alternative pathways leads to hyperlactatemia, hyperuricemia, and hypertriglyceridemia.

Glycogen Storage Disease Type Ia

Diagnosis

Almost all people with GSD Ia have manifestations in the neonatal period. Lethargy, irritability, or tachypnea will often lead newborns to be evaluated by neonatologists, but the diagnosis is rarely made because the manifestations abate with initiation of frequent feeds. Children subsequently are often subclinical until 3 to 6 months of age when the interval between feeds is lengthened. GSD Ia is occasionally diagnosed during a routine physical examination after hepatomegaly and a protuberant abdomen are appreciated (**Table 3**). Usually, however, children are diagnosed when the aforementioned laboratory abnormalities are found during an evaluation for lethargy, seizures, respiratory distress, developmental delay, or failure to thrive.[10,11] Rarely, people receive their diagnosis in adulthood, after evaluations for hyperlipidemia, gout, hepatomegaly, or hepatic tumors.[12,13]

The simplest means of determining the probable defect in a child suspected of having a glycogenosis is to obtain critical blood measurements of glucose, lactate, and ketones during a fasting study (**Table 4**). A brief fasting study (3–4 hours) will result in hypoglycemia and hyperlactatemia. In contrast to the other hepatic forms of GSD, GSD I is hypoketotic (see **Table 3**). Genetic studies have become the recommended test for diagnosing GSD Ia. Assay of G6Pase activity on a liver biopsy should be reserved for those people in whom molecular analysis is nondiagnostic.

Clinical management

The aim of treatment is to prevent hypoglycemia and counter-regulation, thereby minimizing the secondary metabolic derangements and long-term complications. Dietary management may consist of continuous gastric tube feeds or uncooked cornstarch depending on several factors, including the age of the child and child and/or family preferences.[14] Glucose concentrations should remain higher than 75 mg/dL to prevent counter-regulation; hyperglycemia (ie, glucose >100 mg/dL) should be avoided to minimize glycogen storage and decrease insulin production.

Table 2
Overview of the hepatic glycogen storage diseases

GSD Type	Incidence	OMIM#	Enzyme or Protein Deficiency	Gene	Chromosome Location	Mode of Inheritance	High-Risk Populations
GSD 0	Rare	240600	Glycogen synthase	GYS2	12p12.2	Autosomal Recessive	Italians
GSD Ia	1:100,000	232200	Glucose-6-phosphatase-α catalytic subunit	G6PC	17q21.31	Autosomal Recessive	Ashkenazi Jews Mormons Mexicans
GSD Ib	1: 1,000,000	232220	Glucose-6-phosphate transporter	SLC37A4	11q23.3	Autosomal Recessive	Italian Native Americans
GSD III	1:100,000	232400	Glycogen debranching enzyme (includes 4-alpha-glucanotransferase and amylo-1,6-glucosidase activities)	AGL	1p21.2	Autosomal Recessive	Faroe Islanders First Nation (Canada) North African Jews
GSD IV	1:600,000–1:800,000	232500	Glycogen-branching enzyme	GBE	3p12.3	Autosomal Recessive	—
GSD VI	1:100,000	232700	Glycogen phosphorylase (liver)	PYGL	14q22.1	Autosomal Recessive	Scottish
GSD IXa		306000	Phosphorylase kinase, alpha subunit (liver)	PHKA2	Xp22.13	X-linked recessive	—
GSD IXb		261750	Phosphorylase kinase, beta subunit	PHKB	16q12.1	Autosomal Recessive	—
GSD IXc		613027	Phosphorylase kinase, gamma subunit	PHKG2	16p11.2	Autosomal Recessive	—
GSD XI	Rare	227810	GLUT2 transporter	SLC2A2	3q26.2	Autosomal Recessive	—

Table 3
Clinical characteristic of the hepatic glycogen storage diseases

Type	Characteristic Clinical Manifestations
Type 0	• Normal liver size • Fasting ketotic hypoglycemia • Postprandial hyperglycemia without polyuria and polydipsia
Type Ia	• Hepatomegaly • Short stature and failure to thrive • Hypoglycemia • Hepatic adenomas • Renal calcification
Type Ib	• Same as Ia with additional consequences of neutrophilic abnormalities (multiple and recurrent infections) • Severe iron-resistant anemia • Inflammatory bowel disease
Type III	• Firm, very enlarged liver • Hypertrophic cardiomyopathy • Myopathy
Type VI	• Hepatomegaly • Ketotic hypoglycemia • Short stature
Type IX	• Hepatomegaly • Ketotic hypoglycemia (especially in boys) • Short stature • Attention-deficit hyperactivity disorder • Delayed puberty

Due to intestinal immaturity and lack of amylase, cornstarch is rarely tolerated before 6 months of age. Low-dose cornstarch can be initiated between 6 to 12 months, but diarrhea may limit the efficacy of the treatment.[15] Children younger than 2 years of age usually require feeds every 2 to 3.5 hours. Cornstarch feeds can usually be spaced to every 3 to 5 hours in older children and adults.[16] The dose of cornstarch for children younger than 8 years of age can be estimated by calculating the basal glucose production rate using the following formula: $y = 0.0014x^3 - 0.214x^2 + 10.411x - 9.084$, in which y = mg/kg/min of glucose and x = weight in kg.[17] The brain is the major utilizer of glucose. Because the endogenous energy requirements for the brain are stable after 8 years of age, weight-based dosing is not recommended after this age, and a standard of 10 to 11 g of glucose per hour is used to estimate carbohydrate needs.[17] Doses of cornstarch are individualized, based on glucose and lactate

Table 4
Biochemical characteristics of the hepatic glycogenoses

	Fasting Lactate	Postprandial Lactate	Fasting Ketones	Triglycerides	Uric Acid	Other
GSD 0	Normal	+++	+++	+/−	Normal	Low prealbumin
GSD I	+++	Normal	Normal	+++	++	...
GSD III	Normal	+	++	+	Normal	Elevated CK (IIIa)
GSD VI GSD IX	Normal	+/−	+++	+/−	Normal	Low prealbumin

Table 5
Overview of the disorders of gluconeogenesis

Protein Deficiency	FBPase Deficiency	PC Deficiency	Cytosolic PEPCK Deficiency
Gene	*FBP1*	*PC*	*PCK1, PCK2*
Incidence	1:350,000–900,000	1:250,000	Very rare
Hepatomegaly	Yes	Often	No, but liver failure in 1 report
CNS involvement	In case of fasting hypoglycemia	Yes	No
Hypoglycemia	On fasting	Yes	Yes
Hyperlactatemia	On fasting	Depending on the feeding state and subtype of the disorder	Mild

monitoring, to maintain glucose concentrations higher than 75 mg/dL and lactate lower than 2.2 mmol/L. Cornstarch is mixed with water or a sugar-free liquid. Adding glucose is not recommended because it stimulates insulin production and offsets the advantage of the starch.[18] An extended-release cornstarch formulation (Glycosade) is available for night feeds, and it has allowed older children and adults to have a 7 to 10 hour period of coverage without sacrificing metabolic control.[19] In North America, Glycosade is not recommended for daytime coverage or for children younger than 5 years of age.

Restricted intake of galactose, sucrose, and fructose is recommended because these sugars will worsen the hepatomegaly and metabolic derangements.[20] Multivitamin supplementation is required due to the restricted diet. Achieving glucose concentrations between 75 and 100 mg/dL is the key to maximizing metabolic control. In many GSD centers, people are hospitalized annually for titration of the therapy based on intensive glucose and lactate monitoring. Continuous glucose monitoring is used in some centers to identify periods of rapid change.[21] Screening with annual abdominal ultrasounds and urine studies is recommended starting at 5 years of age. Most recommendations for treatment were generated through either the American College of Medical Genetics certified consensus guidelines or the European Study for GSD, which are both based on expert opinion.[22,23]

Disease complications

Complications commonly seen in people with poorly controlled disease are the following:

- Hepatic adenomas (HCAs): HCAs typically develop during puberty and malignant transformation can occur.[24] During malignant transformation, traditional tumor markers can be normal. There is no difference in the rate of HCA formation in people treated with cornstarch when compared with continuous feeds.[16] There is increasing evidence that higher lactate and triglyceride concentrations are associated with adenoma formation.[25] Liver transplantation or surgical resection previously was performed when adenomas exceeded 5 cm. Liver transplantation has been associated with a high rate of secondary renal failure.[26] Beegle and colleagues[27] demonstrated regression of liver lesions if optimal metabolic control is achieved, and medical treatment is now recommended before surgery.

- GSD nephropathy: Hyperfiltration begins early in life and the disease can progress with development of focal segmental glomerulosclerosis, interstitial fibrosis, and renal insufficiency.[28] In 2002, the European Study for GSD reported that 100% of GSD Ia people developed microalbuminuria or proteinuria by 24 years of age.[11] With improved care, the prevalence of GSD nephropathy has decreased and now few adults develop microalbuminuria or proteinuria.
- Osteoporosis: The cause of the abnormal bone mineralization is multifactorial, including insufficient calcium intake, vitamin D deficiency, hypercortisolemia, and hyperlactatemia.[29] When optimal metabolic control is combined with appropriate calcium and vitamin D supplementation, normal bone densities are achieved.[30]
- Renal calcification: This complication previously occurred in 70% of adults. Risk factors for renal calcification include hypercalciuria, elevated urinary uric acid concentrations, and hypocitraturia.[31] Normalization of the urinary citrate has been successful at preventing nephrocalcinosis and nephrolithiasis.
- Other complications: Short stature, delayed puberty, and obesity previously were common in GSD Ia, but growth is now near normal. Pulmonary hypertension, polycystic ovarian disease, and a bleed diathesis rarely occur anymore.

Prognosis

Before the 1970s, most children with GSD I died in infancy or early childhood. Despite having severe hypoglycemia before diagnosis, most people with GSD Ia are neurologically normal because lactate can serve as an alternative fuel for the brain. With advances in medical and dietary management, the prognosis has markedly improved. Currently, children can develop into healthy adults, and more than 100 successful pregnancies have occurred in women with GSD Ia.[32]

Glycogen Storage Disease Type Ib

Diagnosis

Early in life, people with GSD Ib may be clinically identical to those with GSD Ia. With aging, however, most people develop neutropenia, neutrophil dysfunction, and inflammatory bowel disease (IBD).[33] As with all the GSDs, genetic studies are now the preferred method for diagnosing GSD Ib.[34]

Clinical management

Achieving glucose concentrations between 75 and 100 mg/dL is the key to maximizing metabolic control. Gastrointestinal issues may appear early in life, and people frequently do not tolerate cornstarch therapy until 2 years of age. Glycosade has not been well tolerated in GSD Ib. Exacerbations of IBD may occur from the large cornstarch doses, and this has contributed to metabolic instability.[19]

GSD Ib has the unique challenges of neutropenia and IBD. Recombinant human granulocyte-colony-stimulating factor (G-CSF) is used, but this population is prone to untoward effects (massive splenomegaly, splenic sequestration, splenic rupture, portal hypertension, and leukemia). Therefore, a starting dose of 0.5 to 2.5 μg/kg/d is recommended. Daily dosing has been found to result in fewer infections, and the dose should be adjusted based on symptoms and not the absolute neutrophil count.[22] Supplementation with high-dose vitamin E may boost the neutrophil count, improve function, and allow less G-CSF therapy.[35] Bone marrow studies are no longer deemed necessary before commencing the therapy.

Nonabsorbable salicylates (Pentasa, Asacol, and Lialda) are the first-line therapies for IBD. Steroids and immunomodulators must be used with caution because of the metabolic consequences and associated immune dysfunction.

Disease complications

- Neutropenia and recurrent infections: Neutropenia can appear at birth or with aging. It can be permanent or cyclical. Although the severity of neutrophil dysfunction is variable, recurrent bacterial infections (predominantly *Staphylococcus aureus*, *Streptococcus pneumoniae*, and *Escherichia coli*) are common without treatment.[23] *Clostridium difficile* infections are common, and this pathogen should be considered whenever chronic diarrhea is present. Most deaths in the past were due to severe infections; therefore, G-CSF is used by most centers. Recent studies suggest that the bone marrow function may be normal in GSD Ib and that the neutropenia is caused by apoptosis of the white blood cells.[36,37]
- IBD: IBD has been diagnosed as early as 13 months of age, and most people become symptomatic between 5 and 8 years of age.[38] Poor growth and an iron-resistant anemia often are present before abdominal symptomatology.[39] Screening for IBD is performed with a combination of laboratory studies, including assessment of inflammatory makers (sedimentation rate or C-reactive protein), stool calprotectin, and IBD serologic studies. Stool calprotectin requires functioning neutrophils and, therefore, may result in a false-negative result. The disease is usually localized to the small intestine, and a normal colonoscopy does not rule out the complication.[40] Capsule endoscopies can be used to look for evidence of IBD, but some people are treated empirically if they present with the constellation of growth failure, systemic inflammation, anemia, and abdominal symptoms. G-CSF helps decrease the symptoms; however, it is not sufficient by itself to treat the condition.[41]
- Mouth ulcers and periodontal disease: Mouth ulcers and periodontal disease are common likely due to the combination of neutropenia and IBD.[42] Aggressive dental hygiene is recommended with dental visits every 3 to 6 months. Topical therapy with chlorhexidine may help decrease the severity of the mouth ulcers and gum inflammation; however, plaque formation with the medication can be problematic.

Prognosis

Long-term complications in GSD Ib seem to be less frequent than in GSD Ia. Life-threatening infections can occur, but they are uncommon in people who are treated with G-CSF.[22] IBD is the primary cause of morbidity in this population. Many adults with GSD Ib are clinically doing well, and numerous children have been born to mothers with GSD Ib.[43]

Glycogen Storage Disease Type III (Cori or Forbes Disease)

GSD III is caused by deficiency of glycogen debrancher enzyme. The terminal chains of glycogen can be broken down normally; glycogenolysis, however, is arrested when the outermost branch points are reached. As a result of the defect, abnormal glycogen (limit dextrin) accumulates in affected tissues. Type IIIa accounts for 85% of people with GSD III, and involves the liver, heart, and muscles; type IIIb only affects the liver.[44] Both GSD IIIa and IIIb are caused by mutations in the *AGL* gene.[45]

Diagnosis

GSD III has a wide clinical spectrum. Hepatic involvement leads to hepatomegaly and fasting hypoglycemia, which may be indistinguishable in infancy from GSD I.[46] People with GSD III can synthesize glucose via GNG, and energy formation from fatty acid oxidation is intact. As a result, the hypoglycemia often is not as severe as in GSD I, and is typically associated with prominent ketosis. Muscle involvement leads to a chronic myopathy, muscle weakness, and pain, but these manifestations do not present in childhood.[47]

Although fasting hypoglycemia can occur, most people present after failure to thrive, hepatomegaly, or abnormal hepatic transaminases are incidentally found (see **Table 3**). GSD III is often mistaken for a viral hepatitis, and aspartate aminotransferase and alanine aminotransferase concentrations may exceed 1000 U/L. Other common laboratory abnormalities include elevation of creatine kinase (CK), a low prealbumin concentration, and hyperlipidemia. Abnormalities in the muscle enzymes, however, may not be present until children are ambulating.

GSD III can be differentiated from GSD I biochemically by the presence of ketones, lack of fasting hyperlactatemia or nephromegaly, and involvement of the muscles in type IIIa. Genetic studies are the preferred method for diagnosing GSD III. Liver biopsies are no longer recommended if GSD III is suspected. If a biopsy is performed, glycogen-filled hepatocytes with portal fibrosis are characteristic, and abnormal glycogen structure can be identified on electron microscopy. Measurement of enzyme activity in skin fibroblasts or lymphocytes can be used if available.

Clinical management
Treatment is based on avoidance of carbohydrate storage, minimizing ketosis, and preventing muscle damage. Protein can be used both as a substrate for endogenous glucose production and as a fuel for the muscles.[48] Treatment with at least 3 g/kg/d of protein is recommended, and doses are adjusted to normalize prealbumin, total protein, and CK concentrations. Low-dose uncooked cornstarch or continuous feeds are also used to achieve glucose concentrations higher than 75 mg/dL and beta-hydroxybutyrate concentrations lower than 0.3 mmol/L. Glycosade has been used successfully when overnight hypoglycemia or ketosis occurs on traditional therapy.[49] Even though fructose, sucrose, and galactose can be used, total carbohydrate intake is restricted to avoid excessive glycogen storage and to minimize insulin secretion. Because cardiac disease can occur at any age, annual echocardiograms are recommended, and abdominal ultrasounds are obtained every 1 to 2 years to screen for liver disease.[46]

Disease complications
- Failure to thrive: Poor growth is common in early childhood due to a combination of chronic ketosis and protein deficiency. With optimal treatment, growth normalizes.
- Hypertrophic cardiomyopathy: Cardiac hypertrophy can present in the first year of life, but concentric left ventricular hypertrophy most commonly presents in childhood or adolescence. Most people have asymptomatic hypertrophy with relatively normal ventricular function, but severe and potentially lethal cardiac dysfunction, obstruction, and arrhythmias can occur. There are numerous articles documenting reversal of the associated hypertrophic cardiomyopathy using dietary interventions that restrict carbohydrates.[50,51]
- Myopathy: Hypotonia is common at diagnosis, and asymptomatic CK elevation develops in childhood. Decreased stamina and muscle pain often occur in adolescence, and slowly progressive proximal muscle weakness can develop in adulthood. The myopathy is the primary source of morbidity in this population.
- Liver disease: Liver symptoms predominate in childhood, but long-term complications are uncommon. HCAs occur in less than 10% of adults.[52] Hepatic fibrosis is common, but cirrhosis and portal hypertension infrequently occur if

treatment is maximized and alcohol is avoided. Hepatocellular carcinoma is a rare complication in GSD III.[53]

- Type 2 diabetes mellitus: There may be an increased risk for developing type 2 diabetes mellitus. Restriction of carbohydrate intake and regular exercise should be the first measures to manage this complication.

Prognosis

The prognosis for people with GSD III is very good. Complications are rare in childhood if excessive sugar and carbohydrate intake are avoided. Recent studies have demonstrated slowing or prevention of muscle symptoms with a high protein diet, limited intake of carbohydrates, and avoidance of near maximal anaerobic activities.[47]

Glycogen Storage Disease Type VI (Hers Disease) and Glycogen Storage Disease Type IX

Types VI and IX GSDs are considered together because both disorders result in abnormal hepatic phosphorylase activity. GSD VI is caused by a deficiency of liver glycogen phosphorylase.[54] GSD IX is caused by deficiency in glycogen phosphorylase kinase. The phosphorylase kinase enzyme is composed of 4 subunits that are encoded by different genes: alpha, beta, gamma, and delta subunits. The alpha subunit is encoded on the X-chromosome and accounts for the classic condition.[55] Because phosphorylase kinase is required to activate glycogen phosphorylase, GSD VI and IX show significant phenotypic overlap. There is evidence that GSD IX is the most common form of GSD.[56]

Diagnosis

People usually present in infancy or early childhood with growth retardation, hypotonia, and prominent hepatomegaly. Ketotic hypoglycemia, or even ketotic normoglycemia, can occur.[57] However, the hypoglycemia is often unrecognized because the ketones blunt neuroglycopenic symptoms. Hypotonia may lead to delayed motor development. Cognitive and/or speech delays have been reported. Rarely, children present during the school-age years when hepatomegaly is appreciated during an evaluation for attention deficit disorder, hyperlipidemia, short stature, or delayed puberty.[58]

It is possible to diagnose phosphorylase deficiency by assaying the activity of the enzyme in leukocytes and erythrocytes. The blood assay, however, lacks sensitivity because there are tissue-specific isoforms of this enzyme. Biopsies are not required to make the diagnosis, but glycogen-filled hepatocytes with noninflammatory fibrosis are seen. Genetic studies are the preferred method for diagnosing GSDs VI and IX.

Clinical management

Treatment is based on avoidance of carbohydrate storage and minimizing ketosis. A high protein diet (2–2.5 g/kg/d) is used because amino acids can serve as a substrate for GNG. Doses are adjusted to normalize prealbumin concentrations. Although most people with GSD IX can make it through the night with cornstarch and protein, cornstarch feeds in the middle of the night are sometimes required to prevent hypoglycemia and ketosis. For these people, Glycosade can be considered.[49] Carbohydrate restriction is recommended to avoid glycogen storage and to minimize insulin secretion. Due to the risk of liver scarring, annual abdominal ultrasounds are recommended.

Disease complications

- Short stature: Poor growth is common when inadequate protein supplementation or chronic ketosis is present.
- Cirrhosis: People with markedly elevated hepatic transaminases are at higher risk of hepatic fibrosis and cirrhosis.

Prognosis

GSD VI and IX have an outstanding prognosis. It is clear that treatment improves growth, stamina, and prevents complications.[59] Mutations in the gamma subunit, however, may be associated with a more severe phenotype.[60] A small percentage of people with mutations in the alpha subunit are also at risk for cirrhosis.[61] Mutations in the beta subunit are usually associated with mild disease.

Glycogen Storage Disease Type 0

GSD 0 is caused by a deficiency of the hepatic isoform of glycogen synthase, leading to a marked decrease in liver glycogen content.[62] After consumption of carbohydrate, the inability to store glucose as glycogen in the liver results in postprandial hyperglycemia and hyperlactatemia. Fasting can cause severe ketotic hypoglycemia.[63]

Diagnosis

Most children are identified incidentally when ketotic hypoglycemia is documented during a gastrointestinal illness. Postprandial hyperglycemia and fasting ketonuria can be confused as early diabetes, and GSD 0 should be considered in any child with asymptomatic hyperglycemia or glucosuria.[64] There is significant clinical variability, and it can present with seizures, growth failure, or hypoglycemia.[63]

GSD 0 can be diagnosed biochemically. Following consumption of a glucose load or mixed meal, postprandial hyperglycemia and hyperlactatemia occur. Fasting results in ketotic hypoglycemia. Liver biopsies are not recommended, and sequencing of *GYS2* is used to confirm the diagnosis.

Clinical management

The goal of treatment is to prevent hypoglycemia and ketosis. Protein supplementation is recommended, and cornstarch is usually administered 2 to 4 times per day. Blood glucose, lactate, and ketone monitoring are used to determine the cornstarch doses. Protein supplementation is based on symptoms and prealbumin concentrations. Sugar and carbohydrate intake are restricted to avoid hyperglycemia and hyperlactatemia.

Disease complications

Long-term complications are extremely rare in GSD 0. Consumption of sugars leads to hyperglycemia, which can cause elevation of the hemoglobin A1c. Osteoporosis can occur from decreased bone mineralization in the setting of chronic ketosis. Neither liver nor renal disease has been described.

Prognosis

The prognosis for people with GSD 0 is outstanding. Treatment, however, normalizes growth and improves stamina.

INHERITED DISORDERS OF GLUCONEOGENESIS

The formation of glucose from non–hexose metabolic precursors (mainly lactate, pyruvate, glycerol, and alanine) is called GNG. The conversion of pyruvate into glucose is the central pathway for GNG reactions. The glycolysis and GNG pathways are almost identical, but 3 nonreversible enzymatic reactions characterize the disorders of GNG:

1. Glucose-6-phosphate (G6P) is hydrolyzed by glucose-6-phosphatase. The associated inherited disorder is GSD I.
2. Fructose 1,6-bisphosphate is hydrolyzed by FBPase. The associated inherited GNG disorder is FBPase deficiency.

3. Conversion of pyruvate to phosphoenolpyruvate is affected in 2 stages:
   a. Pyruvate must first be carboxylated into oxaloacetate; the associated disorder is the mitochondrial matrix enzyme PC deficiency. In this disorder, there is a combined defect of GNG and the Krebs cycle.
   b. Because oxaloacetate cannot diffuse freely out of the mitochondrion, it is translocated into the cytoplasm via the malate/aspartate shuttle. Synthesis of phosphoenolpyruvate from oxaloacetate is catalyzed by cytoplasmic phosphoenolpyruvate carboxykinase (PEPCK).

The biochemical phenotype of GNG disorders is characterized by fasting intolerance with associated recurrent hypoglycemia with lactic acidosis with or without ketosis (Table 5).

Fructose-1,6-Bisphosphatase Deficiency

FBPase catalyzes hydrolysis of fructose 1,6-bisphosphate into fructose 6-phosphate.

Diagnosis

FBPase deficiency is associated with relatively mild fasting hypoglycemia, severe lactic acidosis, and moderate hepatomegaly during crises. The crucial role of FBPase in the perinatal transition of glucose homeostasis is reflected in that about half of the affected people present as hypoglycemic newborns with severe metabolic acidosis–associated hyperventilation.[65] The remaining people usually present during catabolic periods with ketotic hypoglycemia and hyperlactatemia, hyperalaninemia, hyperketonemia, increased lactate to pyruvate ratio, elevated plasma uric acid concentration, gyceroluria, and pseudohypertriglyceridemia. Lactate concentrations during acute episodes may accumulate up to 25 mmol/L, causing acidosis and necessitating bicarbonate infusions. Upstream to the primary metabolic block, the impaired cytosolic-free NAD to NADH ratio shifts the equilibrium between pyruvate and lactate, which explains the increasing lactate to pyruvate ratio (≤ 40). The diagnosis can be made noninvasively by molecular analysis of the FBP1 gene.[66]

Clinical management

Endogenous carbohydrate requirements are relatively high in newborns and young infants when hepatic glycogen stores are relatively small. Children may be prescribed a late-evening meal with uncooked cornstarch or continuous nocturnal gastric drip feeding. During illness, oral management with glucose polymers is started at home to prevent progressive metabolic derangement. In these conditions, people should not be given fructose or sucrose because the rapidly formed but slowly metabolized fructose-1-phosphate inhibits liver glycogen phosphorylase. People need an emergency protocol ensuring timely intravenous glucose management to correct hypoglycemia. Relatively high infusion rates are needed (10% dextrose at 1.25–1.5 times maintenance) to reverse metabolic derangement and end a metabolic crisis.[67]

Disease complications

Complications are rare except for acute metabolic crises. The condition may be fatal during the neonatal period due to severe hypoglycemia and acidosis. Consumption of glycerol and sorbitol can precipitate a metabolic crisis.

Prognosis

The prognosis is good with proper dietary management.[68]

Pyruvate Carboxylase Deficiency

The chemical reaction of the biotinylated mitochondrial matrix enzyme PC is carboxylation of pyruvate into oxaloacetate. The enzyme is expressed at high levels in liver and kidney. PC is essential for anaplerosis of the Krebs cycle by replenishment of intramitochondrial oxaloacetate. PC also exports acetyl CoA out of mitochondria via the pyruvate-malate shuttle, which is important for lipogenesis.

Diagnosis

PC deficiency presents with failure to thrive, developmental delay, and recurrent seizures. An evaluation reveals hypoglycemia, metabolic acidosis, hyperammonemia, or ketosis.[69] In neonates, a high lactate to pyruvate ratio with a low hydroxybutyrate to acetoacetate ratio is suggestive of the diagnosis. Cystic periventricular leukomalacia associated with lactic acidosis can also be seen. After carbohydrate intake, blood lactate concentrations decrease. PC deficiency is categorized into 3 overlapping phenotypes that probably represent a continuum[69]:

- Type A: infantile or North American form
- Type B: severe neonatal or French form
- Type C: intermittent or benign form.

The serum and urine amino acid profile may reveal hyperalaninemia, low aspartic acid, and increased concentrations of citrulline and lysine. Measurement of PC activity in cultured skin fibroblasts and sequence analysis of the PC gene confirm the diagnosis.

Clinical management

Management aims to prevent catabolism, to correct anaplerosis, and to enhance residual enzyme activity. Treatments include intravenous 10% dextrose infusion; bicarbonate; dietary management; and supplementation of citrate, aspartate, triheptanoin, dichloroacetate, biotin, and thiamine.[70] The ketogenic diet is strictly contraindicated.

Disease complications

Neurologic defects and development delay are the primary complications in PC. Cystic lesions and gliosis in the cortex, basal ganglia, brain stem, and cerebellum can develop. There can be ventricular dilation, cortical and white matter atrophy, and periventricular white mater cysts. Hypomyelination can also occur with type A PC deficiency.[71] There is no consensus regarding the best treatment approach or when to go to liver transplant.[72]

Prognosis

The outcome is poor for severe cases with types A and B PC deficiency. In the most severe cases, neurologic damage already starts prenatally. People with minimal residual PC activity usually do not survive the neonatal period.

Phosphoenolpyruvate Carboxykinase Deficiency

The chemical reaction of PEPCK catalyzes the conversion of oxaloacetate into phosphoenolpyruvate and carbon dioxide. PEPCK deficiency is an extremely rare condition. The first reports on 4 cases with PEPCK deficiency originate from the 1970s[73] and were followed by few publications in the following decades.[74,75] Interpretation of the clinical relevance of PEPCK deficiency has been difficult because the diagnosis has relied solely on enzymatic testing, which was unreliable. Owing to the lack of confirmed cases and rarity of cases, there is a paucity of literature on the natural history and clinical manifestations of PEPCK deficiency.

REFERENCES

1. Duran J, Guinovart JJ. Brain glycogen in health and disease. Mol Aspects Med 2015;46:70–7.
2. Pagliara AS, Karl IE, Haymond M, et al. Hypoglycemia in infancy and childhood. I. J Pediatr 1973;82:365–79.
3. Boden G. Gluconeogenesis and glycogenolysis in health and diabetes. J Investig Med 2004;52:375–8.
4. Adeva-Andany MM, Gonzalez-Lucan M, Donapetry-Garcia C, et al. Glycogen metabolism in humans. BBA Clin 2016;5:85–100.
5. Van den Berghe G. Disorders of gluconeogenesis. J Inherit Metab Dis 1996;19: 470–7.
6. Cano N. Bench-to-bedside review: glucose production from the kidney. Crit Care 2002;6:17–21.
7. Houten SM, Violante S, Ventura FV, et al. The biochemistry and physiology of mitochondrial fatty acid β-oxidation and its genetic disorders. Annu Rev Physiol 2016;78:23–44.
8. Wolfsdorf JI, Weinstein DA. Glycogen storage diseases. Rev Endocr Metab Disord 2003;4:95–102.
9. Chou JY, Jun HS, Mansfield BC. Type I glycogen storage diseases: disorders of the glucose-6-phosphatase transporter complexes. J Inherit Metab Dis 2015;38: 511–9.
10. Chen MA, Weinstein DA. Glycogen storage diseases: diagnosis, treatment and outcome. Transl Sci Rare Dis 2016;1:45–72.
11. Rake JP, Visser G, Labrune P, et al. Glycogen storage disease type I: diagnosis, management, clinical course, and outcome. Results of the European study on glycogen storage disease type I (ESGSD I). Eur J Pediatr 2002;161(Suppl 1): S20–34.
12. Shieh JJ, Lu YH, Huang SW, et al. Misdiagnosis as steatohepatitis in a family with mild glycogen storage disease type 1a. Gene 2012;509:154–7.
13. Cassiman D, Libbrecht L, Verslype C, et al. An adult male patient with multiple adenomas and a hepatocellular carcinoma: mild glycogen storage disease type Ia. J Hepatol 2010;53:213–7.
14. Derks TG, Martens DH, Sentner CP, et al. Dietary treatment of glycogen storage disease type Ia: uncooked cornstarch and/or continuous nocturnal gastric drip-feeding? Mol Genet Metab 2013;109:1–2.
15. Hayde M, Widhalm K. Effects of cornstarch treatment in very young children with type I glycogen storage disease. Eur J Pediatr 1990;149:630–3.
16. Weinstein DA, Wolfsdorf JI. Effect of continuous glucose therapy with uncooked cornstarch on the long-term clinical course of type 1a glycogen storage disease. Eur J Pediatr 2002;161(Suppl 1):S35–9.
17. Bier DM, Leake RD, Haymond MW, et al. Measurement of the "true" glucose production rates in infancy and childhood with 6,6-dideuteroglucose. Diabetes 1977; 26:1016–23.
18. Wolfsdorf JI, Plotkin RA, Laffel LM, et al. Continuous glucose for treatment of people with type 1 glycogen storage disease: comparison of the effects of dextrose and uncooked cornstarch on biochemical values. Am J Clin Nutr 1990;52: 1043–50.
19. Ross KM, Brown LM, Corrado MM, et al. Safety and efficacy of chronic extended release cornstarch for glycogen storage disease I. JIMD Rep 2016; 26:85–90.

20. Shah KK, O'Dell SD. Effect of dietary interventions in the maintenance of normo-glycaemia in glycogen storage disease type 1a: a systemic review and meta-analysis. J Hum Nutr Diet 2013;26:329–39.
21. White FJ, Jones SA. The use of continuous glucose monitoring in the practical management of glycogen storage disorders. J Inherit Metab Dis 2011;34:631–42.
22. Kishnani PS, Austin SL, Abdenur JE, et al. Diagnosis and management of glycogen storage disease type I: a practice guideline of the American College of Medical Genetics and Genomics. Genet Med 2014;16:e1.
23. Rake JP, Visser G, Labrune P, et al. Guidelines for management of glycogen storage disease type I – European Study on Glycogen Storage Disease Type I (ESGSD I). Eur J Pediatr 2002;161(Supp 1):S112–9.
24. Franco LM, Krishnamurthy V, Bali D, et al. Hepatocellular carcinoma in glycogen storage disease type Ia: a case series. J Inherit Metab Dis 2005;28:153–62.
25. Wang DQ, Fiske LM, Carreras CT, et al. Natural history of hepatocellular adenoma formation in glycogen storage disease type I. J Pediatr 2011;159:442–6.
26. Davis MK, Weinstein DA. Liver transplantation in children with glycogen storage disease: controversies and evaluation of the risk/benefit of this procedure. Pediatr Transplant 2008;12:137–45.
27. Beegle RD, Brown LM, Weinstein DA. Regression of hepatocellular adenomas with strict dietary therapy in people with glycogen storage disease type I. JIMD Rep 2015;18:23–32.
28. Chen YT. Type I glycogen storage disease: kidney involvement, pathogenesis, and its treatment. Pediatr Nephrol 1991;5:71–6.
29. Lee PJ, Patel JS, Fewtrell M, et al. Bone mineralization in type 1 glycogen storage disease. Eur J Pediatr 1995;154:483–7.
30. Minarich LA, Kirpich A, Fiske LM, et al. Bone mineral density in glycogen storage disease type Ia and Ib. Genet Med 2012. [Epub ahead of print].
31. Weinstein DA, Somers MJ, Wolfsdorf JI. Decreased urinary citrate excretion in type 1a glycogen storage disease. J Pediatr 2001;138:378–82.
32. Ferrecchia IA, Guenette G, Potocik E, et al. Pregnancy in women with glycogen storage disease types Ia and Ib. J Perinat Neonatal Nurs 2014;28:26–31.
33. Visser G, Rake JP, Fernandes J, et al. Neutropenia, neutrophil dysfunction, and inflammatory bowel disease in glycogen storage disease type Ib: results of the European Study on Glycogen Storage Disease type I. J Pediatr 2000;137:187–91.
34. Chou JY. The molecular basis of type 1 glycogen storage diseases. Curr Mol Med 2001;1:25–44.
35. Melis D, Minopoli G, Balivo F, et al. Vitamin E improves clinical outcome of people affected by glycogen storage disease type Ib. JIMD Rep 2016;25:39–45.
36. Visser G, de Jager W, Verhagen LP, et al. Survival, but not maturation, is affected in neutrophil progenitors form GSD-Ib people. J Inherit Metab Dis 2012;35:287–300.
37. Jun HS, Weinstein DA, Lee YM, et al. Molecular mechanisms of neutrophil dysfunction in glycogen storage disease type Ib. Blood 2014;123:2843–53.
38. Davis MK, Valentine JF, Weinstein DA, et al. Antibodies to CBir1 are associated with glycogen storage disease type Ib. J Pediatr Gastroenterol Nutr 2010;51:14–8.
39. Wang DQ, Carreras CT, Fiske LM, et al. Characterization and pathogenesis of anemia in glycogen storage disease type Ia and Ib. Genet Med 2012;14:795–9.
40. Davis MK, Rufo PA, Polyak SF, et al. Adalimumab for the treatment of Crohn-like colitis and enteritis in glycogen storage disease type Ib. J Inherit Metab Dis 2008;31(Suppl 3):505–9.

41. Melis D, Parenti G, Della Casa R, et al. Crohn's-like ileo-colitis in patients affected by glycogen storage disease Ib: two years' follow-up of patients with a wide spectrum of gastrointestinal signs. Acta Paediatr 2003;92:1415–21.

42. Brinkman C, Adewumi A, Gong Y, et al. Microbial profile of supragingival and subgingival plaque of people with glycogen storage disease. Journal of Inborn Errors of Metabolism & Screening 2016;4:1–6.

43. Dagli A, Lee PJ, Correia CE, et al. Pregnancy in glycogen storage disease type Ib: gestational care and report of first successful deliveries. J Inherit Metab Dis 2010;33(Suppl 3):S151–7.

44. Sentner CP, Hoogeveen IJ, Weinstein DA, et al. Glycogen storage disease type III: diagnosis, genotype, management, clinical course, and outcome. J Inherit Metab Dis 2016;39:697–704.

45. Yang-Feng TL, Zheng K, Yu J, et al. Assignment of the human glycogen de-brancher gene to chromosome 1p21. Genomics 1992;13:931–4.

46. Kishnani PS, Austin SL, Arn P, et al. Glycogen storage disease type III diagnosis and management guidelines. Genet Med 2010;12:446–63.

47. Preisler N, Pradel A, Husu E, et al. Exercise intolerance in glycogen storage disease type III: weakness or energy deficiency? Mol Genet Metab 2013;109:14–20.

48. Derks TG, Smit GP. Dietary management in glycogen storage disease type III: what is the evidence? J Inherit Metab Dis 2015;38:545–50.

49. Ross KM, Brown LM, Corrado MM, et al. Safety and efficacy of long-term use of extended release cornstarch therapy for glycogen storage disease types 0, III, VI, and IX. Journal of Nutritional Therapeutics 2015;4:137–42.

50. Dagli AI, Zori RT, McCune H, et al. Reversal of glycogen storage disease type IIIa-related cardiomyopathy with modification of diet. J Inherit Metab Dis 2009; 32(Suppl 1):S103–6.

51. Sentner CP, Caliskan WB, Vletter WB, et al. Heart failure due to a severe hypertrophic cardiomyopathy reversed by low calorie, high protein dietary adjustments in a glycogen storage disease type IIIa patient. JIMD Rep 2012;5:13–6.

52. Labrune P, Trioche P, Duvaltier I, et al. Hepatocellular adenomas in glycogen storage disease type I and III: a series of 43 people and review of the literature. J Pediatr Gastroenterol Nutr 1997;24:276–9.

53. Demo E, Frush D, Gottfried M, et al. Glycogen storage disease type III-hepatocellular carcinoma a long-term complication? J Hepatol 2007;46:492–8.

54. Burwinkel B, Bakker HD, Herschkovitz E, et al. Mutations in the liver glycogen phosphorylase gene (PYGL) underlying glycogenosis type VI. Am J Hum Genet 1998;62:785–91.

55. Elpeleg ON. The molecular background of glycogen metabolism disorders. J Pediatr Endocrinol Metab 1999;12:363–79.

56. Brown LM, Corrado MM, van der Ende RM, et al. Evaluation of glycogen storage disease as a cause of ketotic hypoglycemia in children. J Inherit Metab Dis 2015; 38:489–93.

57. Hoogeveen IJ, van der Ende RM, van Spronsen FJ, et al. Normoglycemic ketonemia as biochemical presentation in ketotic glycogen storage disease. JIMD Rep 2016;28:41–7.

58. Beauchamp NJ, Dalton A, Ramaswami U, et al. Glycogen storage disease type IX: high variability in clinical phenotype. Mol Genet Metab 2007;92:88–99.

59. Tsilianidis LA, Fiske LM, Siegel S, et al. Aggressive therapy improves cirrhosis in glycogen storage disease type IX. Mol Genet Metab 2013;109:179–82.

60. Burwinkel B, Rootwelt T, Kvittingen EA, et al. Severe phenotype of phosphorylase kinase-deficient liver glycogenosis with mutation in the PHKG2 gene. Pediatr Res 2003;54:834–9.
61. Johnson AO, Goldstein JL, Bali D. Glycogen storage disease type IX: novel PHKA2 missense mutation and cirrhosis. J Pediatr Gastroenterol Nutr 2012;55: 90–2.
62. Orho M, Bosshard NU, Buist NR, et al. Mutations in the liver glycogen synthase gene in children with hypoglycemia due to glycogen storage disease type 0. J Clin Invest 1998;102:105–15.
63. Weinstein DA, Correia CE, Saunders AC, et al. Hepatic glycogen synthase deficiency: an infrequently recognized cause of ketotic hypoglycemia. Mol Genet Metab 2006;87:284–8.
64. Bachrach BE, Weinstein DA, Orho-Melander M, et al. Glycogen synthase deficiency (glycogen storage disease type 0) presenting with hyperglycemia and glucosuria: report of three new mutations. J Pediatr 2002;140:781–3.
65. Kodama H, Okabe I, Gunji Y, et al. Neonatal hyperlactacidemia and hypoglycemia caused by delayed maturation of fructose-1,6-diphosphatase activity. J Pediatr 1988;113:898–900.
66. Santer R, du Moulin M, Shahinyan T, et al. A summary of molecular genetic findings in fructose-1,6-bisphosphatase deficiency with a focus on a common long-range deletion and the role of MLPA analysis. Orphanet J Rare Dis 2016;11:44.
67. Van Hove JL, Myers S, Kerckhove KV, et al. Acute nutrition management in the prevention of metabolic illness: a practical approach with glucose polymers. Mol Genet Metab 2009;97:1–3.
68. Asberg C, Hjalmarson O, Alm J, et al. Fructose 1,6-bisphosphatase deficiency: enzyme and mutation analysis performed on calcitriol stimulated monocytes with a note on long-term prognosis. J Inherit Metab Dis 2010;33(Suppl 3): S113–21.
69. Marin-Valencia I, Roe CR, Pascual JM. Pyruvate carboxylase deficiency: mechanisms, mimics and anaplerosis. Mol Genet Metab 2010;101:9–17.
70. Breen C, White FJ, Scott CA, et al. Unsuccessful treatment of severe pyruvate carboxylase deficiency with triheptanoin. Eur J Pediatr 2014;173:361–6.
71. Garcia-Cazorla A, Rabier D, Touati G, et al. Pyruvate carboxylase deficiency: metabolic characteristics and new neurological aspects. Ann Neurol 2006;59: 121–7.
72. Nyhan WL, Khanna A, Barshop BA, et al. Pyruvate carboxylase deficiency–insights from liver transplantation. Mol Genet Metab 2002;77:143–9.
73. Hommes FA, Bendien K, Elema JD, et al. Two cases of phosphoenolpyruvate carboxykinase deficiency. Acta Paediatr Scand 1976;65:233–40.
74. Clayton PT, Hyland K, Brand M, et al. Mitochondrial phosphoenolpyruvate carboxykinase deficiency. Eur J Pediatr 1986;145:46–50.
75. Leonard JV, Hyland K, Furukawa N, et al. Mitochondrial phosphoenolpyruvate carboxykinase deficiency. Eur J Pediatr 1991;150:198–9.

Inborn Errors of Metabolism with Cognitive Impairment

Metabolism Defects of Phenylalanine, Homocysteine and Methionine, Purine and Pyrimidine, and Creatine

Evgenia Sklirou, MD, Uta Lichter-Konecki, MD, PhD*

KEYWORDS

- Phenylalanine • Homocysteine methionine • Purine pyrimidine
- Creatine metabolism defects

KEY POINTS

- Untreated classic phenylketonuria causes severe intellectual disability. Newborn screening was the logical and necessary consequence of development of a successful treatment.
- Untreated classic homocysteinuria affects the eyes, skeleton, vasculature, and brain. Affected individuals remain asymptomatic, but can later suffer severe thromboembolic episodes.
- Lesch-Nyhan syndrome is an X-linked recessive disorder caused by hypoxanthine-guanine phosphoribosyl transferase deficiency. The result is hypoxanthine accumulation and conversion into uric acid.
- Defects of creatine synthesis: guanidinoacetate methyltransferase deficiency, L-arginine:-glycine amidinotransferase deficiency, and creatine transporter defect, result in cerebral creatine deficiency.

INTRODUCTION

Intellectual disability (ID), according to the definition by the American Association of Intellectual and Developmental Disabilities, is a "disability characterized by significant limitations in both intellectual functioning and in adaptive behavior, which covers many everyday social and practical skills and originates before the age of 18."[1] It has a prevalence of 1% to 3% and it is estimated that the average lifetime cost to society per person is $1 million.[2] After a diagnosis of ID, it is important to try to identify a cause because, although uncommon, a metabolic disease amenable to treatment may be

Division of Medical Genetics, Department of Pediatrics, Children's Hospital of Pittsburgh, University of Pittsburgh, UPMC, 4401 Penn Avenue, Pittsburgh, PA 15224, USA
* Corresponding author.
E-mail address: uta.lichterkonecki@chp.edu

Pediatr Clin N Am 65 (2018) 267–277
https://doi.org/10.1016/j.pcl.2017.11.009
0031-3955/18/© 2017 Elsevier Inc. All rights reserved.
pediatric.theclinics.com

identified. Even if no treatment is available, establishing a diagnosis will help families to understand what to expect, discuss recurrence risks and may also help them to identify appropriate support groups and other resources.

Inborn errors of metabolism (IEMs) account for up to 5% of nonspecific ID.[3] Neurologic manifestations, other than ID, may be part of the IEMs phenotype and include seizures, ataxia, dystonia, spasticity, and psychomotor regression. Multisystem involvement such as hepatosplenomegaly, cardiomyopathy, hearing impairment, eye and skin manifestations, skeletal anomalies, coarse facial features, may indicate a potential metabolic etiology of ID.[3] Unusual body odors, specific food avoidance (eg, protein aversion), and self-injurious behaviors should make pediatricians consider IEMs. History of consanguinity and unexplained fetal or infantile deaths are additional clues toward the diagnosis of a metabolic disorder. Evaluating a child with ID takes a stepwise approach and should start with a detailed personal and family history along with a comprehensive physical examination focusing specifically on neurologic and behavioral findings. IEMs that cause ID include phenylketonuria (PKU), galactosemia, lysosomal storage disorders, urea cycle defects, homocystinuria, cholesterol biosynthesis defects, disorders of purine and pyrimidine metabolism, creatine deficiency syndromes, and congenital disorders of glycosylation. Van Karnebeek and colleagues[4] recommended first- and second-tier metabolic testing to identify individuals with suspected IEMs. A first-tier workup includes serum lactate, ammonia, copper, ceruloplasmin, total plasma homocysteine, plasma amino acids, acylcarnitine profile (whole blood or plasma), creatine metabolites in urine, urine purines and pyrimidines, urine organic acids, and urine oligosaccharides and glycosaminoglycans. Van Karnebeek and colleagues state that these tests can identify 60% of all IEM potentially amenable to treatment. The second tier incorporates specific testing, which is beyond the scope of this article because it requires molecular and invasive testing.

An early diagnosis of treatable metabolic conditions associated with ID can ameliorate if not prevent adverse disease outcomes and reduce the negative disease impact to affected individuals and their families. In this article, we present disorders of phenylalanine metabolism, disorders of homocysteine metabolism, inborn errors of purine and pyrimidine metabolism, and creatine deficiency syndromes that belong in this category.

DEFECTS OF PHENYLALANINE METABOLISM: PHENYLALANINE HYDROXYLASE DEFICIENCY (PHENYLKETONURIA), AND TETRAHYDROBIOPTERIN BIOSYNTHESIS AND REGENERATION DEFECTS
Presenting Symptoms

- Elevated phenylalanine level on newborn screen.
- Depending on the degree of elevation, the pediatrician will be asked to send a repeat newborn screening sample or refer child to a metabolic center immediately.

Clinical Presentation

A. The severe phenotype of PKU is unusual in the United States because successful screening allows early detection and prompt institution of treatment. However, individuals that are under strict dietary control, may still present with attention deficit hyperactivity disorder, anxiety, and academic difficulties.[5] If PKU is left untreated, affected individuals present with the following:
   - Profound ID.
   - Neuropsychiatric and behavioral manifestations: Hypertonia-spastic paraparesis, seizures, dementia, Parkinsonism, behavioral problems, autism, and microcephaly.

- Fair skin and hair pigmentation, eczema.
- Mousy or musty odor.
- Adults with PKU may manifest subtle cognitive sequelae.
B. Clinical manifestations in tetrahydrobiopterin biosynthesis and regeneration defects include:
  - Failure to thrive;
  - Cognitive impairment;
  - Gait abnormalities and dystonia;
  - Drooling, excessive salivation, and swallowing difficulties;
  - Hyperthermia; and
  - Athetosis, cogwheel rigidity, and mood disturbance.

Diagnostic Evaluation

The differential diagnosis of an elevated phenylalanine level includes deficiency of the enzyme phenylalanine hydroxylase (PAH) that converts phenylalanine into tyrosine and deficiency of the cofactor tetrahydrobiopterin, BH4 (**Fig. 1**). The latter accounts for approximately 2% of elevated phenylalanine levels and includes deficiencies in guanosine triphosphate cyclohydrolase, pyruvoyl-tetrahydrobiopterin synthase, dihydropteridine reductase, and pterin-4a-carbinolamine dehydratase. At the metabolic center, analysis of plasma amino acids will confirm the elevated phenylalanine levels, and urine biopterin and dihydropteridine reductase activity measurements, will assess cofactor availability. Disorders of tetrahydrobiopterin synthesis and regeneration have to be ruled out in all newborns with elevated phenylalanine levels. Typically, pterins are measured in urine and dihydropteridine reductase activity in a blood spot. If the phenylalanine level is elevated and cofactor levels are normal, then PAH deficiency is assumed. Depending on the degree of phenylalanine level elevation, individuals are categorized into classic PKU, moderate PKU, mild PKU, and hyperphenylalaninemia.[6] PAH deficiency can be confirmed and the phenotype predicted by determining the mutations in the gene that led to the deficiency.

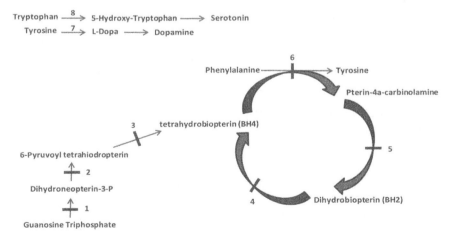

Fig. 1. Phenylalanine hydroxylation and biopterin biosynthesis pathway. Enzymes 7 and 8 require BH4 as cofactor. (1) Guanosine triphosphate cyclohydrolase. (2) Pyruvoyl tetrahydrobiopterin synthase. (3) Sepiapterin reductase (SR). (4) Dihydropteridine reductase (DHPR). (5) Pterin-4a-carbinolamine dehydratase. (6) Phenylalanine 4-hydroxylase (PAH). (7) Tyrosine hydroxylase. (8) Tryptophane Hydroxylase.

Treatment

Diet

If phenylalanine levels are consistently above 6 mg/dL or 360 µmol/L, treatment will be initiated. The level at which treatment was started used to be 600 µmol/L and some centers now use 480 µmol/L as the cutoff level.[7] The mainstay of treatment is a low-phenylalanine diet consisting of a phenylalanine-free formula (medical food) and enough low-protein food so that the natural protein content of the food provides the phenylalanine needed for normal growth and development of the child, yet not too much to increase the phenylalanine level. Lifetime treatment and maintenance of phenylalanine levels between 2 and 6 mg/dL (120 and 360 µmol/L) is the current recommendation. In previous decades, discontinuation or relaxation of therapy was recommended at different ages. As a consequence, still to date insurance companies and state programs will often not cover metabolic formula for affected adults with the exception of women with PKU planning a pregnancy or pregnant.

Chaperone therapy

When the genetic defects are such that a mutant enzyme is made but it is not functional or barely functional, a molecular chaperone may stabilize the enzyme sufficiently enough to improve the enzymatic activity and hence ameliorate the clinical manifestations. The best molecular chaperones for enzymes are typically their cofactors. Sapropterin, a synthetic form of BH4, the natural cofactor of PAH, has been developed for chaperone therapy of PKU and is widely in use. It works in individuals who produce a mutant enzyme that can be stabilized. Typically, these individuals have a milder form of the disease.

In BH4 biosynthesis and regeneration defects, treatment consists of sapropterin and neurotransmitter precursor supplementation, along with low-phenylalanine diet and folinic acid supplementation, depending on the defect.

General Information

- Untreated classic PKU causes most severe ID. Therefore, the introduction of newborn screening was the logical consequence of the development of a successful treatment. Only if affected individuals could be detected and treated before damage had occurred could treatment be truly effective.
- Every child with ID should undergo a plasma amino acid analysis.
- Because BH4, the cofactor of PAH, is also the cofactor of the dopamine synthesizing enzyme tyrosine hydroxylase and the cofactor of the serotonin synthesizing enzyme tryptophan hydroxylase (see **Fig. 1**), individuals with BH4 cofactor deficiency not only have elevated phenylalanine levels, but often also significant movement disorders requiring neurotransmitter precursor supplementation.

Unexpected Consequences of Successful Treatment

Maternal phenylketonuria

- With successful treatment and individuals reaching reproductive age, it became evident that high maternal phenylalanine levels can be teratogenic and result in microcephaly, intrauterine growth restriction, congenital heart defects, and significant ID in the offspring of untreated mothers. Very vigorous dietary control has to be implemented before pregnancy and maintained throughout to prevent adverse fetal effects.

DEFECTS OF HOMOCYSTEINE AND METHIONINE METABOLISM
Presenting Symptoms

- Elevated methionine level on newborn screen or developmental delay and cognitive impairment or characteristic physical findings (see the section on Clinical

Presentation). Depending on the degree of methionine elevation on newborn screen, the pediatrician will be asked to send a repeat newborn screening sample or refer the newborn to a metabolic center immediately. A pediatrician may also refer an older child owing to unexplained cognitive impairment or findings consistent with the diagnosis (Marfanoid habitus, ectopia lentis, etc).

Clinical Presentation in Classic Homocystinuria (Cystathionine ß-Synthase Deficiency)

- Developmental delay of variable severity.
- Psychiatric manifestations include anxiety, personality disorders, depression, and psychotic episodes.
- Skeletal findings include a "Marfanoid" appearance (tall and lean, kyphoscoliosis, arachnodactyly, pectus deformities), vertebral anomalies, genu valgum, and early osteoporosis.
- Eye findings include ectopia lentis, glaucoma, and myopia.
- Cardiovascular findings include thromboembolic events that can affect arteries and veins of any size.
- Skin manifestations include malar flush, livedo reticularis, and thin skin.

Diagnostic Evaluation

- The differential diagnosis of an elevated methionine level is a high-protein diet, liver dysfunction, deficiency of cystathionine ß-synthase (CBS), deficiency of methionine adenosyltransferase I and III, deficiency of glycine N-methyltransferase, and adenosylhomocysteine hydrolase deficiency (**Fig. 2**).[8] In methionine adenosyltransferase I and III deficiency, there is a block in conversion of methionine to s-adenosylmethionine and besides elevated methionine, there may be a slight elevation of total homocysteine. Definitive diagnosis is based on molecular testing. Affected individuals can be clinically asymptomatic or present with manifestations from the central nervous system, depending on the severity of the enzyme deficiency. An unpleasant breath odor can also be present owing to increased dimethylsulfide.[9]

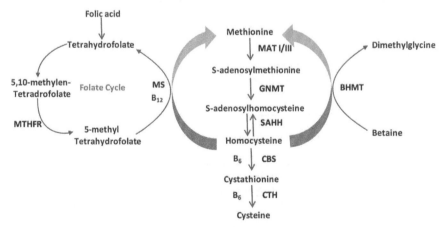

Fig. 2. Homocysteine–methionine metabolism. Enzymes are shown in *red*. B$_{12}$, cobalamin, cofactor for methionine synthase; B$_6$, pyridoxine, cofactor for cystathionine ß-synthase; BHMT, betaine-homocysteine S-methyltransferase; CBS, cystathionine ß-synthase; CTH, cystathionine gamma-lyase; GNMT, glycine N-methyltransferase; MAT I/III, methionine adenosyltransferase I/III; MS, methionine synthase; MTHFR, Methylenetetrahydrofolate reductase; SAHH, S-adenosylhomocysteine hydrolase.

- At the metabolic center, plasma amino acid analysis will be performed to assess the methionine level and a total plasma homocysteine level along with a vitamin B_{12} level will be measured to establish the diagnosis. The differential diagnosis of homocysteine–methionine metabolism defects, based on the biochemical profile, is presented in **Table 1**.

Treatment

In individuals with both, significantly elevated methionine and homocysteine levels, treatment is initiated. Before initiation of treatment, a challenge with vitamin B_6 has to be conducted to assess for vitamin B_6 responsive CBS deficiency versus vitamin B_6 nonresponsive CBS deficiency. Similar to BH4 in PKU, vitamin B_6 is the natural cofactor of CBS and using high doses of natural cofactor can stabilize the mutant enzyme sufficiently to result in a milder phenotype. Treatment consists of diet and medication.

- Diet: A low-methionine diet is implemented consisting of a methionine-free formula and enough natural protein that adequate methionine is available for normal growth.
- Medication: Betaine supplements the dietary therapy by converting homocysteine to methionine, which will increase the methionine level but is less of a concern than an elevated homocysteine level.[8]

General Information

Although untreated classic homocystinuria can impact the eyes, the skeleton, the vascular system, and the brain, there are affected individuals that remain initially asymptomatic, yet can suffer severe thromboembolic episodes later on as adolescents, young adults, or older adults.

Methyltetrahydrofolate reductase deficiency is characterized by high homocysteine and low methionine levels that causes severe ID and is covered in Mohammed Almannai and Ayman W. El-Hattab's article, "Inborn Errors of Metabolism with Seizures: Defects of Glycine and Serine Metabolism and Cofactor Related Disorders," in this issue.

DEFECTS OF PURINE AND PYRIMIDINE METABOLISM

Purines and pyrimidines are not only the building blocks of DNA and RNA, but they also serve as second messengers and conveyors of energy in the cells. They are synthesized either de novo or via a salvage pathway, which is less energy consuming and

Table 1
Biochemical profile in defects of methionine metabolism

Disorder	Total Plasma Homocysteine	Plasma Methionine
CBS deficiency	Elevated	Elevated
MAT I/III deficiency	Normal-slightly elevated	Elevated
GNMT deficiency	Normal-slightly elevated	Elevated
SAAH deficiency	Normal-slightly elevated	Elevated
MTHFR deficiency	Elevated	Low
Vitamin B_{12} defects	Elevated	Low

Abbreviations: CBS, cystathionine β-synthase; GNMT, glycine N-methyltransferase; MAT, methionine adenosyltransferase; MTHFR, methylenetetrahydrofolate reductase; SAAH, S-adenosylhomocysteine hydrolase.

thus preferred.[10] Enzymatic defects affecting their metabolism can practically affect any system and particularly rapidly dividing cells. The huge variability in their presentation, the multisystem involvement, and the imitation of common diseases are common barriers to the diagnosis. More than 30 disorders have been identified and the catalog is still growing.[11] A prompt diagnosis is crucial, especially for diseases amenable to treatment, because successful treatment may delay their progression or alter their course. Only a few disorders of purine metabolism cause cognitive impairment and the mechanism is as yet unknown. Gout is a common manifestation, because uric acid is the final product of purine catabolism. Individuals with IEMs affecting the pyrimidine pathways will most likely present with neurodevelopmental issues. Here, we present 3 disorders that can cause cognitive impairment of variable severity: Lesch-Nyhan syndrome, dihydropyrimidine dehydrogenase deficiency, and dihydropyriminidase deficiency. Adenylosuccinate deficiency, a defect in the pathway for the de novo biosynthesis of purines, can cause profound ID. The disease is covered elsewhere (see Mohammed Almannai and Ayman W. El-Hattab's article, "Inborn Errors of Metabolism with Seizures: Defects of Glycine and Serine Metabolism and Cofactor Related Disorders," in this issue), because seizures are present in the vast majority of affected individuals.

LESCH-NYHAN SYNDROME: A DEFECT OF PURINE SALVAGE
Presenting Symptoms

Lesch-Nyhan syndrome is suspected in a male child who presents with hypotonia along with delayed motor milestones in early infancy, and subsequently develops a movement disorder with dystonia, choreoathetosis, and signs of cerebral palsy with brisk reflexes and spasticity. Cognitive impairment and behavioral problems are also present. In the urine, there is an orange precipitate (uric acid crystals). The hallmark of the disease is self-injurious behaviors that consist of lip, cheek, and finger biting leading to severe mutilation. Significant head injuries owing to head banging are not uncommon. Hyperuricemia is present and, if untreated, symptoms of gout and nephrolithiasis ensue.[12]

Diagnostic Evaluation

A serum uric acid level of greater than 8 mg/dL in combination with the typical clinical symptoms should trigger hypoxanthine guanine phosphoribosyltransferase enzyme activity measurement and/or gene sequencing. Serum uric acid is typically elevated, but not always. The uric acid to creatinine ratio in urine can be used as a sensitive measure to document uric acid overproduction.[12]

Treatment

Allopurinol inhibits the conversion of hypoxanthine and xanthine to uric acid. Hypoxanthine and xanthine are excreted instead. Allopurinol is the key to reducing uric acid levels, preventing stone formation and subsequent gout development. End-stage renal disease owing to urate nephropathy was the rule before the implementation of allopurinol treatment. However, allopurinol does not have any effect on the neurologic symptoms or the behavioral problems. Probenecid and other drugs that lower the uric acid level in plasma by increasing its excretion are contraindicated, because they increase the risk of stone formation.

For symptomatic treatment of the neurologic and behavioral manifestations therapeutic agents like baclofen and benzodiazepines are used. Protective gear to prevent self-harm is also an option.

General Information

Lesch-Nyhan syndrome is an X-linked recessive disorder caused by hypoxanthine guanine phosphoribosyl transferase deficiency. The end result is hypoxanthine accumulation and its conversion into uric acid. Other disorders of purine and pyrimidine metabolism that cause ID are the purine nucleotide synthesis disorders phosphoribosylpyrophosphate synthetase superactivity (X-linked) and adenylosuccinase deficiency (autosomal recessive).[10]

DIHYDROPYRIMIDINE DEHYDROGENASE DEFICIENCY

Dihydropyrimidine dehydrogenase deficiency presents with great phenotypic variation that ranges from asymptomatic to a disorder with developmental delays and seizures [13] Failure to thrive, hypotonia, and eye anomalies (microphthalmia, unusual eye movements, and colobomas) are less frequently present. The variability in the phenotype may imply that other factors play a role in the development of the clinical picture. Dihydropyrimidine dehydrogenase is responsible for catabolizing the widely used chemotherapeutic drug 5-fluorouracil. Dihydropyrimidine dehydrogenase status should be known before the start of therapy with 5-fluorouracil to identify those individuals with a high risk of significant or even fatal toxicity.[14]

DIHYDROPYRIMIDINASE DEFICIENCY (DIHYDROPYRIMIDINURIA)

Dihydropyrimidinase is the second enzyme in the pathway of pyrimidine catabolism. Affected individuals present with ID and seizures, and may have dysmorphic features. Again here, the chemotherapeutic 5-fluorouracil is contraindicated because it may lead to detrimental side effects owing to severe toxicity.

DEFECTS OF CREATINE METABOLISM

Creatine biosynthesis defects or cerebral creatine deficiency syndromes, comprise a group of 3 disorders that disrupt the biosynthesis of creatine and result in creatine deficiency in the brain (**Fig. 3**). Global developmental delays, ID, and seizures are their predominant manifestations. In this article, we will discuss the creatine transporter defect and L-arginine:glycine aminotransferase (AGAT) deficiency. Guanidinoacetate (GAA) methyltransferase deficiency, is discussed in Mohammed Almannai and Ayman W. El-Hattab's article, "Inborn Errors of Metabolism with Seizures: Defects of Glycine and Serine Metabolism and Cofactor Related Disorders," in this issue, because it may present early in life with intractable epilepsy.

L-Arginine:Glycine Aminotransferase Deficiency

Presenting symptoms

ID with a variable spectrum of severity is the most common manifestation. Failure to thrive, hypotonia owing to muscle weakness, behavioral problems, and autistic behaviors may be present as well. Febrile seizures are common.

Diagnostic evaluation

- GAA, creatine, and creatinine measurement in urine and plasma as well as the creatine-to-creatinine ratio in urine[15] are used as screening tests for the differential diagnosis of creatine biosynthesis defects. In AGAT deficiency, GAA is low to low normal in urine and plasma and creatine is low in plasma.[16]

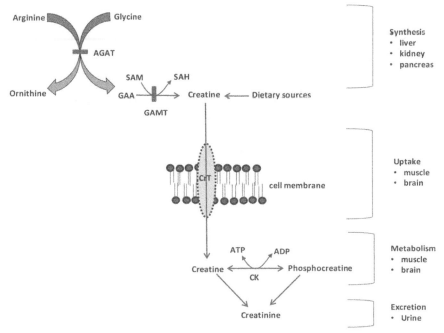

Fig. 3. Creatine biosynthesis pathway. AGAT, L-arginine:glycine amidinotransferase; CK, creatine kinase; CrT, creatine transporter; GAA, guanidinoacetate; GAMT, guanidinoacetate methyltransferase; SAH, S-adenosylhomocysteine; SAM, S-adenosylmethionine.

- Brain magnetic resonance spectroscopy reveals creatine depletion.
- Sequencing of the L-arginine:glycine amidinotransferase gene (*GATM*). If gene sequencing is not diagnostic, measurement of the enzyme activity in lymphoblasts can be used to confirm a diagnosis (low AGAT activity).

Treatment
Creatine supplementation using oral creatine monohydrate is used. Creatine supplementation requires monitoring of renal function. Initiation of treatment before symptoms occur seems to be beneficial. Different creatine compounds are under investigation in therapeutic trials.[17]

General information
The inheritance is autosomal recessive.

Creatine Transporter Defect

Presenting symptoms
Males are typically affected and developmental disabilities may range from mild to severe.[18] Delayed speech and speech disorders (dysarthria, dyspraxia, and echolalia) are prevalent. Attention deficit hyperactivity disorder, autistic behaviors, and other behavioral disorders are common. Neurologic manifestations include hypotonia, spasticity, ataxia, dystonia, ptosis, and seizures. Dysmorphic features such as microcephaly, broad forehead, high palate, and ear anomalies may also be present. Failure to thrive, constipation, and feeding difficulties may occur. Females may have mild ID or be completely asymptomatic.

Diagnostic evaluation

- Screening testing includes measurement of GAA, creatine, and creatinine in plasma and urine. In creatine transporter deficiency, GAA is normal in plasma and urine, creatine is normal in plasma and normal to elevated in urine, and urinary creatine to creatinine ratio is elevated in males and normal to elevated in females.
- Brain magnetic resonance spectroscopy shows decreased creatine signal.
- Molecular genetic analysis of the *SLC6A8* gene is used to confirm the diagnosis.
- If molecular testing is not diagnostic, creatine uptake studies in cultured skin fibroblasts will establish the diagnosis by showing decreased creatine uptake.
- Molecular genetic testing is the preferred approach to establish a suspected diagnosis in females, because both biochemical markers and creatine uptake studies may be normal in affected females.

Treatment

To date, there are not sufficient data regarding the different treatment options. A combination of oral creatine, arginine, and glycine should be considered, based on a systematic literature review. A few affected individuals showed some improvement in their cognitive abilities, especially if treatment had started before 9 years of age.[19] Overall, individuals with creatine transporter deficiency, as compared with AGAT and guanidinoacetate methyltransferase, do not have a successful treatment.

General information

Creatine transporter deficiency is an X-linked recessive disease.

REFERENCES

1. Schalock RL, Luckasson RA, Shogren KA. The renaming of mental retardation: understanding the change to the term intellectual disability. Intellect Dev Disabil 2007;45(2):116–24.
2. Moeschler JB, Shevell M, Committee on Genetics. Comprehensive evaluation of the child with intellectual disability or global developmental delays. Pediatrics 2014;134(3):e903–18.
3. Cleary MA, Green A. Developmental delay: when to suspect and how to investigate for an inborn error of metabolism. Arch Dis Child 2005;90(11): 1128–32.
4. Van Karnebeek CD, Shevell M, Zschocke J, et al. The metabolic evaluation of the child with an intellectual developmental disorder: diagnostic algorithm for identification of treatable causes and new digital resource. Mol Genet Metab 2014; 111(4):428–38.
5. Antshel KM. ADHD, learning, and academic performance in phenylketonuria. Mol Genet Metab 2010;99(Suppl 1):S52–8.
6. Camp KM, Parisi MA, Acosta PB, et al. Phenylketonuria scientific review conference: state of the science and future research needs. Mol Genet Metab 2014; 112(2):87–122.
7. Vockley J, Andersson HC, Antshel KM, et al, American College of Medical Genetics and Genomics Therapeutics Committee. Phenylalanine hydroxylase deficiency: diagnosis and management guideline. Genet Med 2014;16(2):188–200.
8. Picker JD, Levy HL. Homocystinuria caused by cystathionine beta-synthase deficiency. In: Pagon RA, Adam MP, Ardinger HH, et al, editors. GeneReviews® [Internet]. Seattle (WA): University of Washington, Seattle; 2004. p. 1993–2017. Updated November 13, 2014.

9. Mudd SH. Hypermethioninemias of genetic and non-genetic origin. A review. Am J Med Genet C Semin Med Genet 2011;157C:3–32.
10. Sanders LM. Overview of purine and pyrimidine metabolism disorders. 2016. Available at: http://www.merckmanuals.com/professional/pediatrics/inherited-disorders-of-metabolism/overview-of-purine-and-pyrimidine-metabolism-disorders. Accessed April 3, 2017.
11. Jurecka A. Inborn errors of purine and pyrimidine metabolism. J Inherit Metab Dis 2009;32(2):247–63.
12. Nyhan WL, O'Neill JP, Jinnah HA, et al. Lesch-Nyhan syndrome. In: Pagon RA, Adam MP, Ardinger HH, et al, editors. GeneReviews® [Internet]. Seattle (WA): University of Washington, Seattle; 2000. p. 1993–2017. Updated May 15, 2014.
13. Van Kuilenburg AB, Vreken P, Abeling NG, et al. Genotype and phenotype in patients with dihydropyrimidine dehydrogenase deficiency. Hum Genet 1999; 104(1):1–9.
14. Meulendijks D, Cats A, Beijnen JH, et al. Improving safety of fluoropyrimidine chemotherapy by individualizing treatment based on dihydropyrimidine dehydrogenase activity - Ready for clinical practice? Cancer Treat Rev 2016;50:23–34.
15. Verhoeven NM, Salomons GS, Jakobs C. Laboratory diagnosis of defects of creatine biosynthesis and transport. Clin Chim Acta 2005;361(1–2):1–9.
16. Mercimek-Mahmutoglu S, Salomons GS. Creatine deficiency syndromes. In: Pagon RA, Adam MP, Ardinger HH, et al, editors. GeneReviews® [Internet]. Seattle (WA): University of Washington, Seattle; 2009. p. 1993–2017. Updated December 10, 2015.
17. Fons C, Campistol J. Creatine defects and central nervous system. Semin Pediatr Neurol 2016;23(4):285–9.
18. Van de Kamp JM, Mancini GM, Salomons GS. X-linked creatine transporter deficiency: clinical aspects and pathophysiology. J Inherit Metab Dis 2014;37(5): 715–33.
19. Dunbar M, Jaggumantri S, Sargent M, et al. Treatment of X-linked creatine transporter (SLC6A8) deficiency: systematic review of the literature and three new cases. Mol Genet Metab 2014;112(4):259–74.

Inborn Errors of Metabolism with Seizures

Defects of Glycine and Serine Metabolism and Cofactor-Related Disorders

Mohammed Almannai, MD[a], Ayman W. El-Hattab, MD[b],*

KEYWORDS

- Inborn errors of metabolism • Seizures • Epilepsy • Myoclonic epilepsy • Glycine
- Serine • Pyridoxine

KEY POINTS

- Inborn errors of metabolism (IEM) are relatively uncommon causes for seizures in children; however, they should be considered in the differential diagnosis because several IEM are potentially treatable and seizures can be resolved when appropriate treatment is initiated.
- IEM should be particularly considered in neonatal seizures and in the context of refractory seizures. Other clues from clinical presentation, physical examination, laboratory tests, and brain imaging can increase the possibility of IEM.
- Several IEM can present with seizures, either as the main presenting finding or as a part of a more complex phenotype.
- IEM that cause seizures include cofactor-related disorders (eg, pyridoxine-dependent epilepsy, pyridoxal phosphate-responsive epilepsy, and cerebral folate deficiency), glycine and serine metabolism defects (eg, glycine encephalopathy and serine biosynthesis defects), and other disorders (eg, glucose transporter type 1 deficiency, adenylosuccinate lyase deficiency, and guanidinoacetate methyltransferase deficiency).
- When IEM are suspected, diagnosis and treatment should be simultaneous. Early treatment can prevent, or at least minimize, long-term sequelae.

INTRODUCTION

Seizures are frequently encountered in pediatric practice with an estimated prevalence of 1% in children.[1] The etiologic factors of seizures are many, including genetic diseases; structural brain abnormalities; or acquired conditions such as infections, tumors, and trauma. Alternatively, seizures can be secondary to provoking factors such

Declaration of Conflict of Interest: The authors declare that there are no conflicts of interest.
[a] Department of Molecular and Human Genetics, Baylor College of Medicine, Texas Children's Hospital, One Baylor Plaza, Houston, TX 77030, USA; [b] Division of Clinical Genetics and Metabolic Disorders, Pediatrics Department, Tawam Hospital, Tawam Roundabout, Al-Ain 15258, United Arab Emirates
* Corresponding author.
E-mail address: elhattabaw@yahoo.com

as fever and hypoglycemia.[2] Inborn errors of metabolism (IEM) are relatively uncommon causes for seizures in children (**Box 1**). They still should be always considered in the differential diagnosis because several IEM that cause seizures are potentially treatable (**Box 2**) and seizures can be resolved when appropriate treatment is initiated. IEM often require specialized dietary and therapeutic interventions that should be initiated in a timely manner to prevent, or at least minimize, long-term sequelae. Even with

---

Box 1
Inborn errors of metabolism that can present with seizures

- Cofactor-related disorders
  - Pyridoxine-dependent epilepsy
  - Pyridoxal phosphate-responsive epilepsy
  - Cerebral folate deficiency
  - Biotinidase deficiency
  - Holocarboxylase synthetase deficiency
  - Molybdenum cofactor deficiency
  - Severe methylenetetrahydrofolate reductase (MTHFR) deficiency

- Amino acid disorders
  - Glycine encephalopathy
  - Serine biosynthesis defects
  - Sulfite oxidase deficiency
  - Urea cycle disorders
  - Phenylketonuria
  - Organic acidemias
  - Maple syrup urine disease

- Metal transport
  - Menkes disease

- Lysosomal disorders
  - Neuronal ceroid lipofuscinosis
  - Sialidosis type I and type II
  - Metachromatic leukodystrophy
  - GM1 gangliosidosis
  - GM2 gangliosidosis
  - Gaucher disease types 2 and 3
  - Niemann-Pick disease type C

- Disorders of energy metabolism
  - Mitochondrial disorders
  - Guanidinoacetate N-methyltransferase (GAMT) deficiency
  - Disorders of pyruvate metabolism
  - Glucose transporter type 1 (GLUT-1) deficiency
  - Fatty acid oxidation disorders[a]
  - Disorders of gluconeogenesis[a]
  - Glycogen storage disorders[a]

- Disorders of purine and pyrimidine nucleotides metabolism
  - Adenylosuccinate lyase (ADSL) deficiency
  - Lesch-Nyhan syndrome
  - Dihydropyrimidine dehydrogenase deficiency

- Peroxisomal disorders
  - Zellweger syndrome
  - X-linked adrenoleukodystrophy

- Congenital disorders of glycosylation

[a] In these disorders, seizures are secondary to hypoglycemia.

Box 2
Treatable inborn errors of metabolism that can present with seizures
• Phenylketonuria
• Urea cycle disorders
• Organic acidemias
• Maple syrup urine disease
• Pyridoxine-dependent epilepsy
• Pyridoxal phosphate-responsive epilepsy
• Cerebral folate deficiency
• Attenuated glycine encephalopathy
• Serine biosynthesis defects
• Biotinidase deficiency
• GLUT-1 deficiency
• GAMT deficiency
• Severe MTHFR deficiency
• Molybdenum cofactor deficiency type A

untreatable disorders, reaching a diagnosis is essential to direct plans of care and to provide counseling to the family in terms of prognosis and recurrence risk.[3–7]

IEM can cause seizures by different mechanisms, including accumulation of toxic metabolites, energy deficit, cofactor deficiency, abnormal neurotransmission, and brain malformations.[3,4] An example of toxic accumulation is hyperammonemia. Ammonia accumulates in several IEM, including urea cycle disorders and organic acidemias, and is known for its neurotoxicity. Elevated ammonia in the brain results in increased glutamine synthesis that, in turn, induces astrocyte swelling and brain edema.[8] Glucose is the principal source of energy in the brain and, therefore, disorders that cause hypoglycemia (eg, fatty acid oxidation defects) or interfere with glucose transport to the brain (eg, glucose transporter type 1 [GLUT-1] deficiency) can result in brain dysfunction and seizures. In mitochondrial disorders, seizures can also result from energy deficiency and impaired adenosine triphosphate (ATP) production, which is reqred to maintain transmembrane potential.[3] Examples of cofactor-related disorders are pyridoxine-dependent epilepsy and pyridoxal phosphate-responsive epilepsy; both are associated with pyridoxal phosphate deficiency. Pyridoxal phosphate, the active form of pyridoxine, is an important cofactor for many enzymatic reactions, including neurotransmitter metabolism.[9] An example of abnormal neurotransmission is glycine encephalopathy that is associated with elevation in glycine, which is an agonist of N-methyl D-aspartate (NMDA) glutamate receptors. Overstimulation of these excitatory receptors results in seizures. Finally, several IEM are associated with brain malformations that can predispose to seizures. For example, polymicrogyria, which is seen in infants with peroxisomal disorders, is a malformation of cortical development that disrupts the neuronal circuit and leads to epileptic seizures.[10] In fact, the pathophysiology of seizures in IEM is more complex, involving multiple, interrelated mechanisms. Delineating these mechanisms can result in more targeted therapeutic interventions in the future.

More than 200 different IEM are associated with seizures,[4] either as the main presenting finding or, more commonly, as part of a more complex neurologic and metabolic phenotype. Although this seems overwhelming, especially because most IEM are rare, the key point is to maintain a high index of suspicion when working up a child presenting with seizures, particularly in unexplained neonatal seizures and in the context of seizures refractory to standard treatment (**Box 3**). Isolated epilepsy with no other systemic or neurologic features is less likely to be due to IEM.[5]

This article first discusses an approach to IEM that present with seizures, followed by a summary of IEM that cause seizures, including cofactor-related disorders, glycine and serine metabolism defects, and other disorders.

APPROACH TO INBORN ERRORS OF METABOLISM PRESENTING WITH SEIZURES

Approach to a newborn or a child presenting with seizures should include a detailed history and physical examination, followed by comprehensive evaluation, including laboratory work up, electroencephalogram (EEG), and brain imaging if indicated.

History and Physical Examination

Seizures associated with IEM can present at any age (**Table 1**). In general, it is uncommon to have seizures as an isolated presentation of IEM.[5] Usually, there is a variable combination of other manifestations involving different systems. In some disorders, the presentation is nonspecific, in the form of sepsis-like illness or hypoxic ischemic encephalopathy (HIE). In fact, IEM may be accompanied by HIE and this can be misleading and results in delayed diagnosis. Therefore, the possibility of IEM should be considered if a newborn with HIE develops refractory seizures.[6] While taking a history, it is imperative to pay attention to details such as diet history, growth, and development. Children with IEM can have a long-standing history of nonspecific, subtle symptoms, including failure to thrive, recurrent vomiting, aversion to a particular food, or developmental delay. Similarly, a history of unexplained episodes of encephalopathy is alarming. Family history is essential and might be overlooked, especially in acute settings such as emergency rooms and intensive care units. Red flags in family history include previous stillbirth, unexplained neonatal death, and consanguinity.

Different forms of seizures are seen in children with IEM (**Table 2**) with variable EEG abnormalities.[11] For example, early myoclonic epileptic encephalopathy with a burst suppression pattern on EEG is seen in disorders such as glycine encephalopathy, pyridoxine-dependent epilepsy, pyridoxal phosphate-responsive epilepsy,

---

Box 3
Clues raising the suspicion of inborn errors of metabolism in children presenting with seizures

- Refractory seizures
- Unexplained neonatal seizures
- Early myoclonic epileptic encephalopathy
- Unexplained hypoxic ischemic encephalopathy
- History of unexplained episodes of encephalopathy and/or developmental delay
- Seizures related to fasting, food intake, and/or stress
- Aversion or intolerance to particular food, particularly protein
- Recurrent episodes of vomiting and dehydration
- Parental consanguinity
- Positive family history of seizures
- History of unexplained neonatal death in the family

Table 1
Classification of inborn errors of metabolism associated with seizures based on age on onset

Age Group	Disorders
In utero	• Pyridoxine-dependent epilepsy • Pyridoxal phosphate-responsive epilepsy • Glycine encephalopathy • Congenital neuronal ceroid lipofuscinosis
Neonatal period	• Pyridoxine-dependent epilepsy[a] • Pyridoxal phosphate-responsive epilepsy • Holocarboxylase synthetase deficiency • Molybdenum cofactor deficiency • Sulfite oxidase deficiency • Glycine encephalopathy[b] • Urea cycle disorders[c] • Organic acidemias • Maple syrup urine disease[d] • Zellweger syndrome • Serine biosynthesis defects • Congenital neuronal ceroid lipofuscinosis • Disorders of pyruvate metabolism
Infancy	• Organic acidemias • Peroxisomal disorders • Biotinidase deficiency • Serine biosynthesis defects • Molybdenum cofactor deficiency (mild form) • Sulfite oxidase deficiency (mild form) • Phenylketonuria • Menkes disease • Infantile neuronal ceroid lipofuscinosis • Glucose transporter type 1 (GLUT-1) deficiency • Guanidinoacetate N-methyltransferase (GAMT) deficiency • Adenylosuccinate lyase (ADSL) deficiency type I (severe form) • Cerebral folate deficiency • Sialidosis type II • GM2 gangliosidosis (infantile form) • Congenital disorders of glycosylation • Disorders of pyruvate metabolism • GM1 gangliosidosis (infantile variants) • Gaucher disease type 2 • Methylenetetrahydrofolate reductase (MTHFR) deficiency
Early childhood	• Late infantile neuronal ceroid lipofuscinosis • Creatine deficiency syndromes • ADSL deficiency type II (mild-moderate forms) • Mitochondrial disorders • Cerebral folate deficiency • Lesch-Nyhan syndrome • Sialidosis type II • Congenital disorders of glycosylation • X-linked adrenoleukodystrophy • GM1 gangliosidosis (late infantile form) • Metachromatic leukodystrophy (late infantile form)

(continued on next page)

Table 1 (continued)	
Age Group	**Disorders**
Late childhood and adolescence	• Juvenile neuronal ceroid lipofuscinosis • X-linked adrenoleukodystrophy • Gaucher disease type 3 • Niemann-Pick disease type C • Mitochondrial disorders • GM2 gangliosidosis (juvenile form) • Metachromatic leukodystrophy (juvenile form)

[a] Atypical cases can present later (≤3 years).
[b] Atypical forms may have later age of onset.
[c] Later onset is possible. Onset is variable, from infancy to adulthood.
[d] Variable onset in intermediate and intermittent forms.

sulfite oxidase deficiency, and molybdenum cofactor deficiency. Hypsarrhythmia is seen in serine biosynthesis defects, Menkes disease, and untreated phenylketonuria. Epilepsia partialis continua is a common form of seizure in mitochondrial disorders, particularly in Alpers syndrome. In this disorder, an EEG pattern of rhythmic high-amplitude delta with superimposed spikes can help in diagnosis.[12]

On physical examination, findings that suggest IEM include microcephaly, dysmorphic or coarse facial features, abnormal eye examination, unusual odor, hair or skin abnormalities, and organomegaly (**Table 3**).[13]

Table 2 Seizure forms that can be seen in some of the inborn errors of metabolism	
Seizure from	**Disorders**
Myoclonic seizures	• Pyridoxine-dependent epilepsy • Pyridoxal phosphate-responsive epilepsy • Glycine encephalopathy • Neuronal ceroid lipofuscinosis • Biotinidase deficiency • Sialidosis type I and type II • Mitochondrial disorders • Menkes disease (in childhood)
Infantile spasms	• Serine biosynthesis defects • Menkes disease (late infancy) • Mitochondrial disorders • Phenylketonuria • Biotinidase deficiency
Generalized tonic-clonic	• GLUT-1 deficiency • Creatine deficiency syndromes • Mitochondrial disorders • Biotinidase deficiency • Neuronal ceroid lipofuscinosis
Progressive myoclonic epilepsy	• Myoclonic epilepsy with ragged red fibers • Neuronal ceroid lipofuscinosis • Sialidosis type I and type II • Gaucher disease type 3
Epilepsia partialis continua	• Mitochondrial disorders (in particular, Alpers syndrome)
Partial motor seizures	• Zellweger Syndrome

Table 3
Clinical features associated with some metabolic epilepsies

Clinical Feature	Associated Disorders
Microcephaly	• GLUT-1 deficiency • ADSL deficiency • Serine biosynthesis defects • Phenylketonuria • Congenital disorders of glycosylation
Macrocephaly	• GM2 gangliosidosis
Dysmorphic features	• Zellweger syndrome
Coarse features	• GM1 gangliosidosis • Sialidosis type II
Cherry-red spot	• GM1 gangliosidosis • GM2 gangliosidosis • Sialidosis type I and type II • Metachromatic leukodystrophy
Lens dislocation	• Sulfite oxidase deficiency • Molybdenum cofactor deficiency
Supranuclear horizontal ophthalmoplegia	• Gaucher disease type 3
Retinitis pigmentosa	• Neuronal ceroid lipofuscinosis • Congenital disorders of glycosylation • Mitochondrial disorders • Peroxisomal disorders
Inverted nipples	• Congenital disorders of glycosylation
Hepato(spleno)megaly	• Gaucher disease type 2 and 3 • Sialidosis type II • GM1 gangliosidosis • Peroxisomal disorders • Congenital disorders of glycosylation
Dermatitis	• Biotinidase deficiency • Phenylketonuria
Sparse hair	• Biotinidase deficiency (alopecia) • Meknes disease (kinky hair)
Movement disorders	• Organic acidemias • GAMT deficiency • GLUT-1 deficiency
Stroke-like episodes	• Mitochondrial disorders (in particular, mitochondrial encephalomyopathy, lactic acidosis, and stroke-like episodes [MELAS] syndrome) • Congenital disorders of glycosylation
Bone abnormalities	• Sialidosis type II • Gaucher disease type 3 • GM1 gangliosidosis • Peroxisomal disorders (chondrodysplasia punctate)

Laboratory Workup

The aim is to rule out common causes first, such as hypoglycemia, electrolyte disturbances, and central nervous system infections.[14] Although some IEM require detailed testing before diagnosis is made, others can be diagnosed on a clinical basis; for example, by cessation of seizures following administration of pyridoxine in a newborn with pyridoxine-dependent epilepsy. Results of the initial workup can provide some clues (eg, hypoglycemia in fatty acid oxidations defects, metabolic acidosis with organic acidemias, and hyperammonemia in urea cycle disorders). Plasma ammonia and lactate levels should be always considered in the initial workup. Hyperammonemia can be seen in several IEM, including urea cycle disorders and organic acidemias. Seizure by itself can result in significant elevation of lactate but this elevation is transient. Once the seizure has resolved, lactate is rapidly cleared. Therefore, persistently elevated lactate beyond 1 to 2 hours following a seizure should trigger looking for another cause.[15] In the context of IEM, mitochondrial disorders and organic acidemias are examples of disorders that can cause high lactate levels. When available, results of newborn screening can be helpful. Based on the clinical suspicion made from the presentation and initial workup, a second tier of biochemical testing should be ordered, including plasma amino acids, urine organic acids, and plasma acylcarnitine profile, among others. Several IEM can be diagnosed based on a specific pattern of abnormalities in these metabolites. Biochemical tests are of highest diagnostic yield when ordered during acute metabolic decompensations. When obtained, cerebrospinal fluid (CSF) studies should be paired with plasma samples to get informative CSF-to-plasma ratios of metabolites of interest (**Fig. 1**). In several situations, another layer of testing, such as enzyme activity, single gene testing, and functional assays in skin fibroblast samples, might be warranted. In situations in which diagnosis still remains unclear, more comprehensive evaluation with gene panels, global metabolomic profiling, or whole exome sequencing, should be considered.[16]

Neuroimaging

Although neuroimaging is usually nonspecific or normal in IEM presenting with seizures, it can be helpful in limiting diagnostic considerations.[17] For example, glycine encephalopathy and pyridoxine-dependent epilepsy can be associated with dysgenesis of the corpus callosum. Peroxisomal disorders, such as Zellweger syndrome, are associated with cortical gyral abnormalities. Different patterns of signal abnormalities are associated with different IEM.[17]

Magnetic resonance spectroscopy is another imaging modality that allows for noninvasive measurement of central nervous system metabolite levels that can show elevated lactate peak (pyruvate metabolism defects and mitochondrial disorders), elevated glycine peak (glycine encephalopathy), and diminished creatine peak (creatine deficiency syndromes).[18]

Management Considerations

Whenever there is suspicion for IEM, diagnostic workup and treatment should be simultaneous. Early treatment can prevent, or at least minimize, long-term sequelae. Relevant to management of seizures in the context of IEM, there are few principles worth mentioning here. The presentation of early myoclonic epileptic encephalopathy with burst suppression pattern on EEG should trigger a pyridoxine therapeutic trial with EEG monitoring.[7] Similarly, other vitamins and cofactors can be initiated based on the clinical scenario, including pyridoxal phosphate, folinic acid, and biotin.[5] Ketogenic diet can be helpful in children with pyruvate dehydrogenase deficiency and GLUT-1 deficiency. In these disorders, glucose cannot be used as source for energy and with ketogenic diet, energy can be obtained from ketone bodies. Ketogenic diet is also used in children with intractable epilepsy in general.[19] Finally, the underlying suspected diagnosis should be considered when choosing antiepileptic drugs. A good example is valproic acid, which should be avoided in individuals with mitochondrial disorders due to its toxic effects on the mitochondria.[20] Similarly, phenobarbitone inhibits glucose transport and should be avoided in children with GLUT-1 deficiency.[21]

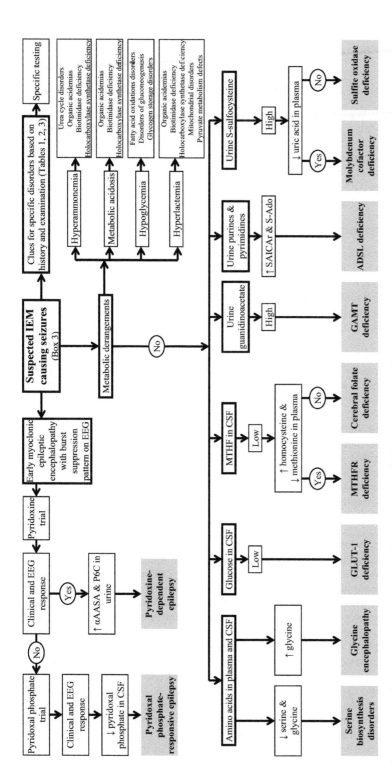

Fig. 1. Approach to IEM presenting with seizures. Decreased (*downward arrows*). Increased (*upward arrows*). ADSL, adenylosuccinate lyase; GAMT, guanidinoacetate N-methyltransferase; GLUT-1, glucose transporter type 1; MTHF, methylenetetrahydrofolate; MTHFR, methylenetetrahydrofolate reductase; P6C, piperideine-6-carboxylate; S-Ado, succinyladenosine; SAICAr, succinylaminoimidazole carboxamide riboside; αAASA, α-aminoadipic semialdehyde.

All of these examples stress the importance of considering IEM in the differential diagnosis of seizures in children because they may influence the choice of antiepileptic drugs.

INBORN ERRORS OF METABOLISM THAT PRESENT WITH SEIZURES

The following IEM associated with seizures are discussed here: cofactor-related disorders (pyridoxine-dependent epilepsy, pyridoxal phosphate-responsive epilepsy, cerebral folate deficiency, methylenetetrahydrofolate reductase [MTHFR] deficiency, biotinidase deficiency, and molybdenum cofactor deficiency), glycine and serine metabolism defects (glycine encephalopathy and serine biosynthesis defects), and other disorders (GLUT-1 deficiency, adenylosuccinate lyase [ADSL] deficiency, and guanidinoacetate methyltransferase [GAMT] deficiency).

PYRIDOXINE-DEPENDENT EPILEPSY

Pyridoxine-dependent epilepsy is an autosomal recessive disorder with prevalence of 1 in 20,000 to 600,000.[9] It occurs due to deficiency of the enzyme antiquitin in the lysine metabolism pathway. Antiquitin functions as a piperideine-6-carboxylate (P6C) and α-aminoadipic semialdehyde (αAASA) dehydrogenase, therefore its deficiency results in the accumulation of αAASA and P6C. The latter binds and inactivates pyridoxal phosphate, which is a cofactor in neurotransmitters metabolism.[9]

Presentation

Pyridoxine-dependent epilepsy usually presents in the first few days of life with 70% of affected children presenting with neonatal seizures. Less commonly, atypical cases can present later, beyond the neonatal period but before the age of 3 years.[22] Seizures can be tonic, clonic, or myoclonic.[23] The hallmark is resistance to standard antiepileptic treatment. Associated clinical features include fetal distress at birth with a low Apgar score, respiratory distress, poor feeding, lethargy, or an encephalopathic picture with irritability and hypotonia.[23] Such presentation can be misinterpreted as HIE. Neuroimages are usually normal. However, some abnormalities may be seen, including hypoplasia or agenesis of the corpus callosum, enlarged ventricles, and mega cisterna magna.[17]

Diagnosis

Pyridoxine-dependent epilepsy should be suspected in a newborn presenting with early myoclonic epileptic encephalopathy with burst suppression pattern on EEG. EEG can evolve into hypsarrhythmia along with multifocal or focal discharges.[5] With such presentation, a trial with pyridoxine, which can be diagnostic and therapeutic, in addition biochemical evaluation is indicated.[7] The diagnosis is established clinically by showing a response to pyridoxine. Administering 100 mg of intravenous pyridoxine with EEG monitoring can result in cessation of the clinical seizures with corresponding EEG changes, generally over a period of several minutes. If a clinical response is not demonstrated, the dose can be repeated up to 500 mg. Oral pyridoxine (30 mg/kg/d) can result in cessation of the seizures within 3 to 5 days.[9] The treatment trial should be initiated in intensive care setting because cessation of seizures might be associated with transient isoelectric EEG along with coma and respiratory depression. Because of the possibility of delayed response to oral pyridoxine, treatment should be continued for at least 7 days[9] or, preferably, until the diagnosis of pyridoxine-dependent epilepsy is confirmed or excluded by biochemical and/or genetic testing.[9] Associated biochemical makers include elevated αAASA levels in urine, plasma, and CSF. Pipecolic acid is another biomarker, but it is not specific. Urinary P6C is also increased.[24] Diagnosis can be confirmed by molecular testing of the *ALDH7A1* gene.

Treatment

Long-term treatment with pyridoxine (15–30 mg/kg/d) is required.[9] The daily dose should not exceed 500 mg because of the risk of peripheral neuropathy.[7]

PYRIDOXAL PHOSPHATE-RESPONSIVE EPILEPSY

Pyridoxal phosphate-responsive epilepsy is an autosomal recessive condition caused by deficiency of pyridox(am)ine phosphate oxidase, an enzyme that converts pyridoxine phosphate and pyridoxamine phosphate into pyridoxal phosphate, the active form of pyridoxine. It is rare condition with only 40 cases reported to date.[25]

Presentation

Presentation is similar to pyridoxine-dependent epilepsy with lethargy, hypotonia, and refractory seizures. Preterm delivery with fetal distress is seen in approximately 50% of affected neonates.[25] Seizures usually present in the first few days of life with more than 80% presenting in the first week.[25] Common forms of seizures are myoclonic, complex partial, and generalized motor.[26] Other forms can also be seen, including tonic-clonic, clonic, tonic, and spasms. EEG usually shows burst suppression.[26] Family history of infertility or fetal loss has been occasionally observed.[27]

Diagnosis

Diagnosis is established clinically by the demonstration of cessation of seizures with pyridoxal phosphate administration (50 mg orally) with corresponding EEG changes, usually within an hour. Some neonates respond to pyridoxine.[27,28] Pyridoxal phosphate in CSF is low. Because pyridoxal phosphate is cofactor for many enzymes, biochemical abnormalities reflecting decreased activity of these enzymes may be seen. These include elevations of glycine and threonine in CSF and plasma, elevation of 3-methoxytyrosine in CSF, and a decrease in the CSF concentrations of 5-hydroxyindolacetic acid and homovanillic acid.[5] Diagnosis can be confirmed by molecular testing of the *PNPO* gene.

Treatment

Seizures can usually be controlled with pyridoxal phosphate (30–50 mg/kg/d).[29] Due to case reports of deranged liver function and cirrhosis, liver function tests should be monitored in children treated with pyridoxal phosphate, especially when high doses are used.[27]

CEREBRAL FOLATE DEFICIENCY

Cerebral folate deficiency is associated with low levels of methyltetrahydrofolate (MTHF) in CSF due to defects in *FOLR1* gene that encodes the folate receptor alpha, a major folate transporter across the blood-brain barrier. This condition, which is inherited in an autosomal recessive manner, is rare and reported in a limited number of families. MTHF is a methyl donor involved in myelin formation and neurotransmitters synthesis.[30]

Presentation

Children with cerebral folate deficiency usually present in early childhood with developmental regression, seizures, movement disorders, and ataxia. Seizures are in the form of myoclonic, tonic, atonic, and generalized tonic-clonic, associated with slow background and multifocal epileptiform activity on EEG.[30] Neuroimaging can show hypomyelination and cerebral and cerebellar atrophy.[31]

Diagnosis

There are very low levels of MTHF in CSF with normal plasma folate levels. Diagnosis can be confirmed by molecular testing of the FOLR1 gene.

Treatment

This condition should be treated with folinic acid (1–5 mg/kg/d), which can restore CSF folate concentrations and improve clinical symptoms.[30,31]

METHYLENETETRAHYDROFOLATE REDUCTASE DEFICIENCY

Severe MTHFR deficiency is a rare, autosomal recessive disorder with an estimated incidence of 1 in 200,000.[32] MTHFR catalyzes the reduction of methylenetetrahydrofolate to MTHF. Deficiency in MTHF, which is a methyl donor in the conversion of homocysteine to methionine, results in elevated total plasma homocysteine and low methionine. Low methionine in turn results in deficiency of S-adenosylmethionine, a methyl donor for several methylation reactions.

Presentation

Severe MTHFR deficiency presents in infancy with hypotonia, lethargy, feeding difficulties, and apnea. Myoclonic, tonic-clonic seizures, and infantile spasms can be seen in the first year of life. At a later age, seizures can evolve into Lennox-Gastaut syndrome.[33] If not identified, the disorder can progress into developmental regression, coma, and death. Later onset forms are seen in individuals with higher residual enzyme activity with features, including psychiatric disorders and gait disturbances.[34] Features on neuroimaging include brain atrophy, delayed myelination, and dilated ventricles.[34]

Diagnosis

Diagnosis can be suspected based on elevated total plasma homocysteine with low methionine. CSF MTHF is significantly low.[33] Blood folate level can be also decreased. Diagnosis can confirmed by measuring enzyme activity or by molecular testing of MTHFR gene.

Treatment

The mainstay of treatment is oral betaine (100–250 mg/kg/d), which is a substrate for betaine methyltransferase, an enzyme that converts homocysteine to methionine, therefore, betaine decreases homocysteine and increases methionine. Early treatment with betaine can improve the outcome.[35]

BIOTINIDASE DEFICIENCY AND HOLOCARBOXYLASE SYNTHETASE DEFICIENCY

Biotin is an essential cofactor for several carboxylase enzymes. Holocarboxylase synthetase is an enzyme that attaches biotin to the carboxylase enzymes, thereby activating them. Biotin is recycled through biotinidase enzyme. Holocarboxylase synthetase and biotinidase deficiencies are autosomal recessive conditions associated with multiple carboxylase enzymes deficiencies. Estimated incidence of biotinidase deficiency is 1 in 60,000,[36] whereas holocarboxylase synthetase deficiency is rarer.

Presentation

Both conditions have overlapping symptoms. Holocarboxylase synthetase deficiency usually present early, before the age of 3 months, with metabolic decompensation in the form of lethargy, hypotonia, vomiting, and hypothermia. Tachypnea, due to acidosis and hyperammonemia is common. Biotinidase deficiency is characterized by more neurologic symptoms, including seizures, hypotonia, ataxia, developmental delay, and hearing and vision problems. The age of onset is variable, depending on the degree of enzyme activity. The average age of onset is 3.5 months in infants with profound deficiency (residual activity <10%).[37] In children with biotinidase deficiency, different forms of seizures can be seen, including myoclonic, generalized tonic-clonic seizures, and infantile spasms. EEG findings are also variable and can vary from normal to sharp, multifocal spikes, and hypsarrhythmia.[38] Both conditions are characterized by skin rash and alopecia, which can be important distinguishing features, although not always present.

Diagnosis

Suggestive findings include metabolic acidosis, elevated lactate, and hyperammonemia. Urine organic acids show a pattern consistent with multiple carboxylase enzymes deficiency with presence of 3-hydroxyisovalerate, 3-methylcrotonylglycine, methylcitrate, hydroxypropionate, and propionylglycine. Diagnosis of biotinidase deficiency can be confirmed by measuring enzyme activity or molecular testing of the *BTD* gene. Diagnosis of holocarboxylase synthetase deficiency can be confirmed by molecular testing of the *HLCS* gene.

Treatment

Both conditions respond to oral biotin with excellent results. In biotinidase deficiency, the dose is 5 to 10 mg/d.[36] Higher doses are usually required for holocarboxylase synthetase deficiency.[39]

MOLYBDENUM COFACTOR DEFICIENCY AND SULFITE OXIDASE DEFICIENCY

Molybdenum is a cofactor for 3 enzymes: xanthine oxidase, aldehyde oxidase, and sulfite oxidase. Deficiency of either molybdenum cofactor or sulfite oxidase results in accumulation of toxic sulfites. Both conditions are inherited in an autosomal recessive manner. More than 100 cases have been reported, although the conditions might be underdiagnosed.

Presentation

Both disorders are clinically indistinguishable. Affected newborns present shortly after birth with feeding difficulties, hypotonia, exaggerated startle response, and seizures.[40,41] Later on, significant developmental delay and spasticity evolve. Lens dislocation is seen in both disorders. Seizures are intractable with burst suppression pattern.[5] Findings on neuroimaging include extensive edema with evolution to encephalomalacia with cystic changes and cortical atrophy in older children.[17] Clinical and radiological presentation can mimic HIE.[17,42]

Diagnosis

Both conditions are associated with increased plasma and urinary S-sulfocysteine levels, and reduced plasma total homocysteine and cystine levels. Molybdenum cofactor deficiency can be differentiated by reduced serum uric acid levels and increased urinary xanthine and hypoxanthine levels because of a secondary deficiency in xanthine oxidase.[40] Diagnosis can be confirmed by molecular testing (MOCS1, MOCS2, and GPHN for molybdenum cofactor deficiency and SUOX for sulfite oxidase deficiency).

Treatment

Newborns with molybdenum cofactor deficiency type A (caused by defects in the MOCS1 gene) can be treated with intravenous cyclic pyranopterin monophosphate, a biosynthetic precursor of the cofactor.[43] To be effective, treatment should be started very early before permanent neurologic damage ensues. There is no treatment for other forms of molybdenum cofactor deficiency. Similarly, the outcome is poor in isolated sulfite oxide deficiency with no effective treatment, although dietary therapy with low cysteine and methionine was reported to be beneficial in some children with the mild, late-onset form of the disease.[44]

GLYCINE ENCEPHALOPATHY

Glycine encephalopathy (nonketotic hyperglycinemia), caused by defects in glycine cleavage enzyme, is an autosomal recessive condition with an estimated incidence of 1 to 60,000.[45] Defects in glycine cleavage enzyme result in accumulation of glycine in body fluids, including the brain. Glycine is an inhibitory neurotransmitter in the brainstem and spinal cord, which can contribute to the apnea and decreased tone observed in affected neonates. Also, glycine is an agonist of NMDA glutamate receptors. Overstimulation of these excitatory receptors results in seizures.[46]

Presentation

Glycine encephalopathy can present in 4 overlapping phenotypes based on age of onset and developmental outcomes. Severe neonatal glycine encephalopathy has an onset during the first week of life and poor long-term outcome as measured by an IQ of less than 20. Attenuated neonatal glycine encephalopathy has an onset during the first week of life but a better long-term outcome (IQ >20). Severe infantile glycine encephalopathy has an onset after the neonatal period and a poor long-term outcome (IQ <20), whereas attenuated infantile glycine encephalopathy has an onset after the neonatal period and a better long-term outcome (IQ >20).[47] Most children (86%) present in the neonatal period, and most of them (92%) have poor outcomes. Presenting symptoms include hypotonia, which is seen in all affected children, seizures, coma, irregular breathing leading to apnea, and hiccups. Children with attenuated forms can have behavioral problems, hyperactivity, and movement disorders. Seizure forms in affected children include myoclonic and generalized seizures. These are often difficult to treat. Findings on EEG include early burst suppression with later progression to hypsarrhythmia or multifocal discharges by the end of first month.[5] Neuroimaging can show hypoplasia or agenesis of the corpus callosum, delayed myelination, brain atrophy, and enlarged ventricles.[17]

Diagnosis

Glycine encephalopathy is associated with elevated glycine in body fluids and this can be documented by measuring plasma and CSF glycine. Plasma levels can be normal though.[45] A CSF-to-plasma glycine ratio of greater than 0.08 is seen in neonatal forms. Ratios less than or equal to 0.08 may predict attenuated outcomes.[48] Plasma and CSF samples should be drawn simultaneously for accurate calculation of the ratio. Diagnosis can be confirmed by molecular testing of the *GLDC*, *AMT*, and *GCSH* genes, which encode glycine cleavage enzyme subunits.[45]

Treatment

Outcomes are poor in children with severe glycine encephalopathy, even with early initiation of treatment.[49] On the other hand, in children with attenuated forms, early treatment can result in improved outcomes.[50] Treatment options include sodium benzoate (250–750 mg/kg/d), which can reduce plasma glycine concentrations, or an NMDA receptor antagonist, such as dextromethorphan, ketamine, or felbamate, which can result in better seizure control.[45]

SERINE BIOSYNTHESIS DEFECTS

Besides protein synthesis, L-serine is a precursor for several compounds, including phosphatidylserine, sphingomyelin, glycine, cysteine, and D-serine.[51] L-serine is synthesized through actions of phosphoglycerate dehydrogenase (PGDH), phosphoserine aminotransferase, and phosphoserine phosphatase. Impairment of any of these enzymes results in serine deficiency that has a broad phenotypic spectrum. At the severe end, infants present with Neu-Laxova syndrome, a lethal multiple malformations syndrome. Less severe forms present in infancy and childhood, mainly with neurologic manifestations, reflecting the important role for serine in neuronal function and development.[52] Serine biosynthesis defects are rare, with PGDH being the most commonly defective enzyme. All the forms are inherited in autosomal recessive manner.

Presentation

Children with infantile serine biosynthesis defects present with intrauterine growth retardation and microcephaly, which is congenital or early in onset. Early onset of seizures in the first few months of life is typical. Infantile spasms are common. Reported other forms of seizures include myoclonic, tonic-clonic, tonic, and atonic.[53] EEG can show hypsarrhythmia, multifocal seizure activity, and Lennox-Gastaut syndrome. Affected children have severe developmental delay. Other reported features include hypertonia, feeding difficulties, congenital cataracts, and hypogonadism.[54] Besides infantile presentation, a milder phenotype is described less frequently in older children with absence and tonic clonic seizures.[55] Neuroimaging can show hypomyelination or delayed myelination, brain atrophy, and ventriculomegaly.

Diagnosis

Serine and, to a lesser extent, glycine are low in CSF and plasma.[53] Plasma serine and glycine values can be normal if samples are drawn in nonfasting state. Therefore, CSF amino acid analysis is the preferred diagnostic test in children with suspected serine biosynthesis defects. Diagnosis can be confirmed by measuring enzyme activity in skin fibroblast or by molecular testing of the *PHGDH*, *PSAT1*, and *PSPH* genes.

Treatment

In the infantile PGDH deficiency, the use of L-serine (200–700 mg/kg/d) and glycine (200–300 mg/kg/d) had beneficial effects on the seizures, irritability, spasticity, and white matter volume and myelination.[54,56] However, there was little improvement of psychomotor development.[55,57] In childhood forms, a lower dose of L-serine

(100–150 mg/kg/d) can be used with improved control of seizures, behavior, and school performance.[55]

GLUCOSE TRANSPORTER TYPE 1 DEFICIENCY

GLUT-1 transports glucose to the brain through blood–brain barrier. Defects in this transporter impair brain energy supply because glucose is the major source of energy in the brain. This condition is inherited in an autosomal dominant pattern in most affected individuals, although recessive inheritance has been described. Incidence is estimated at 1 in 100,000.[58]

Presentation

The classic presentation is in the form of infantile refractory seizures along with developmental delay and movements disorders.[59] Acquired microcephaly can develop. The onset of the seizures is usually before 2 years of age.[59] Different forms of seizures reported include generalized tonic-clonic, absence, complex partial, myoclonic, drop attacks, tonic, simple partial seizures, and infantile spasms. Most affected individuals have mixed types.[60] EEG obtained while fasting can show slowing of background activity with multifocal or generalized high-amplitude irregular spikes and spike-and-waves. Significant difference may be seen between preprandial and postprandial EEG with a decrease in epileptic discharges following a carbohydrate meal.[61] Similarly, clinical symptoms can worse with fasting.

Diagnosis

GLUT-1 deficiency is associated with low CSF glucose, which is typically less than 2.5 mg/dL.[4] The CSF-to-blood glucose ratio is considered superior to the absolute glucose level in the CSF.[62] The normal ratio is greater than 0.6, whereas in GLUT-1 deficiency it is typically less than 0.5 (in the absence of CSF infection or hypoglycemia).[62] Ideally, CSF samples should be obtained while fasting. The diagnosis can be confirmed by molecular testing of the SLC2A1 gene.

Management

Ketogenic diet is the first-line treatment in GLUT-1 deficiency.[63] Ketogenic diet provides an alternative source of energy to the brain in the form of ketone bodies. Initiation of a ketogenic diet leads to seizure control in most affected individuals with less prominent effect on development.[63]

ADENYLOSUCCINATE LYASE DEFICIENCY

ADSL enzyme catalyzes 2 steps in purine nucleotide synthesis. ADSL deficiency is an autosomal recessive disorder that results in the accumulation of succinylpurines that are believed to have toxic effects, particularly on the nervous system. The incidence of ADSL deficiency is not known. To date, fewer than 100 individuals have been reported.

Presentation

ADSL deficiency is associated with a broad clinical spectrum with 3 forms being described. Most affected individuals have type I (severe form), which is characterized by early-onset severe psychomotor retardation, hypotonia, feeding difficulty, growth failure, microcephaly, seizures, and autistic features. Children with the milder form (type II) can present with mild to moderate psychomotor retardation, hypotonia, ataxia, and autistic features.[64] A neonatal fatal form has been reported with intrauterine growth retardation, encephalopathy, severe hypotonia, respiratory failure, intractable seizures, and early mortality.[65] In type I, refractory seizures start early in the first few months of life and are in the form of partial, simple partial motor, myoclonic, tonic seizures, and infantile spasms.[64] Neuroimaging often shows brain atrophy, hypomyelination, and atrophy of the cerebellum, particularly of the vermis.

Diagnosis

ADSL deficiency is characterized by the presence of succinylaminoimidazole carboxamide riboside and succinyladenosine in urine, CSF, and (to a minor extent) plasma. The diagnosis can be confirmed by measuring the ADSL enzyme activity in liver, kidney, blood lymphocytes, or cultured fibroblasts; or molecular sequencing of the *ADSL* gene.

Treatment

Currently, there is no effective treatment available. Seizures in ADSL deficiency are usually refractory and more than 1 antiepileptic agent is required.[64]

GUANIDINOACETATE METHYLTRANSFERASE DEFICIENCY

GAMT mediates the methylation of guanidinoacetate (GAA) that yields creatine. Defects in GAMT result in the deficiency of creatine, which is essential for brain function because of its role in energy storage and transmission, and as neurotransmitter or modulator. GAMT deficiency is an autosomal recessive condition with an estimated prevalence 1 in 500,000.[66]

Presentation

GAMT deficiency is characterized by developmental delay and intellectual disability. Speech and language development tends to be more severely affected. Other features include movement disorders, autism, hyperactivity, and other behavioral problems.[67,68] Onset is between early infancy to the third year of life.[68] Seizures are seen in more than two-thirds of children[67] and reported forms include myoclonic, generalized tonic-clonic, partial complex seizures, and drop attacks.[68]

Diagnosis

GAA is elevated in body fluids and magnetic resonance spectroscopy shows absent or severely reduced creatine peak. Diagnosis can be confirmed by molecular testing of the *GAMT* gene.

Treatment

Creatine deficiency is corrected with creatine-monohydrate (400–800 mg/kg/d) supplementation and GAA accumulation is reduced through L-ornithine supplementation (400–800 mg/kg/d) and arginine restriction, which is achieved through a protein-restricted diet together with arginine-free essential amino acid supplements.[67]

SUMMARY

IEM are relatively uncommon causes for seizures in children; however, they should be considered in the differential diagnosis because several IEM are potentially treatable and seizures can be resolved when appropriate treatment is initiated. Clues from clinical presentation, physical examination, laboratory tests, and neuroimaging can raise the possibility of IEM. Several IEM can present with seizures either as the main presenting finding or as a part of a more complex phenotype. When IEM are suspected, diagnosis and treatment should be simultaneous because early treatment can prevent, or at least minimize, long-term sequelae.

REFERENCES

1. Russ SA, Larson K, Halfon N. A national profile of childhood epilepsy and seizure disorder. Pediatrics 2012;129:256–64.
2. Shorvon SD. The etiologic classification of epilepsy. Epilepsia 2011;52:1052–7.
3. Wolf NI, Bast T, Surtees R. Epilepsy in inborn errors of metabolism. Epileptic Disord 2005;7:67–81.
4. Rahman S, Footitt EJ, Varadkar S, et al. Inborn errors of metabolism causing epilepsy. Dev Med Child Neurol 2013;55:23–36.
5. Wolf NI, Garcia-Cazorla A, Hoffmann GF. Epilepsy and inborn errors of metabolism in children. J Inherit Metab Dis 2009;32:609–17.
6. Campistol J, Plecko B. Treatable newborn and infant seizures due to inborn errors of metabolism. Epileptic Disord 2015;17:229–42.
7. Dulac O, Plecko B, Gataullina S, et al. Occasional seizures, epilepsy, and inborn errors of metabolism. Lancet Neurol 2014;13:727–39.
8. Brusilow SW, Koehler RC, Traystman RJ, et al. Astrocyte glutamine synthetase: Importance in hyperammonemic syndromes and potential target for therapy. Neurotherapeutics 2010;7:452–70.
9. Stockler S, Plecko B, Gospe S, et al. Pyridoxine dependent epilepsy and antiquitin deficiency: clinical and molecular characteristics and recommendations for diagnosis, treatment and follow-up. Mol Genet Metab 2011;104:48–60.
10. Leventer RJ, Guerrini R, Dobyns WB. Malformations of cortical development and epilepsy. Dialogues Clin Neurosci 2008;10:47–62.
11. Pearl PL, Bennett HD, Khademian Z. Seizures and metabolic disease. Curr Neurol Neurosci Rep 2005;5:127–33.
12. Wolf NI, Rahman S, Schmitt B, et al. Status epilepticus in children with Alpers disease caused by POLG1 mutations: EEG and MRI features. Epilepsia 2009;50:1596–607.
13. Enns GM, Packman S. Diagnosing inborn errors of metabolism in the newborn: clinical features. Neoreviews 2001;2:183–91.
14. Pearl PL. New treatment paradigms in neonatal seizures. J Inherit Metab Dis 2009;32:204–13.
15. Andersen LW, Mackenhauer J, Roberts JC, et al. Etiology and therapeutic approach to elevated lactate. Mayo Clin Proc 2013;88:1127–40.
16. Helbig KL, Farwell Hagman KD, Shinde DN, et al. Diagnostic exome sequencing provides a molecular diagnosis for a significant proportion of patients with epilepsy. Genet Med 2016;18:898–905.
17. Poretti A, Blaser SI, Lequin MH, et al. Neonatal neuroimaging findings in inborn errors of metabolism. J Magn Reson Imaging 2013;37:294–312.
18. Rincon SP, Blitstein MB, Caruso PA, et al. The use of magnetic resonance spectroscopy in the evaluation of pediatric patients with seizures. Pediatr Neurol 2016;58:57–66.
19. Barañano KW, Hartman AL. The ketogenic diet: uses in epilepsy and other neurologic illnesses. Curr Treat Options Neurol 2008;10:410–9.
20. Finsterer J, Zarrouk Mahjoub S. Mitochondrial toxicity of antiepileptic drugs and their tolerability in mitochondrial disorders. Expert Opin Drug Metab Toxicol 2012;8:71–9.

21. Gordon N, Newton RW. Glucose transporter type 1 (GLUT-1) deficiency. Brain Dev 2003;25:477–80.
22. Basura GJ, Hagland SP, Wiltse AM, et al. Clinical features and the management of pyridoxine-dependent and pyridoxine-responsive seizures: review of 63 North American cases submitted to a patient registry. Eur J Pediatr 2009;168:697–704.
23. Mills PB, Footitt EJ, Mills KA, et al. Genotypic and phenotypic spectrum of pyridoxine-dependent epilepsy (ALDH7A1 deficiency). Brain 2010;133:2148–59.
24. Struys EA, Bok LA, Emal D, et al. The measurement of urinary Δ^1-piperideine-6-carboxylate, the alter ego of α-aminoadipic semialdehyde, in Antiquitin deficiency. J Inherit Metab Dis 2012;35:909–16.
25. Guerin A, Aziz AS, Mutch C, et al. Pyridox(am)ine-5-Phosphate oxidase deficiency treatable cause of neonatal epileptic encephalopathy with burst suppression: case report and review of the literature. J Child Neurol 2015;30:1218–25.
26. Veerapandiyan A, Winchester S, Gallentine W, et al. Electroencephalographic and seizure manifestations of pyridoxal 5'-phosphate-dependent epilepsy. Epilepsy Behav 2011;20:494–501.
27. Mills PB, Camuzeaux SS, Footitt EJ, et al. Epilepsy due to PNPO mutations: genotype, environment and treatment affect presentation and outcome. Brain 2014; 137:1350–60.
28. Plecko B, Paul K, Mills P, et al. Pyridoxine responsiveness in novel mutations of the PNPO gene. Neurology 2014;82:1425–33.
29. Hoffmann GF, Schmitt B, Windfuhr M, et al. Pyridoxal 5'phosphate may be curative in early onset epileptic encephalopathy. J Inherit Metab Dis 2007;30:96–9.
30. Steinfeld R, Grapp M, Kraetzner R, et al. Folate receptor alpha defect causes cerebral folate transport deficiency: a treatable neurodegenerative disorder associated with disturbed myelin metabolism. Am J Hum Genet 2009;85:354–63.
31. Grapp M, Just IA, Linnankivi T, et al. Molecular characterization of folate receptor 1 mutations delineates cerebral folate transport deficiency. Brain 2012;135: 2022–31.
32. Tortorelli S, Turgeon CT, Lim JS, et al. Two-tier approach to the newborn screening of methylenetetrahydrofolate reductase deficiency and other remethylation disorders with tandem mass spectrometry. J Pediatr 2010;157:271–5.
33. Prasad AN, Rupar CA, Prasad C. Methylenetetrahydrofolate reductase (MTHFR) deficiency and infantile epilepsy. Brain Dev 2011;33:758–69.
34. Huemer M, Mulder-Bleile R, Burda P, et al. Clinical pattern, mutations and in vitro residual activity in 33 patients with severe 5, 10 methylenetetrahydrofolate reductase (MTHFR) deficiency. J Inherit Metab Dis 2016;39:115–24.
35. Huemer M, Diodato D, Schwahn B, et al. Guidelines for diagnosis and management of the cobalamin-related remethylation disorders cblC, cblD, cblE, cblF, cblG, cblJ and MTHFR deficiency. J Inherit Metab Dis 2017;40:21–48.
36. Wolf B. Biotinidase deficiency: if you have to have an inherited metabolic disease, this is the one to have. Genet Med 2012;14:565–75.
37. Wolf B. Biotinidase deficiency. In: Pagon RA, Adam MP, Ardinger HH, et al, editors. GeneReviews® [Internet]. Seattle (WA): University of Washington; 2000. p. 1993–2017. Updated June 9, 2016.
38. Wolf B. The neurology of biotinidase deficiency. Mol Genet Metab 2011;104: 27–34.
39. Baumgartner MR, Suormala T. Biotin responsive disorders. In: Saudubray JM, Baumgartner MR, Walter J, editors. Inborn metabolic diseases. 6th edition. Berlin: Springer; 2016. p. 375–83.

40. Tan WH, Eichler FS, Hoda S, et al. Isolated sulfite oxidase deficiency: a case report with a novel mutation and review of the literature. Pediatrics 2005;116: 757–66.

41. Reiss J, Hahnewald R. Molybdenum cofactor deficiency: mutations in GPHN, MOCS1, and MOCS2. Hum Mutat 2011;32:10–8.

42. Topcu M, Coskun T, Haliloglu G, et al. Molybdenum cofactor deficiency: report of three cases presenting as hypoxic–ischemic encephalopathy. J Child Neurol 2001;16:264–70.

43. Schwahn BC, Van Spronsen FJ, Belaidi AA, et al. Efficacy and safety of cyclic pyranopterin monophosphate substitution in severe molybdenum cofactor deficiency type A: a prospective cohort study. Lancet 2015;386:1955–63.

44. Touati G, Rusthoven E, Depondt E, et al. Dietary therapy in two patients with a mild form of sulphite oxidase deficiency. Evidence for clinical and biological improvement. J Inherit Metab Dis 2000;23:45–53.

45. Van Hove J, Coughlin C II, Scharer G. Glycine encephalopathy. In: Pagon RA, Adam MP, Ardinger HH, et al, editors. GeneReviews® [Internet]. Seattle (WA): University of Washington; 2002. p. 1993–2016. Updated July 11, 2013.

46. Van Hove J, Hennermann JB, Coughlin CR II. Noketotic hyperglycinemia (glycine encephalopathy) and lipoate deficiency disorders. In: Saudubray JM, Baumgartner MR, Walter J, editors. Inborn metabolic diseases. 6th edition. Berlin: Springer; 2016. p. 349–56.

47. Hennermann JB, Berger JM, Grieben U, et al. Predicition of long-term outcome in glycine encephalopathy: a clinical survey. J Inherit Metab Dis 2012;35:253–61.

48. Swanson MA, Coughlin CR, Scharer GH, et al. Biochemical and molecular predictors for prognosis in nonketotic hyperglycinemia. Ann Neurol 2015;78:606–18.

49. Korman SH, Wexler ID, Gutman A, et al. Treatment from birth of nonketotic hyperglycinemia due to a novel GLDC mutation. Ann Neurol 2006;59:411–5.

50. Korman SH, Boneh A, Ichinohe A, et al. Persistent NKH with transient or absent symptoms and a homozygous GLDC mutation. Ann Neurol 2004;56:139–43.

51. De Koning TJ, Snell K, Duran M, et al. L-serine in disease and development. Biochem J 2003;371:653–61.

52. El-Hattab AW, Shaheen R, Hertecant J, et al. On the phenotypic spectrum of serine biosynthesis defects. J Inherit Metab Dis 2016;39:373–81.

53. Van der Crabben SN, Verhoeven-Duif NM, Brilstra EH, et al. An update on serine deficiency disorders. J Inherit Metab Dis 2013;36:613–9.

54. El-Hattab AW. Serine biosynthesis and transport defects. Mol Genet Metab 2016; 118:153–9.

55. Tabatabaie L, Klomp LWJ, Rubio-Gozalbo ME, et al. Expanding the clinical spectrum of 3-phosphoglycerate dehydrogenase deficiency. J Inherit Metab Dis 2011; 34:181–4.

56. de Koning TJ, Jaeken J, Pineda M, et al. Hypomyelination and reversible white matter attenuation in 3-phosphoglycerate dehydrogenase deficiency. Neuropediatrics 2000;31:287–92.

57. de Koning TJ, Duran M, Van Maldergem L, et al. Congenital microcephaly and seizures due to 3-phosphoglycerate dehydrogenase deficiency: outcome of treatment with amino acids. J Inherit Metab Dis 2002;25:119–25.

58. Coman DJ, Sinclair KG, Burke CJ, et al. Seizures, ataxia, developmental delay and the general paediatrician: glucose transporter 1 deficiency syndrome. J Paediatr Child Health 2006;42:263–7.

59. Leen WG, Klepper J, Verbeek MM, et al. Glucose transporter-1 deficiency syndrome: the expanding clinical and genetic spectrum of a treatable disorder. Brain 2010;133:655–70.
60. Pong AW, Geary BR, Engelstad KM, et al. Glucose transporter type I deficiency syndrome: epilepsy phenotypes and outcomes. Epilepsia 2012;53:1503–10.
61. von Moers A, Brockmann K, Wang D, et al. EEG features of glut-1 deficiency syndrome. Epilepsia 2002;43:941–5.
62. De Giorgis V, Veggiotti P. GLUT1 deficiency syndrome 2013: current state of the art. Seizure 2013;22:803–11.
63. Klepper J. Glucose transporter deficiency syndrome (GLUT1DS) and the ketogenic diet. Epilepsia 2008;49(Suppl 8):46–9.
64. Jurecka A, Zikanova M, Kmoch S, et al. Adenylosuccinate lyase deficiency. J Inherit Metab Dis 2015;38:231–42.
65. Mouchegh K, Zikanova M, Hoffmann GF, et al. Lethal fetal and early neonatal presentation of adenylosuccinate lyase deficiency: observation of 6 patients in 4 families. J Pediatr 2007;150:57–61.
66. Desroches CL, Patel J, Wang P, et al. Carrier frequency of guanidinoacetate methyltransferase deficiency in the general population by functional characterization of missense variants in the GAMT gene. Mol Genet Genomics 2015; 290:2163–71.
67. Stockler-Ipsiroglu S, van Karnebeek C, Longo N, et al. Guanidinoacetate methyltransferase (GAMT) deficiency: outcomes in 48 individuals and recommendations for diagnosis, treatment and monitoring. Mol Genet Metab 2014;111:16–25.
68. Mercimek-Mahmutoglu S, Stoeckler-Ipsiroglu S, Adami A, et al. GAMT deficiency: features, treatment, and outcome in an inborn error of creatine synthesis. Neurology 2006;67:480–4.

Inborn Errors of Metabolism with Movement Disorders

Defects in Metal Transport and Neurotransmitter Metabolism

Trishna Kantamneni, MD, Lileth Mondok, MD, Sumit Parikh, MD*

KEYWORDS

- Metal transport • Neurotransmitter metabolism • Pediatric movement disorders

KEY POINTS

- Movement disorders in pediatric age group are largely of the hyperkinetic type.
- Metal ion accumulation in the central nervous system presents predominantly with movement disorders and over time leads to psychomotor decline.
- Abnormalities in monoamine and amino acidergic neurotransmitter metabolism present in individuals with a combination of abnormal movements, epilepsy, and cognitive and motor delay.
- Detailed clinical history, careful examination, appropriate diagnostic work-up with metabolic screening, CSF neurotransmitters, and targeted genetic testing help with accurate diagnosis and appropriate treatment.

INTRODUCTION

Movement disorders in the pediatric age group are a diverse group of conditions that lead to abnormal involuntary movements usually associated with abnormalities or injury to the basal ganglia and its connections and are seen in a variety of neurologic disorders. Movement disorders in children are usually divided into two main groups: hyperkinetic/dyskinetic (chorea, athetosis, tremor, ballismus, myoclonus, tics, and stereotypies)[1] movement disorders (**Table 1**); and hypokinetic movement disorders, which include the parkinsonian phenotypes. Hypokinetic disorders are uncommon in the pediatric population but are seen with select genetic conditions, such as mitochondrial disease. Abnormal movements can be the main presenting feature of a disease or can occur as a late manifestation.

A broad approach to evaluating movement disorders in children is dividing them into acquired and hereditary causes. Abnormal involuntary movements secondary to

Disclosure Statement: No disclosures.
Department of Neurology, Neurological Institute, Center for Pediatric Neurology, Cleveland Clinic, 9500 Euclid Avenue, S60, Cleveland, OH 44195, USA
* Corresponding author.
E-mail address: parikhs@ccf.org

Table 1
Hyperkinetic movements
Dystonia	Involuntary sustained or intermittent muscle contractions cause twisting and repetitive movements, abnormal postures, or both.
Chorea	Ongoing random-appearing sequence of one or more discrete involuntary movements or movement fragments.
Athetosis	Slow, continuous, involuntary writhing movement that prevents maintenance of a stable posture.
Myoclonus	Sequence of repeated, often nonrhythmic, brief shock-like jerks caused by sudden involuntary contraction or relaxation of one or more muscles.
Tremor	Rhythmic back-and-forth or oscillating involuntary movement about a joint axis.

From Sanger TD, Chen D, Fehlings DL, et al. Definition and classification of hyperkinetic movements in childhood. Mov Disord 2010;25(11):1538–49; with permission.

medications, infectious or postinfectious etiology, or other structural neurologic lesions (stroke, neonatal hypoxic ischemic encephalopathy, kernicterus) are more common causes and should be evaluated thoroughly especially in acute or subacute presentations. A progressive disease course with prominent developmental delays, cognitive decline, and psychiatric features combined with an abnormal neurologic examination is highly suspicious for an underlying metabolic disorder as the primary cause of a movement disorder. Almost all categories of inborn errors of metabolism can potentially have a type of movement disorder as a symptom. **Box 1** lists some of the common inborn errors of metabolism that present predominantly with abnormal movements. This article in particular provides an overview of inborn errors of metal transport and neurotransmitter metabolism that have movement disorder as the primary manifestation of disease.

A meticulous history and physical examination, especially proper identification of the presenting movement disorder, are the essential tools in arriving at the correct diagnosis. Ancillary testing with neuroimaging, cerebrospinal fluid (CSF) studies, and genetic testing is largely dependent on the degree of clinical suspicion and should be used as such to provide the highest diagnostic yield.

DISORDERS OF METAL TRANSPORT

Movement disorders in the pediatric population secondary to metallic ions are primarily caused by excessive accumulation and deposition of the substance in the brain leading to a disruption of normal anatomy and physiology. Deficiency states of these metals can also cause neurologic symptoms but typically not primarily movement disorders. The most common conditions involve an abnormal increase in iron, copper, and manganese.

Iron

Iron deposition in the basal ganglia, specifically the globus pallidus and substantia nigra, can cause either a hypokinetic or hyperkinetic movement disorder. These disorders have been termed neurodegeneration with brain iron accumulation (NBIA) and share the key feature of iron accumulation in the brain on pathology with associated dystonia, spasticity, parkinsonism, and psychiatric symptoms. NBIA disorders include several different conditions with pantothenate kinase–associated neurodegeneration (PKAN; previously known as Hallervorden-Spatz disease) being the most common.

PKAN was initially described by Hallervorden and Spatz in 1922. The disorder was later renamed to PKAN as Dr. Hallervorden and Spatz had actively collected and

Box 1
Inborn errors of metabolism presenting with abnormal movements based on age of initial presentation

Age of onset: birth to early infancy

Sepiapterin reductase deficiency

6-Pyruvoyl tetrahydropterin synthase deficiency

Dihydropteridine reductase deficiency

Aromatic amino acid decarboxylase deficiency

Dopamine transporter deficiency syndrome

Tyrosine hydroxylase deficiency

Pyruvate dehydrogenase deficiency

Crigler-Najjar syndrome

Early onset of Pelizaeus-Merzbacher disease

Leigh disease

Age of onset: late infancy to early childhood

Glutaric aciduria type I

Creatine deficiency

Autosomal-recessive guanine triphosphate cyclohydrolase deficiency

Lesch-Nyhan syndrome

Mucolipidosis type IV

Congenital folate malabsorption

Gaucher disease type III

Niemann-Pick disease type C

GM1 gangliosidosis

Hypermanganesemia with dystonia 1

Hypermanganesemia with dystonia 2

Pelizaeus-Merzbacher disease

Leigh disease

Biotin-thiamine responsive basal ganglia disease

Age of onset: late childhood to adulthood

Autosomal-dominant guanine triphosphate cyclohydrolase deficiency

Classic homocystinuria

Pantothenate kinase-associated neurodegeneration

Neuroferritinopathy

Aceruloplasminemia

Wilson disease

Leigh disease

Biotin-thiamine responsive basal ganglia disease

studied brain samples from victims of the T4 killings, the Nazi program to gas psychiatric (and developmentally disabled) individuals at "euthanasia" centers.[2] In the classic form, it presents in early childhood (usually before 6 years of age) with predominant dystonia, rigidity, and choreoathetosis. There is rapid progression to nonambulation and presence of cognitive decline. Corticospinal tracts are involved causing spasticity, hyperreflexia, and extensor toe sign on examination. Atypical presentations include older age of onset, a primary parkinsonian presentation, and predominant psychiatric symptoms (personality changes and emotional lability). Dilated eye examination may reveal retinal pigmentary changes.[3]

Radiologic features of PKAN on brain MRI show bilateral areas of hyperintensity within a region of hypointensity in the medial globus pallidus on T2-weighted images, a pattern known as "eye of the tiger" (**Fig. 1**).[4]

The disease is inherited in an autosomal-recessive manner and is caused by mutations in *PANK2* gene. The *PANK2* gene codes for enzyme pantothenate kinase that regulates coenzyme A production. Coenzyme A is involved in fatty acid metabolism and it has been postulated that dysfunction of this system causes increased oxidative stress in vulnerable areas, primarily the basal ganglia.[5] Diagnosis of PKAN includes demonstration of typical brain MRI findings and genetic testing. Treatment is largely supportive with novel studies looking into pantothenic acid replacement therapy.

Another childhood-onset NBIA disorder is phospholipase A$_2$ group 6–associated neurodegeneration or phospholipase A$_2$–associated neurodegeneration, which has infantile and childhood forms. The infantile onset form is also known as infantile neuroaxonal dystrophy and accounts for most presentations. Affected children present at around 6 months to 2 years of age with predominant psychomotor regression and then less prominent dystonia, choreoathetosis, or parkinsonism. Central hypotonia and cerebellar ataxia are other common findings, as is visual impairment. There is rapid progression of the disease and shortened lifespan (death within the first decade).[6]

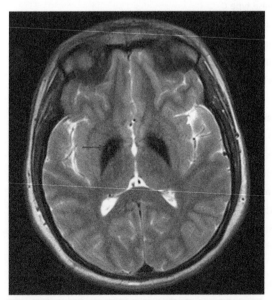

Fig. 1. Axial MRI T2-weighted image of the brain showing bilateral areas of hyperintensity (*arrow*) within a region of hypointensity in the medial globus pallidus known as "eye of the tiger" sign. (*Courtesy of* Dr Neil Friedman, Cleveland Clinic, Cleveland, OH.)

Childhood phospholipase A_2–associated neurodegeneration (also known as atypical neuroaxonal dystrophy) presents around 1 to 6 years of age and is characterized by a more insidious gait disturbance, speech delay, and diminished social interaction. Both forms are caused by mutations in the *PLA2G6* gene, which codes for the phospholipase enzyme required for phospholipid remodeling and fatty acid metabolism.[7]

Brain MRI may show iron accumulation and cerebellar atrophy.[8] Electromyogram studies demonstrate a distal sensory axonal neuropathy. Diagnosis is made with genetic testing. Treatment is largely supportive.

There are several other NBIA disorders with onset in late adolescence to adulthood with key features summarized in **Box 1**.

Manganese

Primary disorders of manganese metabolism causing movement disorder are rare. There is an autosomal-recessive disorder of manganese metabolism caused by mutations in *SLC30A10*. The gene product is a manganese transporter and as a result of its dysfunction, cells exposed to excessive manganese generate reactive oxygen species causing neuronal injury.[9] Hypermanganesemia with dystonia 1 is characterized by gait and speech disturbances, dystonia, and central hypotonia within the first 5 years of life. There may also be a phenotype associated with later-onset parkinsonism. In a study describing five Indian children with the mutation, T1-weighted MRI brain findings showed severe bilateral hyperintensities at the level of the basal ganglia, dorsal midbrain, and cerebellum.[10]

Presence of severe hypermanganesemia is the primary metabolic abnormality in this disease, resulting from loss of SLC30A10 protein function, and the resulting deficiency of manganese excretion at the level of the liver and the biliary system. There is associated polycythemia and liver cirrhosis.[11]

Early recognition is important because therapeutic strategies are available with manganese-chelating agents (disodium calcium edetate), oral iron supplementation, or both.[10]

There is another disorder of manganese metabolism recently described that has been termed hypermanganesemia with dystonia 2 with a handful of subjects described to date.[12] Key features of manganese metabolism disorders are summarized in **Table 2**.

Copper

A well-known disorder of copper metabolism is Wilson disease (hepatolenticular degeneration). It should be suspected in individuals with liver disease presenting with any movement disorder. In some cases, psychiatric and neurologic manifestations precede liver disease, thus high index of suspicion is warranted for new progressive movement disorder in young individuals. Wilson disease is an autosomal-recessive condition caused by mutations in the *ATP7B* gene. *ATP7B* encodes for a liver- and brain-specific ATP-dependent copper exporter and mutations result in abnormal copper excretion into plasma and bile and subsequent toxic accumulation of the metal. Hepatic copper is bound to apoceruloplasmin to be transported in the blood as ceruloplasmin, and without bound copper, apoceruloplasmin is preferentially degraded leading to the low levels detected in Wilson disease.[15]

Neurologic symptoms usually develop in the second or third decade, but can happen as young as 8 years old. Those with a primarily hepatic presentation generally have an earlier age at presentation, 11 to 15 years of age, than those with a primarily neurologic presentation, mean age at onset from 15 to 21 years of age.[16] Common symptoms

Table 2
Disorders of metal transport presenting as movement disorders

Disorder	Age of Onset	Presentation	Other Features	Gene
Iron				
PKAN	Childhood (before age 6)	Dystonia, rigidity, and choreoathetosis	"Eye of the tiger" sign on brain MRI Retinal pigmentary changes	PANK2
Phospholipase A₂–associated neurodegeneration	Infantile (6 mo–2 y) Atypical/childhood (1–6 y)	Psychomotor regression, central hypotonia, dystonia, choreoathetosis, parkinsonism Gait disturbance, dystonia, speech delay, diminished social interaction	Brain MRI with iron accumulation in globus pallidus and substantia nigra, and cerebellar atrophy Visual impairment with optic atrophy Electromyogram shows distal sensory axonal neuropathy	PLA2G6
Aceruloplasminemia[13]	Adulthood (25–60 y)	Facial and neck dystonia, tremors, chorea, ataxia, and cognitive dysfunction Triad of retinal degeneration, diabetes, and neurologic disease	MRI brain with iron accumulation in striatum and thalamus Evidence of iron accumulation in liver Absence of serum ceruloplasmin Treatment with iron-chelating agents	CP[a]
Neuroferritinopathy[14]	Adulthood (20–50)	Chorea and dystonia, less often tremor and parkinsonism	Brain MRI with basal ganglia cavitation	FTL1[b]
Manganese				
Hypermanganesemia with dystonia 1	Childhood (before 5 y)	Gait and speech disturbances, dystonia, central hypotonia, late-onset parkinsonism	Brain MRI with bilateral T1 hyperintensities at the level of the basal ganglia, dorsal midbrain, and cerebellum Associated with liver cirrhosis and polycythemia Serum hypermanganesemia	SLC30A10

	Age of onset	Clinical features	Diagnostic findings	Gene
Hypermanganesemia with dystonia 2	Infancy/childhood (6 mo–3 y)	Loss of motor milestones, dystonia, spasticity, bulbar dysfunction, parkinsonism	Brain MRI with T1-hyperintensity of the cerebral white matter, globus pallidus, and striatum Hypointensity of the globus pallidus is also evident on T2-weighted imaging Serum hypermanganesemia	*SLC39A14*
Copper				
Wilson disease (hepatolenticular degeneration)	Childhood–adulthood (8–35 y)	Neurologic: tremor, dystonia, dysarthria, gait disturbance, chorea Psychiatric: personality changes, psychosis, depression Hepatic failure	Brain MRI may show T2-weighted hyperintensity in putamen and thalami, and the midbrain can show "face of panda sign" Kayser-Fleischer rings on slit lamp examination Low serum ceruloplasmin or copper Elevated 24-h urine copper values	*ATP7B*

a CP gene codes for ceruloplasmin, autosomal-recessive inheritance.
b FTL1 gene codes for ferritin light chain involved in iron transport, autosomal-dominant inheritance.

include dysarthria and hyperkinetic movement disorder. An early sign is abnormal handwriting.

Reduced excretion of copper to bile results in accumulation in liver; kidney; eye; and brain, especially basal ganglia. This deposition leads to movement disorders of dystonia, parkinsonism, tremor, and choreoathetosis. In a study of 119 individuals with neurologic Wilson disease, dysarthria (91%) and gait disturbance (75%) are most common. In children less than 10, focal and multifocal dystonias are frequently observed. Dystonic involvement in Wilson disease sometimes emerges only during walking or performance of other tasks. Proximal tremor of high amplitude with arms lifted to shoulder level is one of the characteristic symptoms and is frequently termed "wing beating tremor."[17] Chorea and athetosis have been reported to occur in 6% to 16% of those with neurologic Wilson disease. Chorea is more common in young-onset disease (16 years of age and younger) where it has been reported in 20%.[18]

The most common screening method for Wilson disease is a blood ceruloplasmin determination, although this is inadequate for either ruling in or ruling out Wilson disease. A 24-hour urine copper test is more sensitive. Slit-lamp examination should be done to examine for Kayser-Fleischer rings. Brain MRI shows T2-weighted hyperintensity in putamen and thalami, and the midbrain can show "face of panda sign" characterized by preservation of normal signal intensity in the red nucleus and lateral portion of the substantia nigra, high signal in the tegmentum, and hypointensity of the superior colliculus.[19]

Early recognition is key because of available treatment. Pharmacologic agents include penicillamine, trientine, and zinc acetate.[20] Neurologic worsening following initiation of penicillamine therapy is a concern. The risk of neurologic worsening may be approximately 50% when penicillamine is used as initial treatment of neurologic Wilson disease because of mobilization of large hepatic copper stores leading to increased toxic copper exposure to the brain, and subsequent worsening of symptoms.[20]

Symptomatic treatment of the movement disorders found in individuals with Wilson has not been carefully studied and response to treatment is inconsistent. L-Dopa and dopamine agonists do not seem to provide reliable relief of parkinsonism. β-Blockers and primidone, medications used to treat essential tremor, can be tried in those with limiting essential tremor-like tremor, but their benefit is limited.[21]

Menkes disease is an X-linked recessive disorder with mutation in *ATP7A* gene resulting in copper deficiency but does not primarily manifest as a movement disorder.

DISORDERS OF NEUROTRANSMITTER METABOLISM

Neurotransmitter disorders are a group of genetic diseases caused by abnormal synthesis, metabolism, or transport of the neurotransmitters. Aberrations affecting the monoamine neurotransmitters, which includes serotonin and catecholamines (dopamine, epinephrine and norepinephrine), and inhibitory amino acidergic (γ-aminobutyric acid [GABA] and glycine) neurotransmitters can present in individuals with a combination of abnormal movements, abnormal tone, epilepsy, and cognitive and motor delay.

Disorders of Monoamine Metabolism

Monoamine neurotransmitters (dopamine and serotonin) related diseases are divided into disorders of cofactor tetrahydrobiopterin (BH4) metabolism with normal or elevated plasma phenylalanine levels and disorders of monoamine synthesis, transport, and degradation (**Fig. 2**). Tryptophan and tyrosine are converted to serotonin and dopamine, respectively. BH4 is a necessary cofactor for the enzymes that catalyze the previously mentioned steps (**Fig. 3**). Therefore, enzymatic deficiencies that lead to decreased

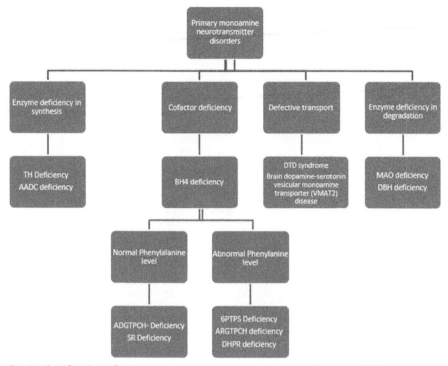

Fig. 2. Classification of primary monoamine neurotransmitter disorders. 6PTPS, 6-pyruvoyl tetrahydropterin synthase; AADC, aromatic L-aminoacid decarboxylase; ADGTPCH, autosomal-dominant guanosine triphosphate cyclohydrolase 1; ARGTPCH, autosomal-recessive guanosine triphosphate cyclohyd; BH4, tetrahydrobiopterin; DBH, dopamine β-hydroxylase; DHPR, dihydropteridine reductase; DTD, dopamine transporter deficiency; MAO, monoamine oxidase; SR, sepiapterin reductase; TH, tyrosine hydroxylase.

BH4 levels ultimately interfere with the synthesis of monoamine neurotransmitters (**Fig. 4**). The diagnosis for this group of disorders is established based on clinical history, physical examination, and CSF neurotransmitters, and confirmed via genetic testing. A few select disorders are discussed here and the rest are summarized in **Table 3**.

Autosomal-dominant guanosine triphosphate cyclohydrolase deficiency
Guanosine triphosphate cyclohydrolase (GTPCH) deficiency was first described in 1971 by Segawa and coworkers[22] as a hereditary progressive dystonia with diurnal fluctuation. The other names for it include Segawa disease and autosomal-dominant dopa-responsive dystonia.

Symptoms typically manifest in the first decade of life, but many cases may present in the adult years. Foot dystonia causing a gait disturbance is the most common presenting symptom. Diurnal fluctuation with improvement after sleep is common.[23] Cognition is usually normal. Other symptoms, such as tremor, asymmetric limb dystonia, or spastic diplegia, can also be seen. There is significant improvement of symptoms with low-dose levodopa/carbidopa, hence a trial of levodopa is diagnostic.

In 1994, autosomal-dominant GTPCH-I deficiency was identified as the cause of dopa-responsive dystonia.[24] GTPCH-I is the initial and rate-limiting step in the biosynthesis of BH4, which is an essential cofactor of tyrosine hydroxylase. GTPCH-I deficiency results in defective biosynthesis of serotonin and catecholamines.[25]

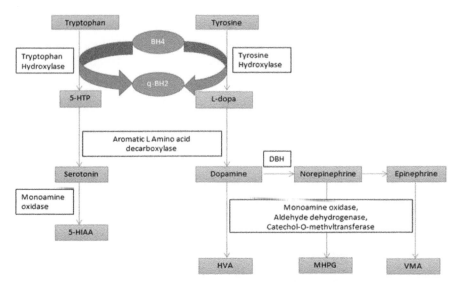

Fig. 3. Monoamine synthesis pathway. BH4 is a required cofactor for tryptophan and tyrosine hydroxylases. AADC deficiency impairs synthesis of serotonin and dopamine. 5-HIAA, 5-hydroxyindoleacetic acid; 5-HTP, 5-hydroxytryptophan; BH4, tetrahydrobiopterin; DBH, dopamine β-hydroxylase; HVA, homovanillic acid; L-dopa, levodihydroxyphenylalanine; MHPG, 3-methoxy-4-hydroxyphenylglycol; q-BH2, (quinonoid) dihydrobiopterin; VMA, vanillylmandelic acid.

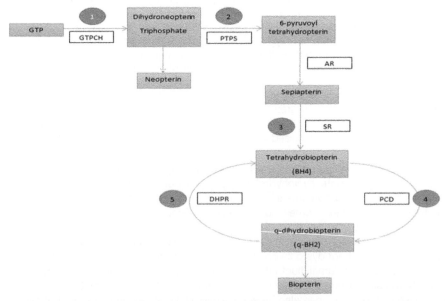

Fig. 4. Terahydrobiopterin biosynthesis and degradation pathway. 1. Autosomal-dominant and autosomal-recessive GTPCH deficiency. 2. 6-PTPS deficiency. 3. Sepiapterin reductase deficiency. 4. PCD deficiency. 5. DHPR deficiency. AR, aldose reductase; BH4, tetrahydrobiopterin; DHPR, dihydropteridine reductase; GTP, guanine triphosphate; GTPCH, GTP cyclohydrolase; PCD, pterin-4α-carbinolamine dehydratase; PTPS, 6-pyruvoyl tetrahydropterin synthase; q-BH2, (quinonoid) dihydrobiopterin; SR, sepiapterin reductase.

Table 3
Monoamine neurotransmitter disorders presenting as movement disorders

Disorder	Age of Onset	Presentation	Other Features	Gene
Autosomal-dominant GTP cyclohydrolase deficiency	Childhood (but can occur at any age)	Dystonia, gait disorder, tremor, parkinsonism	Trial of levodopa diagnostic	GCH 1
Sepiapterin reductase deficiency	Infancy	Parkinsonism, oculogyric crisis, dystonia, behavioral disturbances "Cerebral palsy mimic"	Low dose L-DOPA/carbidopa is helpful with motor symptoms	SPR
6-Pyruvoyl tetrahydropterin synthase deficiency	Infancy	Hyperkinetic/hypokinetic movements, hypotonia, oculogyric crisis, seizures, developmental delay	Hyperphenylalaninemia on newborn screen Elevated urine and CSF neopterin	PTS
Autosomal-recessive GTP cyclohydrolase deficiency	Infancy/early childhood	Dystonia, developmental delay, seizures	Hyperphenylalaninemia on newborn screen Low urine and CSF neopterin	GCH 1
Dihydropteridine reductase deficiency	Neonatal/early Infancy	Microcephaly, global developmental delay, hyperkinetic movements, seizures	Hyperphenylalaninemia on newborn screen White matter abnormalities, basal ganglia calcification on MRI brain Elevated CSF biopterin	QDPR
Aromatic L- amino acid decarboxylase deficiency	Infancy/childhood	Hypotonia, oculogyric crisis, dyskinesia, developmental delay	Low dopamine, HVA, serotonin, norepinephrine in CSF Plasma AADC markedly reduced	DDC
Dopamine transporter deficiency syndrome	Infancy	Hyperkinetic/hypokinetic movements, orolingual dyskinesia Progressive generalized dystonia "Cerebral palsy mimic"	Elevated CSF HVA	SLC6A3

Abbreviations: 6PTPS, 6-pyruvoyl-tetrahydropterin synthase; AADC, aromatic L-aminoacid decarboxylase; GTP, guanine triphosphate; HVA, homovanillic acid.

CSF neurotransmitter studies before the initiation of levodopa can show decreased biopterin, neopterin, and homovanillic acid. Neuroimaging is usually normal. Gene sequencing is now available for diagnostic confirmation. Identification and treatment of this disorder is often rewarding because affected individuals often show a complete to near complete motor response to a combination of low-dose levodopa (4–5 mg/kg/d) and a dopa decarboxylase inhibitor.

Autosomal-recessive guanosine triphosphate cyclohydrolase deficiency

Autosomal-recessive GTPCH deficiency accounts for less than 10% of all the GTPCH deficiency cases.[26] Unlike the autosomal-dominant form, these individuals may have complete absence of GTPCH. Onset is usually during infancy and the disorder can present with developmental delay, pyramidal tract signs, dystonia, athetosis, tremor, seizures, and autonomic dysfunction. Some affected individuals are identified by the presence of hyperphenylalaninemia on newborn screening. CSF neurotransmitter analysis shows low levels of neopterin, biopterin, and monoamines. Treatment with tetrahydrobiopterin is usually not sufficient and supplementation with precursors of the monoamines (levodopa and 5-hydroxytryptophan) is required.

Sepiapterin reductase deficiency
Sepiapterin reductase catalyzes the final two-steps in tetrahydrobiopterin synthesis. Deficiency of this enzyme results in tetrahydrobiopterin depletion, which leads to deficient dopamine and serotonin synthesis. It is inherited as an autosomal-recessive trait. Sepiapterin reductase deficiency can present in infancy with progressive psychomotor retardation, abnormal tone, seizures, oculogyric crisis, diurnal fluctuations of dystonia, choreoathetosis, tremor, behavioral and psychiatric features, and hypersomnolence.[27] Low-dose levodopa/carbidopa can improve some of the motor symptoms.

6-Pyruvoyl-tetrahydropterin synthase deficiency
6-Pyruvoyl-tetrahydropterin synthase deficiency is the most commonly seen disorder of tetrahydrobiopterin metabolism. Clinical phenotype can vary from mild peripheral disease to severe generalized disease. Severe phenotypes present typically in early infancy with significant neurologic impairment (initial hypotonia, subsequent hypertonia, different hyperkinetic movements, seizures, irritability, and developmental delay). Hyperphenylalaninemia is found on newborn screening. CSF neurotransmitter analysis shows decreased levels of biopterin with elevated neopterin. Most affected individuals with the severe phenotype despite early diagnosis and supplementation with tetrahydrobiopterin and levodopa/carbidopa continue to have delays in development.

Disorders of Glycine Metabolism

Glycine is a simple amino acid that functions as a neurotransmitter with excitatory (cortical) and inhibitory (spinal cord and brainstem) effects.[28]

Hereditary hyperekplexia
In 1966, Suhren and colleagues[29] investigated members of a large Dutch pedigree with exaggerated startle reflexes and sudden violent falls, and named the disorder "hyperekplexia." Hereditary hyperekplexia is a rare disorder that has been identified in about 70 families. It has an autosomal-dominant mode of inheritance.[30]

Diagnosis requires three cardinal features: (1) generalized stiffness immediately after birth, normalizing during the first years of life; (2) excessive startle reflex; and (3) short period of generalized stiffness following the startle.[31] The pathophysiology is still unclear; however, hypothesis of brainstem abnormalities versus a primary cortical abnormality have been proposed. All laboratory tests and neuroimaging studies are normal. Eighty percent of the hereditary hyperekplexia is caused by mutations in genes encoding the alpha 1 subunit of glycine receptor GLRA1 resulting in defective inhibitory glycine neurotransmission. Genetic confirmation by DNA sequencing is available. Clonazepam seems to be the most effective treatment. Other medications, such as carbamazepine, phenytoin, diazepam, valproate, 5-hydroxytryptophan, and phenobarbital, have been described to variable benefits in case reports.

Glycine encephalopathy
Glycine encephalopathy, previously known as nonketotic hyperglycinemia, is an autosomal-recessive disorder that results in defective glycine cleavage causing

accumulation of large quantities of glycine in all body tissues including the brain. It is characterized by a rapidly progressive course in neonatal period or early infancy. The classical neonatal phenotype can often present with in utero seizures. Other clinical features include neonatal encephalopathy, hypotonia, myoclonic jerks, and apneas. Electroencephalography reveals a burst suppression pattern. MRI brain findings are nonspecific and can include agenesis of the corpus callosum. The other clinical phenotypes include an infantile pattern that presents after 6 months with partial seizures, and a childhood variant with mild intellectual disability, vertical gaze palsies, and abnormal movements.[28]

Elevated levels of glycine in serum and CSF are diagnostic. Genetic testing is available for confirmation. The outcome is generally poor; sodium benzoate and dextromethorphan have been used with some reported benefits.[32]

Disorders of γ-Aminobutyric Acid Metabolism

GABA is the major inhibitory neurotransmitter of the brain. It is synthesized from glutamate via glutamic acid decarboxylase. GABA is then metabolized to succinic acid by GABA transaminase and succinic semialdehyde dehydrogenase (SSADH) (**Fig. 5**). Disorders of glutamic acid decarboxylase, GABA-transaminase, and SSADH have all been identified. SSADH deficiency is an autosomal-recessive disorder and is the most common disorder of GABA metabolism. In the absence of SSADH, GABA is converted to γ-hydroxybutyric acid (GHB). The clinical phenotype of SSADH deficiency includes a wide spectrum of neurologic manifestations (global developmental delay, cognitive impairment, hypotonia, generalized epilepsy, psychiatric problems, and sleep disturbances). When compared with the other neurotransmitter disorders the course of SSADH deficiency is not intermittent or episodic thus making it difficult to differentiate from other static encephalopathies.

Neuroimaging is usually abnormal with increased T2 signal involving the bilateral globus pallidus, subcortical white matter, cerebellar dentate nucleus, and brainstem.[33] The condition can sometimes be identified with urine organic acids, which show elevated GHB; however, this peak may sometimes be obscured by a large normal urea peak. The GHB peak is detected when the laboratory is performing specific ion monitoring. Otherwise specialized testing of GHB in CSF is sometimes needed. GABA levels in urine and CSF are also elevated. Currently there is no standard treatment available. Valproate is often avoided because it inhibits any residual SSADH resulting in further increase in concentrations of GHB.

SUMMARY

Many of the conditions discussed are complex and affected individuals often present with different movement phenotypes with cognitive and motor delays in addition to

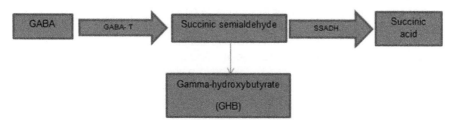

Fig. 5. GABA metabolism pathway. GABA-T, GABA transaminase; GHB, γ-hydroxybutyrate.

other neurologic symptoms. Detailed clinical history, careful examination, appropriate diagnostic work-up with metabolic screening, CSF neurotransmitters, and targeted genetic testing help with accurate diagnosis and appropriate treatment.

REFERENCES

1. Sanger TD, Chen D, Fehlings DL, et al. Definition and classification of hyperkinetic movements in childhood. Mov Disord 2011;25(11):1538–49.
2. Shevell M. Racial hygiene, active euthanasia, and Julius Hallervorden. Neurology 1992;42:2214–9.
3. Hayflick SJ, Westaway SK, Levinson B, et al. Genetic, clinical, and radiographic delineation of Hallervorden-Spatz syndrome. N Engl J Med 2003;348:33–40.
4. Sethi KD, Adams RJ, Loring DW, et al. Hallervorden-Spatz syndrome: clinical and magnetic resonance imaging correlations. Ann Neurol 1988;24:692–4.
5. Zhou B, Westaway SK, Levinson B, et al. A novel pantothenate kinase gene (PANK2) is defective in Hallervorden-Spatz syndrome. Nat Genet 2001;28:345–9.
6. Kurian MA, McNeill A, Lin JP, et al. Childhood disorders of neurodegeneration with brain iron accumulation (NBIA). Dev Med Child Neurol 2011;53:394–404.
7. Gregory A, Polster BJ, Hayflick SJ. Clinical and genetic delineation of neurodegeneration with brain iron accumulation. J Med Genet 2009;46:73–80.
8. Kurian MA, Morgan NV, MacPherson L, et al. Phenotypic spectrum of neurodegeneration associated with mutations in the PLA2G6 gene (PLAN). Neurology 2008;70:1623–9.
9. Lechpammer M, Clegg MS, Muzar Z, et al. Pathology of inherited manganese transporter deficiency. Ann Neurol 2014;75:608–12.
10. Quadri M, Kamate M, Sharma S, et al. Manganese transport disorder: novel SLC30A10 mutations and early phenotypes. Mov Disord 2015;30:996–1001.
11. Quadri M, Federico A, Zhao T, et al. Mutations in SLC30A10 cause parkinsonism and dystonia with hypermanganesemia, polycythemia, and chronic liver disease. Am J Hum Genet 2012;90:467–77.
12. Tuschl K, Meyer E, Valdivia LE, et al. Mutations in SLC39A14 disrupt manganese homeostasis and cause childhood-onset parkinsonism-dystonia. Nat Commun 2016;7:11601.
13. Miyajima H. Aceruloplasminemia, an iron metabolic disorder. Neuropathology 2003;23:345–50.
14. Kumar N, Rizek P, Jog M. Neuroferritinopathy: pathophysiology, presentation, differential diagnoses and management. Walker R, ed. Tremor Other Hyperkinet Mov (N Y) 2016;6:355.
15. De Bie P, Muller P, Wijmenga C, et al. Molecular pathogenesis of Wilson and Menkes disease: correlation of mutations with molecular defects and disease phenotypes. J Med Genet 2007;44:673–88.
16. Brewer GJ. Wilson's disease: a clinician's guide to recognition, diagnosis, and management. Boston: Kluwer Academic; 2001.
17. Machado A, Chien HF, Deguti MM, et al. Neurological manifestations in Wilson's disease: report of 119 cases. Mov Disord 2006;21:2192–6.
18. Lorincz MT. Neurologic Wilson's disease. Ann N Y Acad Sci 2010;1184:173–87.
19. Hitoshi S, Iwata M, Yoshikawa K. Mid-brain pathology of Wilson's disease: MRI analysis of three cases. J Neurol Neurosurg Psychiatry 1991;54:624–6.
20. Brewer GJ, Terry CA, Aisen AM, et al. Worsening of neurologic syndrome in patients with Wilson's disease with initial penicillamine therapy. Arch Neurol 1987;44(5):490–3.

21. Lorincz MT. Recognition and treatment of neurologic Wilson's disease. Semin Neurol 2012;32:538–43.
22. Segawa M, Hosaka A, Miyagawa F, et al. Hereditary progressive dystonia with marked diurnal fluctuation. Adv Neurol 1976;14:215–33.
23. Segawa M. Autosomal dominant GTP cyclohydrolase I (AD GCH 1) deficiency (Segawa disease, dystonia 5; DYT 5). Chang Gung Med J 2009;32(1):1–11.
24. Ichinose H, Ohye T, Takahashi E, et al. hereditary progressive dystonia with marked diurnal fluctuation caused by mutations in the GTP cyclohydrolase I gene. Nat Genet 1994;8:236–42.
25. Saudubray J-M, Van den Berghe G, Walter JH. Inborn metabolic diseases. Berlin: Springer; 2012. p. 579–89.
26. Thöny B, Blau N. Mutations in the BH4-metabolizing genes GTP cyclohydrolase I, 6-pyruvoyl tetrahydropterin synthase, sepiapterin reductase, carbinolamine-4a-dehydratase, and dihydropteridine reductase. Hum Mutat 2006;27:870–8.
27. Leuzzi V, Carducci C, Tolve M, et al. Very early pattern of movement disorders in sepiapterin reductase deficiency. Neurology 2013;81(24):2141–2.
28. Pearl PL, Taylor JL, Trzcinski S, et al. The pediatric neurotransmitter disorders. J Child Neurol 2007;22(5):606–16.
29. Suhren O, Bruyn GW, Tuynman A. Hyperexplexia, a hereditary startle syndrome. J Neurol Sci 1966;3:577–605.
30. Bakker MJ, van Dijk JG, van den Maagdenberg AMJM, et al. Startle syndromes. Lancet Neurol 2006;5(6):513–24.
31. Tijssen MAJ, Rees MI. Hyperekplexia. In: Pagon RA, Adam MP, Ardinger HH, et al, editors. GeneReviews®. Seattle (WA): University of Washington, Seattle; 2007 [updated 2012]. p. 1993–2017. Available at: https://www.ncbi.nlm.nih.gov/books/NBK1260/.
32. Korman SH, Boneh A, Ichinohe A, et al. Persistent NKH with transient or absent symptoms and a homozygous GLDC mutation. Ann Neurol 2004;56:139–43.
33. Pearl PL, Gibson KM. Clinical aspects of the disorders of GABA metabolism in children. Curr Opin Neurol 2004;17:107–13.

Inborn Errors of Metabolism with Myopathy

Defects of Fatty Acid Oxidation and the Carnitine Shuttle System

Areeg El-Gharbawy, MD[a,b], Jerry Vockley, MD, PhD[a,*]

KEYWORDS

- Fatty acid oxidation defects • Carnitine shuttling defects • Cardiomyopathy
- Rhabdomyolysis

KEY POINTS

- Inherited metabolic myopathies should be considered in the differential diagnosis of any individual with muscle pain, fatigue, and recurrent rhabdomyolysis, particularly when triggered by physiologic stress, such as strenuous exercise, intercurrent illnesses, or prolonged fasting.
- Metabolic myopathies, including fatty acid oxidation disorders (FAODs) and carnitine shuttle defects, are heterogeneous disorders that are mostly detected by newborn screening. Because of wide phenotypic variability, diagnostic and treatment challenges remain.
- Referral to a metabolic specialist allows establishing the diagnosis in a timely, cost-effective manner.
- Early recognition of inherited metabolic myopathies allows appropriate choice of therapies conditions and the opportunity to provide genetic counseling to families.

INTRODUCTION

Muscle tissue (heart and skeletal) has a high energy demand to perform essential functions such as ionic homeostasis and contractility. Metabolic fuels for the generation of adenosine triphosphate (ATP) come from different sources, including glucose, free fatty acids, pyruvate, lactate, and ketone body metabolism, and to a lesser extent from amino acids.[1,2] Fatty acids are used as an alternative energy source when glucose is not available. In fetal heart and immediately after birth,

Disclosure Statement: Dr J. Vockley receives research funding from Ultragenyx Pharmaceuticals and the NIH (R01 DK78775).

[a] Department of Pediatrics, Division of Medical Genetics, University of Pittsburgh School of Medicine, Children's Hospital of Pittsburgh, 4401 Penn Avenue, Pittsburgh, PA 15224, USA;
[b] Cairo University, Kasr Al-Aini, Cairo, Egypt
* Corresponding author.
E-mail address: Gerard.vockley@chp.edu

acetyl-CoA derived from pyruvate metabolism and glycolysis provides reducing equivalents for energy generation. In adult hearts, the main source of ATP is oxidative phosphorylation, with 50% to 70% of the reducing equivalents coming from fatty acid oxidation (FAO).[3] The remaining ATP in the heart is derived from glycolysis and the tricarboxylic acid (TCA) cycle. In skeletal muscle, red muscle fibers rich in mitochondria are used for slow and prolonged contractions, whereas white skeletal muscle fibers depend on anaerobic glycolysis for "fast and short twitch" movements. During rest, glycolysis and oxidative phosphorylation using reducing equivalents from a low basal rate of FAO are the main source of ATP production in skeletal muscle. During fasting or physiologic stress, FAO is upregulated and becomes a major source of energy.[2-4] FAO is regulated by the availability of competing substrates (eg, glucose, lactate, ketones, and amino acids), hormonal influences, contractility, blood supply, and restrictions in oxygen supply. FAO rates are ultimately modulated by transcriptional control of the genes for enzymes involved in fatty acid metabolism and mitochondrial biogenesis.[3,5]

Long-chain fatty acyl-CoAs cross the inner mitochondrial membrane via the carnitine shuttle. Acyl-CoA molecules are first conjugated to carnitine by carnitine-palmitoyl transferase I (CPT1). Acylcarnitines are then transported across the highly impermeable inner mitochondrial membrane by the carnitine-acylcarnitine translocase (CACT). Free acyl-CoAs are then released into the mitochondrial matrix via the action of carnitine-palmitoyl transferase 2 (CPT2) with transport of free carnitine back to the cytoplasm (**Fig. 1**).[3-5] Medium- and short-chain acyl-CoAs enter mitochondria

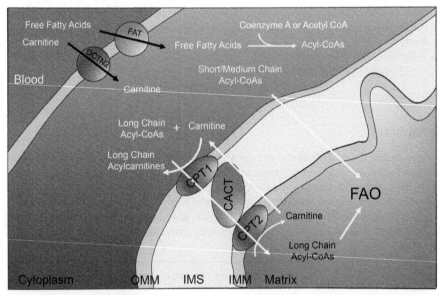

Fig. 1. Fatty acid transport and carnitine shuttle. Carnitine is imported into cells by the carnitine transporter (OCTN2). Free fatty acids enter the cell through dedicated transferases (FAT). Carnitine acyltransferases reversibly transfer an acyl group from an acyl-CoA to carnitine for long-chain substrates. The carnitine shuttle system facilitates the transport of long-chain fatty acids from the cytosol into the mitochondrial matrix, where FAO takes place. This system is made up of CPT1 on the outer mitochondrial membrane (OMM), CACT an inner-mitochondrial membrane space (IMS) protein, and CPT2 on the inner membrane of the mitochondria (IMM).

directly. Oxidation of acyl-CoAs occurs through sequential metabolism of acyl-CoAs by 4 enzymatic steps catalyzed by enzymes varying in chain length specificity: acyl-CoA dehydrogenases (ACADs), enoyl-CoA hydratases, L-3-hydroxyacyl-CoA dehydrogenases, and 3-ketoacyl-CoA thiolases.[3–5] Three ACADs are primarily used for energy production in muscle and heart: very long-chain, medium-chain, and short-chain acyl-CoA dehydrogenases (VLCAD, MCAD, and SCAD). The subsequent 3 steps for long-chain substrates are catalyzed by trifunctional protein (TFP), a heterooctomer encompassing all 3 remaining enzymatic activities. Each cycle of oxidation shortens the carbon chain length by 2, generating 1 molecule of acetyl-CoA, reduced flavin adenine dinucleotide ($FADH_2$), and reduced nicotinamide adenine dinucleotide ($NADH^+$). Reducing equivalents from the flavoenzyme ACADs are channeled to complex III of the respiratory chain by sequential redox reactions with electron transfer flavoprotein (ETF) and ETF:CoQ oxidoreductase (ETF:CoQO; also known as ETF dehydrogenase, ETFDH).[6–8] $NADH^+$ from the 3-hydroxyacyl-CoA dehydrogenase reaction serves as substrate for complex I of the respiratory chain.

During times of high energy demand, acetyl-CoA in the mitochondrial matrix is channeled into the TCA cycle, leading to the production of additional redox equivalents ($FADH_2$, $NADH^+$) that enter the respiratory chain. Proton pumping by respiratory chain complexes I, III, and IV leads to the establishment of an electrochemical proton gradient across the inner mitochondrial membrane that can subsequently be used to synthesize ATP via the mitochondrial ATP synthase (complex V) or drive transmembrane transport processes directly.[2,9] Insufficient fuel reserves are associated with the risk of developing cardiomyopathy and/or rhabdomyolysis during periods of physiologic stress and illness.[2,10–12]

Multiple inborn errors of metabolism (IEMs) have been associated with variable forms of myopathy and/or cardiomyopathy. **Table 1** includes a nonexhaustive list of more frequently encountered disorders. Metabolic myopathies associated with energy defects involve primarily defects in FAO, glycogenolysis, glycolysis, oxidative phosphorylation, and mitochondrial disorders. Long-chain FAODs, including CPT2 deficiency, VLCAD deficiency, long-chain hydroxyacyl-CoA dehydrogenases (LCHAD) deficiency and TFP deficiency, and glycogen metabolism disorders, including glycogen storage diseases (GSDs) types V, VII, and IXd, are associated with an increased risk of rhabdomyolysis induced by exercise. Rhabdomyolysis is less likely to occur in mitochondrial disorders, including oxidative phosphorylation defects, or in GSD types II, IIIa, and IV.[12] Other disorders speculated to cause primarily toxic accumulation of metabolites, and possibly secondary energy defects, and carnitine depletion if not supplemented include organic acidemias as propionic and methylmalonic acidemias where low muscle tone and motor developmental delay may be noted. Posttranslational defects such as those detected in congenital disorders of glycosylation (N-, O-linked and combined) constitute an expanding group of disorders that cause multiple forms of muscular dystrophy. Myopathy is common in O-mannosylation defects leading to muscle eye brain disease, and limb girdle muscular dystrophy.[13] Only defects of FAO and the carnitine shuttle system are discussed in this review.

CARNITINE SHUTTLE DEFECTS AND FATTY ACID OXIDATION DISORDERS
General Concepts

Mitochondrial FAO is essential for energy supply in all tissues. In skeletal muscle, FAO is active during sustained periods of low-intensity exercise, prolonged fasting, and times of physiologic stress, such as intercurrent illness. Cardiac muscle preferentially

Table 1
Inborn errors of metabolism associated with myopathy

IEMs Associated with Myopathy	Inheritance	Clinical Phenotype
Defects in energy metabolism		
Carnitine shuttle defects		
Primary systemic carnitine deficiency	AR	HCM, hypotonia, muscle weakness, fatigue
Carnitine palmitoyl transferase deficiency type 2 (CPT2) deficiency[b]	AR	Muscle weakness, rhabdomyolysis, exercise intolerance (isolated muscle phenotype), CM, hepatomegaly, hypoglycemia, seizures, cystic kidneys (severe infantile)
Carnitine acylcarnitine translocase (CACT) deficiency	AR	CM, arrhythmias, muscle damage, hepatomegaly, hypoglycemia
FAODs		
VLCAD deficiency[b]	AR	HCM, arrhythmias, sudden death, muscle weakness, exercise intolerance, recurrent rhabdomyolysis, hypoketotic hypoglycemia, "Reye-like" hepatic syndrome
LCHAD deficiency[b]	AR	Sudden death, "Reye-like" hepatic syndrome, hypoketotic hypoglycemia, myopathy, recurrent rhabdomyolysis, CM, retinopathy
TFP deficiency[b]	AR	Sudden death, "Reye-like" hepatic syndrome, hypoketotic hypoglycemia, CM, recurrent, rhabdomyolysis, peripheral neuropathy
MAD deficiency	AR	Muscle weakness, CM, hypoglycemia, hepatopathy, respiratory dysfunction, encephalopathy, acidosis
Mitochondrial respiratory chain defects		
Respiratory chain complexes I–V	AR	Myopathy, CM, hepatopathy, Leigh syndrome, epilepsy, developmental delay ± lactic acidosis
Coenzyme Q deficiency		Myopathy, proteinuria, ataxia, low tissue Coenzyme Q, corrected by Coenzyme Q supplementation
Mitochondrial disorders with mt DNA mutations		
Mitochondrial encephalomyopathy with lactic acidosis and strokelike episodes (MELAS)	Mitochondrial	MELAS
Myoclonic epilepsy with ragged-red fibers (MERRF)		MERRF
Neurogenic muscular weakness, ataxia, retinitis pigmentosa (NARP)		NARP
Kearns-Sayre syndrome		CHB, muscle weakness, ataxia, ophthalmoplegia

(continued on next page)

Table 1
(continued)

IEMs Associated with Myopathy	Inheritance	Clinical Phenotype
Disorders of glycogen metabolism		
Glycogen storage disease type 3a (Cori disease; debrancher deficiency)	AR	Hepatomegaly, ketotic hypoglycemia, muscle weakness, CM, growth retardation, liver cirrhosis, hepatocellular carcinoma (adulthood)
Glycogen storage disease type 5 (McArdle disease; myophosphorylase deficiency)[b]	AR	Exercise intolerance (2nd wind phenomena), muscle weakness, exercise-induced rhabdomyolysis
Glycogen storage disease type 7 (Tarui disease; phosphofructokinase deficiency)[b]	AR	Exercise intolerance (out of wind), muscle weakness, rhabdomyolysis, infantile CM, mild macrocytic anemia
Glycogen storage disease type 9d (muscle phosphorylase kinase deficiency)[b]	XL	Exercise intolerance, muscle weakness and atrophy, hepatomegaly
IEMs with possible secondary energy defect, carnitine deficiency		
Propionic aciduria	AR	DCM, long QT, abnormal respiratory complex in cardiac and skeletal muscle, lactic acidosis, hyperammonemia, DD, low carnitine if not supplemented, hypotonia
Methylmalonic aciduria	AR	Hypotonia, lactic acidosis, hyperammonemia, DD, low carnitine if not supplemented
Other IEMs with myopathy		
GSD II (Pompe disease; acid maltase deficiency)[a]	AR	Infantile DCM, myopathy, atrophy, diaphragmatic weakness (lysosomal storage defect)
GSD IV (Anderson disease; brancher deficiency)	AR	Hepatomegaly, CM, muscle weakness, atrophy, neuromuscular disease, adult isolated myopathy
Danon disease (*LAMP2*-related)[a]	XD	HCM, DCM, short PR, WPW, isolated cardiac variants, proximal muscle weakness (85%)
Congenital disorders of glycosylation N- and O-linked disorders	AR	Multisystem disorder, including brain muscle eye disease, CM, limb girdle muscular dystrophy (O-mannosylation defects), hypotonia, liver disease, (N-linked)

Abbreviations: AR, autosomal recessive; CHB, congenital heart block; CHF, congestive heart failure; CM, cardiomyopathy; DCM, dilated cardiomyopathy; DD, developmental delay; HCM, hypertrophic cardiomyopathy; RCM, restrictive cardiomyopathy; WPW, Wolff-Parkinson-White; XD, X-linked dominant; XL, X-linked recessive.

[a] Classified also as a lysosomal storage disease.

[b] Conditions associated with the risk of recurrent rhabdomyolysis.

oxidizes fatty acids for energy generation even under nonstress conditions and has a limited ability to rely completely on glucose during periods of stress.[10,11] Carnitine is a trimethylated amino acid derived from the diet (especially red meat, fish, and dairy products) and is biosynthesized from lysine and methionine in the liver, kidney, and brain. It is ubiquitously distributed in tissues, but is especially in high concentration in muscle.[14] Importantly, carnitine is necessary for import of long-chain fatty acyls-CoAs into mitochondria as acylcarnitines for FAO. It also facilitates oxidation of branched-chain ketoacids, transports acyl moieties from degraded fatty acids out of peroxisomes, and modulates intramitochondrial acyl CoA/CoA sulfhydryl ratio.[15] Enzymatic defects in FAO and the carnitine shuttling pathway are associated with impaired energy production during times of increased demand. Fatty acid oxidation disorders (FAODs) are collectively one of the most common groups of disorders identified through newborn screening.[6,7] Carnitine shuttle defects and mitochondrial long-chain FAODs have similar clinical findings and are among the most frequent IEMs associated with myopathy and/or cardiomyopathy (**Table 2**). In this review, the authors focus primarily on long-chain FAODs and carnitine shuttle defects associated with myopathy.

There likely are multiple mechanisms of pathogenesis in FAO and carnitine shuttle defects. An insufficient ATP supply to meet energetic demands of heart and muscle

Table 2
Carnitine shuttle and fatty acid oxidation disorders

Disorder (Prevalence)	Acylcarnitine Profile	Cardiac and Muscle Disease
Carnitine shuttle defects		
Primary systemic carnitine deficiency; carnitine transporter defect (1:200,000)	↓ C0, C2	HCM, DCM, CHF, arrhythmias, sudden death hypotonia, muscle weakness
Carnitine palmitoyl transferase deficiency type 2 (1:50–100,000)	↑ C16, C18, C18:1	Cardiomyopathy (infantile form), CHF, muscle weakness, rhabdomyolysis, exercise intolerance
Carnitine acylcarnitine translocase deficiency	↑ C16, C18, C18:1	Cardiomyopathy, CHF arrhythmias, muscle damage
Fatty acid oxidation pathway defects		
VLCAD deficiency (1:40–80,000)	↑ C14:1, C14:2, C14, C12:1	HCM, DCM, CHF arrhythmias, sudden death, muscle weakness, exercise intolerance, rhabdomyolysis
LCAD deficiency (1:80,000)	↑ OH-C16, OH-C18:1, OH-C18:2	CM, CHF myopathy, muscle weakness, retinitis pigmentosa, exercise intolerance, rhabdomyolysis
TFP deficiency (1:200,000)	↑ OH-C16, OH-C18:1, OH-C18:2	CM, DCM, CHF, muscle weakness, exercise intolerance, peripheral neuropathy-myopathy, rhabdomyolysis
MAD deficiency (1:200,000)	Complex ↑ in chains of variable lengths	CM, muscle weakness, rhabdomyolysis
MCAD deficiency (1:10–15,000)	↑ C6, C8, C10, C12	Muscle weakness, exercise intolerance, rhabdomyolysis

cells has clear adverse effects. Although all cellular functions are susceptible to the reduced availability of ATP, its hydrolysis by myosin is essential for muscle cell-specific sarcomere contraction. Thus, defects in any enzyme involved in energy generation and homeostasis will affect cardiac and skeletal muscle, especially during times of physiologic stress, such as fasting and acute illness.[2,8] Depletion of TCA cycle intermediates has been postulated to exacerbate the primary enzyme deficiency.[16,17] Accumulated toxic metabolites from compromised FAO (long-chain CoA-esters, or their free long-chain fatty acids) may cause adverse cellular effects because of altered pH (acid accumulation), inhibition of intermediary metabolism (acyl-CoA deficit), or cell damage due to free radical production.[2,8]

Depending on the severity of the underlying enzymatic defect, clinical manifestations vary from one disorder to another and are clinically heterogeneous within each disorder. In infants, FAODs typically present during periods of acute illness or when oral intake is poor. Hypoglycemia, liver disease, and cardiomyopathy occur in more severe infantile forms of the disease, whereas exercise intolerance and rhabdomyolysis may manifest later in toddlers or older children.[10,11,18] Exercise is the most common trigger of rhabdomyolysis in late-onset CPT2 deficiency, the most common inherited metabolic cause of rhabdomyolysis in adults.[12] Symptoms associated with these defects typically appear after prolonged, moderate-intensity exercise, such as jogging or swimming. Viral infections, fasting, cold, general anesthesia, and sleep deprivation are also trigger factors for metabolic decompensation.[7,11,12,18]

Most FAODs and carnitine shuttle defects are detected by newborn screening using tandem mass spectrometry of blood spots. Morbidity and mortality can be reduced in most of these conditions when identified early and treated before symptoms appear.[19] However, newborn screening has not been successful in reducing the poor prognosis associated with some severe phenotypes such as neonatal/severe infantile forms of CPT2 and CACT deficiencies, or preventing the development of neuropathy and retinal complications in severe mitochondrial TFP deficiency.[7,19,20]

Positive newborn screening results require follow-up studies, including a blood acylcarnitine profile (see **Table 2**), urine organic acids, functional/enzyme testing, or molecular analysis.[6,7,11,15] In the absence of newborn screening, these disorders pose a diagnostic challenge because of the intermittent nature of clinical symptoms and biochemical abnormalities, many of which are present only during times of physiologic distress and catabolism. In this setting, analysis of blood and urine samples obtained during an acute illness or episode of decompensation is critical to unmask the biochemical defect.

Outcome is variable from one disorder to the other, typically depending on the severity of the underlying metabolic defect and residual enzymatic activity. Affected individuals with more severe defects presenting early in the neonatal period, infancy, or early childhood have a poorer prognosis, especially if diagnosed in a symptomatic child rather than through newborn screening. Milder forms presenting later in life may still be life threatening, especially if cardiomyopathy is present.[7,19,20]

Specific Disorders

The following FAODs will be discussed in detail: systemic primary carnitine deficiency (carnitine transporter deficiency; CTD), CACT deficiency, CPT2 deficiency, VLCAD deficiency, MCAD deficiency, mitochondrial TFP deficiency, LCHAD deficiency, and multiple acyl-CoA dehydrogenase (MAD) deficiency (glutaric aciduria type 2; GA II).

Systemic primary carnitine deficiency (carnitine transporter deficiency)

Free carnitine is freely filtered by renal glomeruli, and 95% is reabsorbed by the renal tubules by a high-affinity carnitine transporter in the cellular plasma membrane, whereas most esterified carnitine is excreted in the urine. Carnitine is not catabolized in humans, and its only metabolic conversion is through ester formation.[15,21] Active carnitine transport from blood into cells is mediated by the same transporter that functions in the kidney. Active transport of carnitine into tissue takes place against a concentration gradient, permitting tissue carnitine concentrations to be 20- to 50-fold higher than plasma levels.[22] The carnitine transporter OCTN2 is encoded by the SLC22A5 gene on chromosome 5q31.2-3 and transports carnitine in a sodium-dependent manner.[22,23] CTD (OMIM 212120) is inherited as an autosomal recessive trait. As a result of its deficiency, carnitine is not reabsorbed in the kidney, leading to urinary loss and depletion of blood and tissue levels.

Clinical manifestations and complications Loss of carnitine in the kidney results in very low concentration in other tissues, resulting in severe impairment of long-chain FAO, which leads to hypoketotic hypoglycemia with fasting and stress. Age of presentation may range from infancy to adulthood, but neonatal hypoglycemia and sudden death may occur.[24,25] Clinical manifestations in early-onset disease include chronic or acute skeletal and cardiomyopathy, typically exacerbated by metabolic decompensation. Untreated, cardiac disease proceeds to dilated cardiomyopathy with reduced left ventricular ejection fraction or restrictive mild interventricular septal hypertrophy. Electrocardiogram findings include abnormal T waves, ventricular hypertrophy, and atrial arrhythmias.[25–27] Life-threatening arrhythmias can also occur, including nonsustained ventricular tachycardia with periods of sinus rhythm and ventricular premature beats, even in the presence of only borderline left ventricular hypertrophy.[27] During episodes of metabolic decompensation, glucose and ketone bodies are inappropriately low. Transaminases and ammonia may be moderately elevated, and metabolic acidosis, prolonged prothrombin time, and elevated creatine kinase (CK) can occur.[25,28] Later-onset disorders can present with milder skeletal muscle manifestations, including hypotonia, myopathy, and exercise intolerance. A founder mutation has led to an extremely high incidence of CTD in the Faroe Islands, often manifesting as sudden death in adults due to previously undetected disease.[29] Secondary systemic carnitine deficiency can be caused by lack of dietary intake usually in strict vegans, prolonged total parenteral nutrition without carnitine supplementation, defective intestinal uptake, or renal loss due to a more general renal tubulopathy.[30] It can also be seen in FAODs or organic acidurias, and can be iatrogenically induced by valproate intake leading to carnitine depletion.[31]

Diagnosis CTD deficiency should be suspected by the finding of very low free plasma carnitine concentrations (<10 μmol/L) accompanied by increased fractional excretion of carnitine in urine. Mutation analysis of the SLC22A5 gene confirms the diagnosis, but fibroblast carnitine uptake can also be measured if a functional assay is needed. Maternal carnitine deficiency has been identified through newborn screening of an unaffected baby, emphasizing the need to check a plasma carnitine level in mothers of newborns with a critically low free carnitine level.

Treatment Carnitine supplementation should be provided at a dose of 200 to 300 milligrams per kilogram body weight divided throughout the day.[2,26] Affected individuals can develop a "fishlike" body odor due to bacterial metabolism of excess carnitine in sweat or urine, but no serious adverse effects are described. This side effect can be minimized by intermittent treatment with metronidazole.

Carnitine-acylcarnitine translocase deficiency

CACT, located in the inner mitochondrial membrane, facilitates transfer of long-chain acylcarnitine species from CPT1 to CPT2. Mutations in the *SLC25A20* on chromosome 3p21.31 are responsible for CACT deficiency (OMIM 212138).

Clinical manifestations and complications Because neonates depend largely on metabolism of long-chain fatty acids for energy, neonatal presentation is typically severe, with hypoketotic hypoglycemia, hyperammonemia, hypertrophic cardiomyopathy and/or arrhythmia, apnea, hepatic dysfunction, skeletal muscle weakness, and encephalopathy. Unexpected death has also been reported.[32] Children with severe CACT deficiency have a poor prognosis, with most dying before 1 year of age, although longer-term survival is now being reported.[17]

Diagnosis Free carnitine is low in blood, with marked elevations of C16, C18, and C18:1 carnitine species. This acylcarnitine profile is identical to that seen in CPT2 deficiency, and genetic or enzymatic testing is needed to differentiate the 2 disorders.[33] Urine organic acids may show dicarboxylic aciduria. Newborn screening by tandem mass spectrometry will identify CACT deficiency in most cases.

Treatment Avoidance of fasting with continuous feeds for neonates (or every 2–3 hours during the day and continuous at night) is the only available treatment of CACT deficiency. Formula should have reduced long-chain fat plus medium-chain triglyceride (MCT) supplementation. Triheptanoin, an odd chain, MCT with anaplerotic properties, has been reported to successfully treat cardiomyopathy in a limited number of affected individuals.[17] Carnitine supplementation remains controversial because of a theoretic risk of accumulation of long-chain acylcarnitine species, although no proof of toxicity has been reported. Regardless, it is probably not useful unless carnitine levels are low.[34] During an acute episode, intravenous glucose should be administered at a rate of 8 to 12 mg/kg/min in order to inhibit lipolysis and promote anabolism.

Carnitine palmitoyl tansferase 2 deficiency

CPT2 is located on the inner surface of the inner mitochondrial membrane and catalyzes conversion of long-chain acylcarnitines back into long-chain acyl-CoA species with return of carnitine to the cytoplasm. The *CPT2* gene is located on chromosome 1p32.[35]

Clinical manifestations and complications Individuals with CPT2 deficiency (OMIM 600650) present with heterogeneous clinical symptoms based on the severity of the underlying enzymatic defect and are really represent a nearly continuous spectrum.[28] Missense mutations that allow production of some functional enzyme activity are usually associated with milder phenotypes, whereas complete inactivating and protein-truncating mutations produce the more severe forms.[28,36,37] A severe neonatal form presents in the first few days after birth with cardiomyopathy, hypoketotic hypoglycemia, multiorgan dysfunction and failure (including liver and heart), neuronal migration defects, and cystic kidneys. Later-onset, infantile disease is characterized by liver failure, cardiomyopathy, myopathy, and ketotic hypoglycemia in the first year of life.[37] Partial deficiency of CPT2 activity typically leads to episodes of recurrent rhabdomyolysis in adolescence or adulthood, the most common phenotype in this disorder. Affected individuals present with exercise intolerance and recurrent attacks of rhabdomyolysis triggered by fasting, rigorous exercise, cold, and acute illness. Cardiomyopathy and liver disease are not seen.[38–41] Prognosis in neonatal or infantile onset disease is poor[37] with near uniform mortality. Longevity is not affected in late-onset disease, and affected individuals are usually well or minimally symptomatic between acute episodes.

Diagnosis The plasma acylcarnitine profile shows elevated C16, C18:1, and C18:2 carnitine species. CK levels are high during rhabdomyolysis but may return to normal or be only mildly elevated when affected individuals are well. Carnitine levels are usually normal.[38,39] Persistent elevation of serum CK level is observed in approximately 10% of affected individuals.[38] Diagnosis is confirmed by DNA mutation analysis that detects mutations in roughly 80% of affected individuals. A c.338C>T (p.Ser113Leu) mutation is found in 60% to 75% of mutant alleles and is associated with late-onset disease.[40,41] This mutation leads to a thermolabile protein in cells, likely resulting in degradation of the protein during fever or muscular exercise accompanied by elevated body temperature.[41,42] Enzyme analysis of fibroblasts or muscle tissue is possible.

Treatment Individuals with CPT2 deficiency should be instructed to avoid prolonged fasting (>10 hours) and sustained, intensive exercise. Carbohydrate intake before and during exercise may prevent attacks.[12,43] Dietary supplementation with MCT provides an alternative substrate for FAO.[43] General measures to treat acute rhabdomyolysis include intravenous hydration, alkalization of the urine, and close monitoring of CK, kidney function, and electrolytes. Treatment of electrolyte imbalances and electrocardiogram monitoring is important to reduce the risk of arrhythmias. Hemodialysis and hemofiltration may be indicated to prevent progressive renal failure.[44] Carnitine supplementation is probably not useful but may be given if levels are persistently low.

Very long-chain acyl-CoA dehydrogenase deficiency

VLCAD is bound to the inner mitochondrial membrane and catalyzes the first intramitochondrial step of the long-chain FAO spiral.[45] It is encoded by the *ACADVL* gene on chromosome 17p13. VLCAD deficiency (OMIM 201475) is inherited as an autosomal recessive condition.

Clinical manifestations and complications The clinical presentation of VLCAD deficiency is a spectrum from severe neonatal symptoms to late-onset muscle disease and probably relates to residual enzyme activity.[46–48] Early, severe, infantile disease presents shortly after birth with hypertrophic or dilated cardiomyopathy, arrhythmias, pericardial effusion, hypoglycemia, and liver failure. Early childhood disease may manifest with hypoketotic hypoglycemia, hyperammonemia, lactic acidosis, and elevated transaminases. Regardless of age of onset, affected individuals typically transition to muscular symptoms later in childhood as seen in affected individuals with late onset, characterized by exercise intolerance, and muscle cramps and recurrent episodes of rhabdomyolysis triggered by prolonged exercise or fasting. Hypoglycemia is unusual beyond the first few years of life, but the risk remains. Genotype-phenotype correlations have been reported but are imperfect.[46–49] VLCAD deficiency may be asymptomatic at birth, and thus, newborn screening is critical to identify affected infants. Abnormal newborn screening results should be followed by confirmatory functional and molecular testing.[50,51]

Diagnosis Plasma acylcarnitine profile shows characteristic elevation of C14:1, C14:2, C14, and C12:1 species.[49–51] Urine organic acids are notable for extremely reduced or absent ketones, with elevated long-chain carboxylic and dicarboxylic acids. Diagnostic abnormalities may disappear when affected individuals are well, making analysis of samples obtained during acute episodes critical. Individuals diagnosed with VLCAD deficiency require baseline and follow-up measurements of blood CK, liver transaminases, echocardiography, and an electrocardiogram. In the setting of acute disease, measurement of blood glucose concentration, lactic acid, and blood ammonia concentration are indicated. Molecular testing with gene sequencing is currently the least invasive and easiest confirmatory test.[46,47,49] If 2 known deleterious *ACADVL* mutations are identified, a presumptive diagnosis of VLCAD deficiency is confirmed. A c.848T>C mutation (V283L) represents ~20% of all mutant alleles in infants detected by newborn screening and is predictive of milder disease.[49–51] Measurement of VLCAD enzyme activity in leukocytes and cultured fibroblasts is available. Flux through the FAO pathway can be demonstrated in cultured fibroblasts by supplementing the growth medium with stable isotope-labeled palmitic acid (C16) and analyzing acylcarnitines in the medium. An abnormal profile is diagnostic and can distinguish VLCAD deficiency from other FAODs.[2,11,49] In addition, the pattern of metabolites provides some insight into clinical phenotype, with excess tetradecanoyl (C14) carnitine correlating with more severe disease, and dodecanoyl (C12) carnitine correlating with milder disease.

Treatment Individuals with VLCAD deficiency should avoid fasting and receive high caloric glucose containing fluids during acute illness to prevent catabolism. A glucose infusion rate of 8 to 12 mg/kg/min is recommended to prevent lipolysis and reverse catabolism.[52,53] General measures for treatment of rhabdomyolysis should be initiated as indicated, but alkalization of the urine and dialysis are usually not necessary. Cardiac dysfunction is usually reversible with early, intensive supportive care, pharmacologic treatment, and diet modification. Frequent, small meals with a snack before bed and with activity may provide greater metabolic stability. Infant formulas optimized for long-chain fatty acid disorders are available. Supplemental fat calories provided through MCT (15%–18% of total calories) provide a fat source that bypasses long-chain FAO.[52–54] MCT oil (0.5 g/kg lean body weight) has been demonstrated to improve exercise tolerance in individuals with long-chain FAODs if administered 20 minutes before exercise.[43,52–54] Use of an odd chain, MCT, triheptanoin, has been reported to improve exercise tolerance and heart function and reduce the frequency and severity of episodes of metabolic decompensation.[16,17] Dietary restriction of long-chain fats in asymptomatic and mild cases and the use of carnitine supplementation are controversial.[53,55,56] Affected individuals with low carnitine levels and myopathic symptoms may benefit from low-dose carnitine supplementation, but concern has been raised (unsupported by clinical data) about the arrhythmogenic potential of long-chain acylcarnitines.

Medium-chain acyl CoA dehydrogenase deficiency
MCAD is the first enzyme in mitochondrial FAO of CoA esters of medium-chain fatty acids. MCAD deficiency (OMIM 201450) is an autosomal recessive condition and is the most common FAO disorder detected by newborn screening.[57]

Clinical manifestations and complications Presentation can occur at any age. Neonates may present with "Reye-like" hepatic syndrome, hypoglycemia, or sudden infant death syndrome (more frequent in breast-fed than bottle-fed infants). Infants with MCAD deficiency usually have normal development but present with hypoglycemia, lethargy, and seizures, during physiologic stress due to intercurrent illness or fasting. Sudden infant death may also occur. Prepubertal children show a tendency toward obesity. Symptoms in adults usually occur after prolonged fasting or alcohol intoxication; sudden death may be the first presentation in undiagnosed cases. Affected individuals have reported complaints of fatigue, exercise intolerance, and muscle aches; elevated CK and rhabdomyolysis have also been reported.[57–60]

Accumulation of toxic metabolites and impaired gluconeogenesis during acute metabolic decompensation result in hypoketotic hypoglycemia. Lactic acidosis and hyperammonemia may also occur.

Diagnosis Newborn screening using tandem mass spectrometry effectively identifies MCAD deficiency, showing elevated C6-C12 species. The diagnosis may be confirmed by molecular analysis, cellular function studies, or plasma acylcarnitine. Urine organic acid analysis may show dicarboxylic aciduria, but may also be normal when an affected individual is well.[11] Some medications and supplements such as valproate and formulas containing MCT oil may falsely elevate medium-chain species.[57] Urine acylglycine analysis is the preferred test in persons who are clinically asymptomatic showing urinary hexanoylglycine, 3-phenylpropionylglycine, and suberylglycine.[61] A c.985A>G mutation is the most common mutation identified in individuals of Northern European decent, followed by the c.233T>C mutation.[57]

Treatment Prevention is the mainstay of therapy and includes educating the family about avoidance of fasting and seeking medical care during acute illness or poor oral intake. Frequent feeding is recommended in infants, starting at every 4 hours until 6 months of age and then increasing to 8 hours after 1 year of age. A low-fat diet (eg, 30% of total energy from fat) may be beneficial.[57] All affected individuals should have an updated "emergency" letter that includes a detailed explanation of the management of acute metabolic decompensation, emphasizing the importance of intravenous glucose infusion and hospitalization, even if glucose level is normal because hypoglycemia is an end-stage event in this condition. Treatment of symptomatic individuals entails reversing catabolism by provision of carbohydrate orally or intravenously. If intravenous fluids are necessary, they should contain at least 10% dextrose with appropriate electrolytes beginning at a rate of 10 to 12 mg glucose per kg/min, with adjustment based on the affected individual's age and needs to maintain normoglycemia.[56,57] The use of L-carnitine supplementation is controversial. Carnitine supplementation (50 mg/kg/d in 2 or 3 divided doses) is not harmful and may be administered when carnitine levels are low, but its need is not proven.

Mitochondrial trifunctional protein deficiency and long-chain 3-hydroxyacyl-CoA dehydrogenase deficiency

TFP is an enzyme that catalyzes the second through fourth steps of FAO for substrates with chain lengths of C12 to C18. TFP enzyme activities include 2-enoyl-CoA hydratase, LCHAD, and 3-ketoacyl-CoA thiolase. TFP is a hetero-octamer, made up of 4 α-subunits encoded by the nuclear gene *HADHA* containing the LCHAD and 2-enoyl-CoA hydratase domains, and 4 β-subunits encoded by *HADHB* containing 3-ketoacyl-CoA thiolase activity. Both genes are located in tandem in opposite directions relative to gene transcription on chromosome 2p23. Isolated LCHAD deficiency (OMIM 609015) is more common than TFP deficiency (OMIM 609016).[62–64]

Clinical manifestations and complications Clinical symptoms in TFP deficiency are usually more severe than in isolated LCHAD deficiency, with earlier onset and a higher risk for mortality.[63,64] However, in either disorder, presentation is variable. Neonates and infants many present with sudden death, hepatopathy (Reye-like disease), hypoketotic hypoglycemia, rhabdomyolysis, myopathy, cardiomyopathy, and pulmonary edema. Long-term complications, such as cardiomyopathy, peripheral neuropathy, and pigmentary retinopathy, and retinal degeneration leading to progressive visual loss also occur.[64–66] A late-onset neuromyopathic form is characterized by progressive peripheral neuropathy and intermittent exercise-induced myoglobinuria. Although individuals with isolated LCHAD deficiency usually lose deep tendon reflexes in the first few years of life, progressive neuropathy is predominantly seen in individuals with TFP deficiency. Retinopathy is typically more severe in LCHAD deficiency. Individuals with complete TFP deficiency often do not survive the second decade of life.

Diagnosis The blood acylcarnitine profile is abnormal but does not distinguish LCHAD from TFP deficiency; long-chain hydroxyl acylcarnitines (OH-C16, OH-C18:1, and OH-C18:2) are elevated in both. These abnormalities can usually be identified at birth by newborn screening of dried blood spots with tandem mass spectrometry. Urine organic acids under stress are notable for minimal ketones and the presence of dicarboxylic acids. Enzyme analysis, fibroblast FAO flux studies, and gene sequencing will differentiate LCHAD from TFP deficiency.[62–64] Affected individuals require routine monitoring of blood CK, liver transaminases, electrocardiography, and echocardiography. In acute decompensation, measurement of blood glucose concentration, lactic acid, and blood ammonia concentration is also indicated. Mutations in the *HADHA* gene usually cause isolated LCHAD deficiency, and a common mutation in *HADHA* (c.1528G>C; E474Q) accounts for ~80% of the mutant alleles in LCHAD deficiency. Defects in the *HADHB* gene invariably affect all 3 enzymatic activities causing complete TFP deficiency. Molecular studies in individuals with TFP deficiency show a wide range of "private" mutations in both genes. *HADHB* RNA level and the rate of thiolase degradation correlate with the severity of clinical manifestations.[62–64,66]

Treatment Therapy is similar to VLCAD deficiency and includes avoiding the physiologic triggers of fasting and illness. Diet should be modified to decrease long-chain fat intake along with supplementation of the diet with MCT oil and essential fatty acids. Docosahexaenoic acid is recommended at a dose of 60 mg/d in children weighing less than 20 kg and a dose of 120 mg per day in children greater than 20 kg body weight in an attempt to delay or prevent retinal disease.[43,52,53] Carnitine supplementation remains controversial, but low doses do not cause harm. Intravenous supplementation of carnitine in high doses during decompensation is not recommended.[52]

Multiple acyl-CoA dehydrogenase deficiency (glutaric aciduria type 2)
MAD deficiency (OMIM 231680) is an autosomal recessive combined disorder of fatty acid, amino acid, and choline metabolism. It results from deficiency of one of the subunits of ETF (ETFA and ETFB), or ETF;CoQO (ETFDH), located on chromosomes 15q23-q25, 19q13.3, and 4q32-qter, respectively.[66,67] The broad effect of these defects is due to a global inability to reoxidize all of the primary mitochondrial flavin adenine dinucleotide (FAD)-dependent dehydrogenases, which are involved in multiple catabolic pathways. The clinical picture is variable, based on the severity of the underlying enzymatic defect. In its most severe form, affected individuals have congenital anomalies, including cystic dysplastic kidneys and abnormal brain findings, and die in the newborn period of hypoglycemia, hyperammonemia, and metabolic acidosis. Individuals with less severe disease show less dramatic hypoglycemia, encephalopathy, muscle weakness, or cardiomyopathy.[68] Respiratory dysfunction may be present.[69] Some affected individuals may present with only late-onset myopathy. There is significant genetic heterogeneity in MAD deficiency with some genotype-phenotype correlations.[68] Specific mutations in ETFDH have been associated with riboflavin-responsive symptoms as well as a myopathic form related to secondary CoQ10 deficiency.[68,70–72] Furthermore, disorders of FAD synthesis and transport have been described, with overlapping clinical and laboratory findings to classical MAD deficiency.

Diagnosis A diagnosis of MAD deficiency can be made through blood acylcarnitine profiling and characterization of urine organic acids. The secondary deficiency of all primary mitochondrial FAD-dependent dehydrogenases leads to a complex and variable accumulation of metabolites, including glutaric acid (thus the alternative name of GA II), ethylmalonic, butyric, isobutyric, 2-methylbutyric, and isovaleric acids. Lactic acid and ammonia may be secondarily elevated, and hypoglycemia may be present.[2,68] Confirmation of diagnosis is accomplished by direct DNA sequence of the *ETFA*, *ETFB*, and *ETFDH* genes. If variants of unknown significance are found, functional assays, including enzyme activity and acylcarnitine profiling, can be performed on fibroblasts.[2,68,70–73] Newborn screening will identify many, but not all cases.

Treatment During an episode of acute metabolic decompensation, affected individuals should receive a high-glucose infusion rate, similar to other FAODs. Chronically, treatment of severe MAD deficiency is difficult because of multiple affected metabolic pathways. Avoidance of fasting and conjugation of toxic metabolites with L-carnitine and glycine are indicated, and a low-fat diet may be helpful.[68] A general restriction of protein may be helpful but is difficult because of the large number of amino acids whose metabolism is affected. MCT oil should be avoided, because oxidation of all chain length fats is impaired. D,L-3-hydroxybutyrate has been shown to be of benefit in a limited number of case reports, especially in treating cardiomyopathy.[74] For riboflavin-responsive *ETFDH* mutations, resolution of symptoms occurs with riboflavin supplementation (up 150 mg daily). Coenzyme Q_{10} supplementation may also be of some benefit in some individuals with riboflavin-responsive MAD deficiency and may augment riboflavin response.[68,70–73]

THERAPIES UNDER INVESTIGATION FOR LONG-CHAIN FATTY ACID OXIDATION DISORDERS

Triheptanoin is a source of 7-carbon fatty acids proposed to be superior to MCT because its metabolism provides an anaplerotic 3-carbon product (propionyl-CoA).[75] Studies to date suggest an improvement in glucose homeostasis and cardiomyopathy along with a residual but reduced risk for rhabdomyolysis.[16,17,75] The drug is currently in a US Food and Drug Administration approval trial.

Bezafibrate, a PPAR pan-agonist, has been shown to increase CPT2 and VLCAD enzyme activity in cultured fibroblasts from some individuals with missense mutations in this gene.[76,77] However, one clinical trial in individuals with CPT2 or VLCAD deficiency failed to demonstrate efficacy, and thus, further study is needed.[78]

SUMMARY

Disorders of carnitine transport and long-chain FAO are a heterogenous group of disorders with a common end pathophysiology related to reduced mitochondrial energy production. Identification through newborn screening is possible for most of the disorders, but in those regions where it is not performed, a high index of clinical suspicion is necessary because diagnostic metabolites may normalize when affected individuals are well. Prognosis in general is good with early diagnosis and treatment, and new therapies currently in clinical trials are likely to improve therapeutic options in the near future.

REFERENCES

1. Rodrigues B, McNeill JH. The diabetic heart: metabolic causes for the development of a cardiomyopathy. Cardiovasc Res 1992;26:913–22.

2. Das AM, Steuerwald U, Illsinger S. Inborn errors of energy metabolism associated with myopathies. J Biomed Biotechnol 2010;2010;340849.
3. Lopaschuk GD, Ussher JR, Folmes CDL, et al. Myocardial fatty acid metabolism in health and disease. Physiol Rev 2010;90:207–58.
4. Wanders RJA, Vreken P, den Boer MEJ, et al. Disorders of mitochondrial fatty acyl-CoA β-oxidation. J Inherit Metab Dis 1999;22:442–87.
5. Stanley WC, Recchia FA, Lopaschuk GD. Myocardial substrate metabolism in the normal and failing heart. Physiol Rev 2005;85:1093–129.
6. Spiekerkoetter U, Haussmann U, Mueller M, et al. Tandem mass spectrometry screening for very long-chain acyl-CoA dehydrogenase deficiency: the value of second-tier enzyme testing. J Pediatr 2010;157:668–73.
7. Spiekerkoetter U, Mayatepek E. Update on mitochondrial fatty acid oxidation disorders. J Inherit Metab Dis 2010;33:467–8.
8. Cox GF. Diagnostic approaches to pediatric cardiomyopathy of metabolic genetic etiologies and their relation to therapy. Prog Pediatr Cardiol 2007;24:15–25.
9. Mitchell P. Chemiosmotic coupling in energy transduction: a logical development of biochemical knowledge. J Bioenerg 1972;3:5–24.
10. Jeukendrup AE, Saris WH, Wagenmakers AJ. Fat metabolism during exercise: a review—part II: regulation of metabolism and the effects of training. Int J Sports Med 1998;19:293–302.
11. Rinaldo P, Matern D, Bennett MJ. Fatty acid oxidation disorders. Annu Rev Physiol 2002;64:477–502.
12. Smith EC, El-Gharbawy A, Koeberl DD. Metabolic myopathies: clinical features and diagnostic approach. Rheum Dis Clin North Am 2011;37:2201–17.
13. Martin P, Freeze HH. Glycobiology of neuromuscular disorders. Glycobiology 2003;13:67R–75R.
14. Sharma S, Black SM. Carnitine homeostasis, mitochondrial function, and cardiovascular disease. Drug Discov Today Dis Mech 2009;6:1–4.
15. Tein I, De Vivo DC, Bierman F, et al. Impaired skin fibroblast carnitine uptake in primary systemic carnitine deficiency manifested by childhood carnitine-responsive cardiomyopathy. Pediatr Res 1990;28:247–55.
16. Vockley J, Marsden D, McCracken E, et al. Long-term major clinical outcomes in patients with long chain fatty acid oxidation disorders before and after transition to triheptanoin treatment - a retrospective chart review. Mol Genet Metab 2015;116:53–60.
17. Vockley J, Charrow J, Ganesh J, et al. Triheptanoin treatment in patients with pediatric cardiomyopathy associated with long chain-fatty acid oxidation disorders. Mol Genet Metab 2016;119:223–31.
18. Byers SL, Ficicioglu C. The infant with cardiomyopathy: when to suspect inborn errors of metabolism? World J Cardiol 2014;26:1149–55.
19. Spiekerkoetter U, Bastin J, Gillingham M, et al. Current issues regarding treatment of mitochondrial fatty acid oxidation disorders. J Inherit Metab Dis 2010;33:555–61.
20. Spiekerkoetter U. Mitochondrial fatty acid oxidation disorders: clinical presentation of long-chain fatty acid oxidation defects before and after newborn screening. J Inherit Metab Dis 2010;33:527–32.
21. Winter SC, Buist NRM. Cardiomyopathy in childhood, mitochondrial dysfunction and the role of L-carnitine. Am Heart J 2000;139:S63–9.
22. Tang NLS, Ganapathy V, Wu X, et al. Mutations of OCTN2, an organic cation/carnitine transporter, lead to a deficient cellular carnitine uptake in primary carnitine deficiency. Hum Mol Genet 1999;8:655–60.

23. Tein I. Carnitine transport: pathophysiology and metabolism of known molecular defects. J Inherit Metab Dis 2003;26:147–69.
24. Rinaldo P, Stanley CA, Hsu BYL, et al. Sudden neonatal death in carnitine transporter deficiency. J Pediatr 1997;131:304–5.
25. Stanley CA, DeLeeuw S, Coates PM, et al. Chronic cardiomyopathy and weakness or acute coma in children with a defect in carnitine uptake. Ann Neurol 1991;30:709–16.
26. Lamhonwah AM, Olpin SE, Pollitt RJ, et al. Novel OCTN2 mutations: no genotype–phenotype correlations: early carnitine therapy prevents cardiomyopathy. Am J Med Genet 2002;111:271–84.
27. Rijlaarsdam RS, van Spronsen FJ, Bink-Boelkens MTHE, et al. Ventricular fibrillation without overt cardiomyopathy as first presentation of organic cation transporter 2 deficiency in adolescence. Pacing Clin Electrophysiol 2004;27:675–6.
28. Longo N, di San Filipo CA, Pasquali M. Disorders of carnitine transport and the carnitine cycle. Am J Med Genet C Semin Med Genet 2006;142C:77–85.
29. Lund AM, Joensen F, Hougaard DM, et al. Carnitine transporter and holocarboxylase synthetase deficiencies in the Faroe Islands. J Inherit Metab Dis 2007;30: 341–9.
30. Bremer J, Buist NRM. Carnitine-metabolism and functions. Physiol Rev 1983;63: 1420–80.
31. Silva MFB, Aires CCP, Luis PBM, et al. Valproic acid metabolism and its effect on mitochondrial fatty acid oxidation: a review. J Inherit Metab Dis 2008;31:205–16.
32. Rubio-Gozalbo ME, Bakker JA, Waterham HR, et al. Carnitine acylcarnitine translocase deficiency, clinical, biochemical and genetic aspects. Mol Aspects Med 2004;25:521–32.
33. Brivet M, Slama A, Ogier H, et al. Diagnosis of carnitine acylcarnitine translocase deficiency by complementation analysis. J Inherit Metab Dis 1994;17:271–4.
34. Al Aqeel AI, Rashed MS, Wanders RJA. Carnitine-acylcarnitine translocase deficiency is a treatable disease. J Inherit Metab Dis 1999;22:271–5.
35. Gellera C, Verderio E, Floridia G, et al. Assignment of the human carnitine palmitoyltransferase II gene (CPT11) to chromosome 1p32. Genomics 1997;24:195–7.
36. Thuillier L, Rostane H, Droin V, et al. Correlation between genotype, metabolic data and clinical presentation in carnitine palmitoyl transferase 2 (CPT2) deficiency. Hum Mutat 2003;21:493–501.
37. Isackson PJ, Bennett MJ, Lichter-Konecki U, et al. CPT2 gene mutations resulting in lethal neonatal or severe infantile carnitine palmitoyl transferase II deficiency. Mol Genet Metab 2008;94:422–7.
38. Wieser T, Deschauer M, Olek K, et al. Carnitine palmitoyltransferase II deficiency: molecular and biochemical analysis of 32 patients. Neurology 2003;60:1351–3.
39. Di Mauro S, Di Mauro PMM. Muscle carnitine palmityl transferase deficiency and myoglobinuria. Science 1973;182:929–31.
40. Vladutiu GD. The molecular diagnosis of metabolic myopathies. Neurol Clin 2000; 18:53–104.
41. Deschauer M, Wieser T, Zierz S. Muscle carnitine palmitoyltransferase II deficiency: clinical and molecular genetic features and diagnostic aspects. Arch Neurol 2005;62:37–41.
42. Olpin SE, Afifi A, Clark S, et al. Mutation and biochemical analysis in carnitine palmitoyltransferase type II (CPT II) deficiency. J Inherit Metab Dis 2003;26:543–57.
43. Gillingham MB, Scott B, Elliott D, et al. Metabolic control during exercise with and without medium-chain triglycerides (MCT) in children with long-chain 3 hydroxyl

acyl-CoA dehydrogenase (LCHAD) or trifunctional protein (TFP) deficiency. Mol Genet Metab 2006;89:58–63.

44. Huerta-Alardín AL, Varon J, Marlk PE. Bench-to-bedside review: rhabdomyolysis – an overview for clinicians. Crit Care 2005;9:158–69.

45. Uchida Y, Izai K, Orii T, et al. Novel fatty acid beta-oxidation enzymes in rat liver mitochondria. I. Purification and properties of very-long-chain acyl-coenzyme A dehydrogenase. J Biol Chem 1992;267:1027–33.

46. Andresen BS, Olpin S, Poorthuis BJ, et al. Clear correlation of genotype with disease phenotype in very-long chain acyl-CoA dehydrogenase deficiency. Am J Hum Genet 1999;64:479–94.

47. Andresen BS, Vianey-Saban C, Bross P, et al. The mutational spectrum in very long-chain acyl-CoA dehydrogenase deficiency. J Inherit Metab Dis 1996;19: 169–72.

48. Bertrand C, Largilliere C, Zabot MT, et al. Very long chain acyl-CoA dehydrogenase deficiency: identification a new inborn error of mitochondrial fatty acid oxidation in fibroblasts. Biochim Biophys Acta 1993;1180:327–9.

49. Vianey-Saban C, Divry P, Brivet M, et al. Mitochondrial very-long-chain acyl-coenzyme A dehydrogenase deficiency: clinical characteristics and diagnostic considerations in 30 patients. Clin Chim Acta 1998;269:43–62.

50. Boneh A, Andresen BS, Gregersen N, et al. VLCAD deficiency: pitfalls in newborn screening and confirmation of diagnosis by mutation analysis. Mol Genet Metab 2006;88:166–70.

51. McHugh DM, Cameron CA, Abdenur JE, et al. Clinical validation of cutoff target ranges in newborn screening of metabolic disorders by tandem mass spectrometry: a worldwide collaborative project. Genet Med 2011;13:230–54.

52. Solis JO, Singh RH. Management of fatty acid oxidation disorders: a survey of current treatment strategies. J Am Diet Assoc 2002;102:1800–3.

53. Spiekerkoetter U, Lindner M, Santer M, et al. Treatment recommendations in long-chain fatty acid oxidation defects: consensus from a workshop. J Inherit Metab Dis 2009;32:498–505.

54. Behrend AM, Harding CO, Shoemaker JD, et al. Substrate oxidation and cardiac performance during exercise in disorders of long chain fatty acid oxidation. Mol Genet Metab 2012;105:110.

55. Arnold GL, Van Hove J, Freedenberg D, et al. Delphi clinical practice protocol for the management of very long chain acyl-CoA dehydrogenase deficiency. Mol Genet Metab 2009;96:81–2.

56. Saudubray JM, Martin D, De Lonlay P, et al. Recognition and management of fatty acid oxidation defects : a series of 107 patients. J Inherit Metab Dis 1999;22: 488–502.

57. Derks TG, Reijngoud DJ, Waterham HR, et al. The natural history of medium-chain acyl CoA dehydrogenase deficiency in the Netherlands: clinical presentation and outcome. J Pediatr 2006;148:665–70.

58. Iafolla AK, Thompson RJ Jr, Roe CR. Medium-chain acyl-coenzyme A dehydrogenase deficiency: clinical course in 120 affected children. J Pediatr 1994;124:409–15.

59. Ruitenbeek W, Poels PJE, Tumbull DM, et al. Rhabdomyolysis and acute encephalopathy in late onset medium chain acyl-CoA dehydrogenase deficiency. J Neurol Neurosurg Psychiatry 1995;58:209–14.

60. Lang TF. Adult presentations of medium-chain acyl-CoA dehydrogenase deficiency (MCADD). J Inherit Metab Dis 2009;32:675–83.

61. Rinaldo P, O'Shea JJ, Coates PM, et al. Medium-chain acyl-CoA dehydrogenase deficiency. Diagnosis by stable-isotope dilution measurement of urinary

n-hexanoylglycine and 3-phenylpropionylglycine. N Engl J Med 1988;319: 1308–13.

62. Wanders RJA, Ijlst L, Poggi F, et al. Human trifunctional protein deficiency: a new disorder of mitochondrial fatty acid β-oxidation. Biochem Biophys Res Commun 1992;188:1139–45.

63. Das AM, Illsinger S, Lucke T, et al. Isolated mitochondrial long-chain ketoacyl-CoA thiolase deficiency resulting from mutations in the HADHB gene. Clin Chem 2006;52:530–4.

64. Scheuerman O, Wanders RJA, Waterham HR, et al. Mitochondrial trifunctional protein deficiency with recurrent rhabdomyolysis. Pediatr Neurol 2009;40:465–7.

65. Den Boer MEJ, Dionisi-Vici C, Chakrapani A, et al. Mitochondrial trifunctional protein deficiency: a severe fatty acid oxidation disorder with cardiac and neurologic involvement. J Pediatr 2003;142:684–9.

66. Spiekerkoetter U, Khuchua Z, Yue Z, et al. General mitochondrial trifunctional protein (TFP) deficiency as a result of either α- or β-subunit mutations exhibits similar phenotypes because mutations in either subunit alter TFP complex expression and subunit turnover. Pediatr Res 2004;55:190–6.

67. Christensen E, Kolvraa S, Gregersen N. Glutaric aciduria type II: evidence for a defect related to the electron transfer flavoprotein or its dehydrogenase. Pediatr Res 1984;18:663–7.

68. Frerman FE, Goodman SI. Defects of electron transfer flavoprotein and electron transfer flavoprotein ubiquinone oxidoreductase: glutaric acidaemia type II. In: Scriver CR, Beaudet AL, Sly WS, et al, editors. The metabolic and molecular bases of inherited disease. New York: McGraw-Hill; 2001. p. 2357–65.

69. Olsen RKJ, Pourfarzam M, Morris AAM, et al. Lipid-storage myopathy and respiratory insufficiency due to ETFQO mutations in a patient with late-onset multiple acyl-CoA dehydrogenation deficiency. J Inherit Metab Dis 2004;27:671–8.

70. Olsen RKJ, Olpin SE, Andresen BS, et al. ETFDH mutations as a major cause of riboflavin-responsive multiple acyl-CoA dehydrogenation deficiency. Brain 2007; 130:2045–54.

71. Wen B, Dai T, Li W, et al. Riboflavin-responsive lipid storage myopathy caused by ETFDH gene mutations. J Neurol Neurosurg Psychiatry 2010;81:231–6.

72. Gempel K, Topaloglu H, Talim B, et al. The myopathic form of coenzyme Q10 deficiency is caused by mutations in the electron-transferring-flavoprotein dehydrogenase (ETF-DH) gene. Brain 2007;130:2037–44.

73. Gregersen N, Andresen BS, Pedersen CB, et al. Mitochondrial fatty acid oxidation defects remaining challenges. J Inherit Metab Dis 2008;31:643–57.

74. Van Hove JLK, Grunewald S, Jaeken J, et al. D,L-3-Hydroxybutyrate treatment of multiple acyl-CoA dehydrogenase deficiency (MADD). Lancet 2003;361: 1433–5.

75. Roe CR, Sweetman L, Roe DS, et al. Treatment of cardiomyopathy and rhabdomyolysis in long-chain fat oxidation disorders using an anaplerotic odd-chain triglyceride. J Clin Invest 2002;110:259–69.

76. Djouadi F, Aubrey F, Schlemmer D, et al. Bezafibrate increases very-long-chain acyl-CoA dehydrogenase protein and mRNA expression in deficient fibroblasts and is a potential therapy for fatty acid oxidation disorders. Hum Mol Genet 2005;14:2695–703.

77. Gobin-Limballe S, Djouadi F, Aubey F, et al. Genetic basis for correction of very-long-chain acyl-coenzyme A dehydrogenase deficiency by bezafibrate

in patient fibroblasts: toward a genotype-based therapy. Am J Hum Genet 2007;81:1133–43.

78. Orngreen MC, Madsen KL, Preisler N, et al. Bezafibrate in skeletal muscle fatty acid oxidation disorders: a randomized clinical trial. Neurology 2014;82: 607–13.

Inborn Errors of Metabolism with Hepatopathy
Metabolism Defects of Galactose, Fructose, and Tyrosine

Didem Demirbas, PhD, William J. Brucker, MD, PhD,
Gerard T. Berry, MD*

KEYWORDS

- Galactosemia • Fructose intolerance • Tyrosinemia • Nitisinone • Liver
- Liver disease • Inborn errors of metabolism • Hepatopathy

KEY POINTS

- If you think of galactosemia as a diagnostic possibility, eliminate the ingestion of lactose immediately.
- The elimination of sucrose, fructose, and sorbitol usually allows for normal growth and development in children with hereditary fructose intolerance.
- Diagnosis of tyrosinemia type I and the institution of nitisinone (NTBC) therapy are imperative to start early in the first year to eliminate the risk of hepatocellular carcinoma.

INTRODUCTION

As the largest internal organ of the body, the liver performs numerous vital functions and regulates many biochemical processes, including metabolism and the distribution of nutrients; interconversion of metabolites from ingested food; synthesis and secretion of biomolecules such as serum proteins, blood clotting factors, cholesterol, and bile acids; storage of glucose in glycogen form, as well as storing minerals and vitamins; and clearance of ammonia, bilirubin, toxins, and drug metabolites. Being in the center of the anabolic and catabolic pathways, the liver is affected by many inborn errors of metabolism. Common features of the hepatic pathophysiology involve inflammation, necrosis, cholestasis, and steatosis. Cholestasis can be seen in many metabolic disorders. Defects in bile acid metabolism, peroxisomal disorders, cholesterol biogenesis disorders, Neimann-Pick disease type C, and citrin deficiency

Division of Genetics and Genomics, Boston Children's Hospital, Harvard Medical School, Center for Life Science Building, 3 Blackfan Circle, Boston, MA 02115, USA
* Corresponding author.
E-mail address: gerard.berry@childrens.harvard.edu

Pediatr Clin N Am 65 (2018) 337–352
https://doi.org/10.1016/j.pcl.2017.11.008
0031-3955/18/© 2017 Elsevier Inc. All rights reserved.

(citrullinemia type 2) can present with cholestatic liver disease. Hepatocellular necrosis can result as a pathology of catabolic errors. The diseases of galactose, fructose, and tyrosine metabolism described in this article cause hepatocellular necrosis and liver failure. The manifestations of hepatocellular necrosis include jaundice caused by unconjugated hyperbilirubinemia, edema, ascites, hepatic synthetic failure, and hepatic encephalopathy. Elevated serum transaminases, hypoglycemia, hyperammonemia, hypofibrinogenemia, and hypoprothrombinemia can also be observed.[1] It should also be noted other inborn errors of metabolism may have liver involvement. For example, hepatomegaly or hepatosplenomegaly is observed in hepatic glycogen storage disorders, gluconeogenesis disorders, lysosomal disorders, and glucose transporter 2 deficiency (Fanconi-Bickel syndrome); Reye-like syndrome is associated with fatty acid oxidation and carnitine disorders. The diseases that may cause liver dysfunction are listed in **Boxes 1** and **2**.

GALACTOSEMIA OWING TO GALACTOSE-1-PHOSPHATE URIDYLTRANSFERASE DEFICIENCY

Key points

- Galactosemia is a medical emergency in the newborn period and ingestion of lactose should be eliminated immediately.

- Acute complications of the newborn period are resolved with dietary restriction of lactose.

- Despite dietary lactose and galactose restriction, long-term neurologic complications and primary ovarian insufficiency may be observed.

Clinical Description

Galactosemia is a metabolic disease associated with the failure of the interconversion of galactose to glucose (**Fig. 1**).[2] The first observation of classic galactosemia is described as "breastmilk induced neonatal nutritional toxicity" in 1908,[3] followed by a description of a similar infant with galactosuria in 1917.[4] Although the biochemical basis of the disease was still not identified, Mason and Turner[5] described the responsiveness of an infant with galactosuria and hypergalactosemia to a lactose-restricted diet. Two decades later, the enzyme defect was identified to be galactose-1-phosphate uridyltransferase (GALT) deficiency.[6] GALT is a critical enzyme in the Leloir pathway, the pathway responsible for the interconversion of galactose to glucose, and is responsible for the uridylation of galactose-1-phosphate so that it may undergo its final conversion to UDPglucose, performed by epimerase.

The pathology of GALT deficiency is directly related to the amount of residual GALT activity. Different common pathologic sequence variants in the GALT gene produce symptoms of galactosemia to varying degrees, which depend on the aspect of protein structure that they impair. As a result, galactosemia owing to GALT enzyme deficiency can be categorized into 3 groups based on residual enzyme activity: (1) classic galactosemia (0%–1% enzyme activity), (2) clinical variant galactosemia (1%–10% enzyme activity), and (3) biochemical variant (Duarte) galactosemia (15%–35% enzyme activity). In the clinical variant of galactosemia, the erythrocyte GALT activity may be around 1% to 10%, but certain genotypes (such as S135L/S135L) manifest absent or barely detectable enzyme activity in red blood cells; however, they have some enzyme activity (approximately 10% of controls) in the liver.[2] Classic galactosemia is very severe and Duarte galactosemia is often an incidental biochemical finding

Box 1
Metabolic disorders that cause liver disease

Carbohydrate metabolism defects

Galactosemia

Hereditary fructose intolerance

Fructose 1,6-biphosphatase deficiency

Glycogen storage disease (Ia, Ib, III, IV, VI, IXa, IXb, and IXc)

Fanconi Bickel syndrome

Transaldolase deficiency

Glycerol-3-phosphate dehydrogenase I deficiency

Citrullinemia type 2

Congenital disorders of glycosylation

Amino acid disorders

Tyrosinemia, type I

Urea cycle and related disorders

Carbamyl phosphate synthase 1 deficiency

Ornithine transcarbamylase deficiency

Citrullinemia

Arginosuccinic acidemia

N-Acetyl glutamate synthase deficiency

Hyperornithinemia–hyperammonemia–homocitrulllinuria syndrome

Lysinuric protein intolerance

Fatty acid oxidation defects

Carnitine palmitoyltransferase-I deficiency

Carnitine palmitoyltransferase-II deficiency

Primary carnitine deficiency

Carnitine-acylcarnitine translocase deficiency

Very long chain acyl-CoA dehydrogenase deficiency

Long chain 3- hydroxyl acyl-CoA

3-Hydroxy-3-methyl-glutaryl-coenzyme A lyase deficiency

Multiple acyl-coenzyme A dehydrogenase deficiency

Mitochondrial disorders

LARS disease

Electron transport chain deficiencies

POLG1

MPV17

TWINKLE

Deoxyguanosine kinase

GRACILE syndrome

Succinyl-coenzyme A synthetase deficiency

Phosphoenolpyruvate carboxykinase deficiency

Storage disorders

Gaucher, types I, II, and III

Niemann-Pick syndrome (types A, B, and C)

Sandhoff disease

Sialidosis (type II)

Galactosialidosis

Sialic acid transporter disorder

I-cell disease

GM1 gangliosidosis

Multiple sulfatase deficiency

Wolman disease fetalis

Farber disease (type I)

Mucopolysaccharidosis (type VII)

Sterol synthesis defects

Mevalonic acidemia

Peroxisomal biosynthesis and function defects

Zellweger disease

Infantile Refsum disease

Bile salt metabolic defects

Metal metabolism disorders

Juvenile hemochromatosis

Hemochromatosis, other

Wilson disease

Idiopathic copper toxicosis

Other disorders

Glycine-*N*-methyltransferase

Progressive familial intrahepatic cholestasis syndromes 4, including Byler disease (progressive familial intrahepatic cholestasis syndrome 1)

that may require no treatment. The clinical impact is that it is important to understand not only that galactosemia may be present, but the sequence variant can in some cases predict the course of the disease. As sequencing becomes more readily available, the clinical course of variants will be characterized more thoroughly, making their practical understanding more important in the primary care setting.

Classic galactosemia (OMIM 230400) is associated with absent or barely detectable enzyme activity and is potentially a life-threatening multiorgan disorder in the newborn period when untreated. Complications observed in infants with classic galactosemia on a lactose-unrestricted diet include growth failure, increased red blood cell turnover, bleeding, hepatocellular disease or cholestasis, renal tubular disease, cataracts, encephalopathy, cerebral edema, and *Escherichia coli* sepsis. Newborn screening programs have largely eliminated the acute neonatal deaths

---

Box 2
Inborn errors of metabolism listed according to the type of liver involvement

Liver failure

Galactosemia

Hereditary fructose intolerance

Tyrosinemia type 1

Mitochondrial disorders: electron transport chain deficiencies (eg, neonatal cytochrome C oxidase deficiency), POLG1, MPV17, TWINKLE, deoxyguanosine kinase, LARS mutations, GRACILE syndrome, phosphoenolpyruvate carboxykinase deficiency

Transaldolase deficiency

Glycogen storage disorders (eg, brancher deficiency, glycogen storage disease type IV)

Wilson disease

Niemann-Pick disease type C

Fatty acid oxidation disorders (eg, carnitine palmitoyltransferase II deficiency, primary carnitine deficiency, carnitine-acylcarnitine translocase deficiency, very long chain acyl-coenzyme A dehydrogenase deficiency, long chain 3- hydroxyl acyl-coenzyme A deficiency)

Congenital disorders of glycosylation (eg, congenital disorder of glycosylation type 1a)

Cholestasis

Galactosemia

Alpha-1-antitrypsin deficiency

Progressive familial intrahepatic cholestasis syndromes 4, including Byler disease (progressive familial intrahepatic cholestasis syndrome 1)

Defects in bile acid metabolism

Citrin deficiency (citrullinemia type 2)

Peroxisomal disorders (eg, Zellweger disease, infantile Refsum disease)

Neimann-Pick type C

Sterol synthesis disorders (eg, mevalonic acidemia)

Steatosis

Fatty acid oxidation disorders

Urea cycle disorders (eg, ornithine transcarbamylase deficiency)

Hepatomegaly

Fructose 1,6-bisphosphatase deficiency

Glycogen storage disease (eg, glycogen storage disease types I, III, IV, VI, and IX)

Fanconi Bickel syndrome (glucose transporter 2 deficiency)

Glycerol-3-phosphate dehydrogenase I deficiency

Arginosuccinic aciduria

Hepatosplenomegaly

Niemann-Pick type A

Sialidosis (type II)

I-cell disease

Galactosialidosis

GM1 gangliosidosis

Lysinuric protein intolerance

Mevalonic acidemia

Mucopolysaccharidosis (type VII)

Gaucher

Sandhoff disease

Reye-like syndrome

Fatty acid oxidation defects

Isovaleric acidemia

3-Hydroxy-3-methyl-glutaryl coenzyme A lyase deficiency

Carnitine palmitoyltransferase I deficiency

observed in classic galactosemia. Upon implementation of a lactose-restricted diet, the acute complications of classic galactosemia resolve and the severe complications of liver failure, sepsis, and death are prevented. However, despite dietary galactose restriction, even when diet treatment started on day 1 of life, individuals with classic galactosemia remain at risk of chronic complications involving the brain and the ovary. Long-term, diet-independent complications of classic galactosemia are developmental delay, delayed language development, speech defects

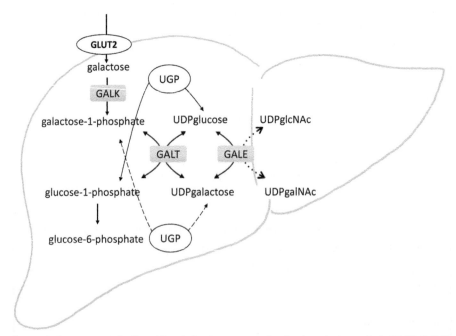

Fig. 1. Galactose metabolism. The defective enzyme in classic galactosemia is GALT. GALE, UDP-galactose 4′-epimerase; GALK, galactokinase; GALT, galactose-1-phosphate uridyltransferase; UDPgalactose, uridine diphosphate galactose; UDPglcNAc, uridine diphosphate N-acetylglucosamine; UDPgalNAc, uridine diphosphate N-acetylgalactosamine; UGP, UDP-glucose pyrophosphorylase.

(childhood apraxia of speech and dysarthria), learning difficulties, cognitive deficits, tremor, ataxia, dystonia, low bone density, and premature ovarian insufficiency or hypergonadotropic hypogonadism, which is observed in almost all females with classic galactosemia.[2,7–9]

Similar to classic galactosemia, the clinical variant of galactosemia can result in life-threatening illness in the newborn period. In untreated infants, feeding problems, failure to thrive, and hepatocellular damage can be observed. The implementation of a galactose-restricted diet induces resolution of the neonatal signs and allows for normal growth and development. Most females with the clinical variant of galacto-semia do not manifest premature ovarian insufficiency.

The biochemical variant (Duarte) of galactosemia is recognized as a likely benign va-riety. Newborns with Duarte galactosemia may be recognized by an abnormal newborn screening result and may have increased galactose metabolites. Infants with Duarte galactosemia typically do not present with clinical disease while on a reg-ular diet; however, there are no prospective, long-term, evidence-based studies to rule out the association of the Duarte genotype with a disease state, such as a higher prevalence of speech abnormalities. The requirement and/or efficiency of dietary lactose restriction for individuals affected with Duarte galactosemia is an area of debate. Some specialists recommend no dietary restriction, whereas others recom-mend lactose restriction only in the first year of life.[2,10]

Enzyme Defect

Classic galactosemia is due to deficiency of GALT, the second enzyme of the Leloir pathway of the galactose metabolism (see **Fig. 1**). This enzyme functions as a homodimer and reversibly converts galactose-1-phosphate and UDPglucose to UDPgalactose and glucose-1-phosphate.[11] In the absence of GALT activity, galactose-1-phosphate and galactose build up, and galactose is also converted to galactitol and galactonate. The accumulation of galactitol in the lens is clinically signif-icant because it often leads to cataract formation. Galactitol accumulation in the brain was detected in individuals with galactosemia on an unrestricted diet.[12]

Molecular Genetics

GALT enzyme is encoded by the *GALT* gene, which is located on chromosome 9 in the p13 region. The mode of inheritance for GALT deficiency is autosomal reces-sive. The incidence of GALT deficiency is 1 in 40,000 to 60,000 in the United States. More than 300 mutations have been reported (Associated Regional and University Pathologists [ARUP] GALT database[13]), and the majority of them are missense mu-tations. The most common classic galactosemia mutations that cause absence of enzyme activity are Q188R, K285N, L195P, and a 5.2-kb deletion. Q188R is the most common GALT mutation in Northern Europeans and the 5.2-kb deletion is mostly seen in the Ashkenazi Jewish population. The S135L variant that causes nondetectable activities in red blood cells but contributes to approximately 10% enzyme activity in liver, and thus is considered a clinical variant, is mostly seen in African American and native South African patients. The mutation associated with biochemical variant galactosemia is N314D, also known as Duarte (D2) variant. This variant is in *cis* with a 4-bp deletion in the promoter region (c.-119_116delGTCA) and causes a reduction in the GALT activity. The homozygous state for the D2 allele results in approximately 50% enzyme activity. The asparagine to aspartate substitution at amino acid 314 (N314D) can also be linked to p.Leu218-Leu in *cis* configuration (D1, LA variant) and this causes increased GALT activity of about 117% in the heterozygous state.[10]

Treatment

The treatment for galactosemia is the immediate restriction of lactose from the diet. All milk products should be replaced with lactose-free formulas (eg, Isomil or Prosobee). The elimination of lactose from the diet usually prevents death and allows for the disappearance of acute complications such as poor growth, poor feeding, emesis, jaundice, and the liver enlargement and dysfunction that includes hyperbilirubinemia, transaminasemia, hypofibrinogenemia with a bleeding diathesis, cataracts, encephalopathy (including lethargy, irritability, and hypotonia), hyperchloremic metabolic acidosis, albuminuria, generalized aminoaciduria, and anemia. The recently released international guidelines for the management of classic galactosemia recommends a life-long galactose-restricted diet by the elimination of sources of lactose from milk and dairy products, although galactose from nonmilk sources including legumes, fruits, and vegetables are considered minimal and are permitted; certain mature cheeses with a low galactose content are also allowed.[14]

Erythrocyte galactose-1-phosphate levels are usually greater than 10 mg/dL in the newborn period in the clinical variant of galactosemia and in classic galactosemia. It can be as high as 120 mg/dL in classic galactosemia. Normal levels are less than 1 mg/dL. For individuals on a lactose-free diet, the levels are 1 mg/dL or greater in classic galactosemia and less than 1 mg/dL in the clinical variant.[2]

To address the long-term complications of galactosemia, evaluation by a psychologist or developmental pediatrician starting at age 1 years as well as by a pediatric endocrinologist for females during the pubertal period are recommended.[14] Early intervention by a speech therapist is usually very effective in resolving speech problems.

UDP-GALACTOSE 4′-EPIMERASE DEFICIENCY GALACTOSEMIA

Key points

- Similar to GALT deficiency, the elimination of lactose from the diet resolves acute complications of UDP-galactose 4′-epimerase (GALE) deficiency.
- Generalized GALE deficiency is treated with a lactose-restricted diet.
- Individuals with peripheral and intermediate form of GALE deficiency are largely asymptomatic.

Clinical Description

GALE deficiency galactosemia (OMIM 230350) presents with elevated galactose-1-phosphate levels in newborn screening and reduced activity of GALE in red blood cells (see **Fig. 1**).[15] Generalized GALE deficiency is a very rare condition; only 6 cases from 3 consanguineous Pakistani families are described so far.[9,16,17] The first report of the generalized form presented with clinical symptoms similar to classic galactosemia in the newborn period.[16] The acute clinical symptoms associated with severe or generalized GALE deficiency include hypotonia, poor feeding, vomiting, weight loss, jaundice, hepatomegaly, and liver dysfunction. Similar to GALT deficiency, eliminating galactose from the diet and switching to a milk-free formula resolves these acute complications. Owing to its ultrarare status, our knowledge on the long-term complications of GALE deficiency is limited. Although it is difficult to dissect the sole effect of GALE deficiency owing to the consanguineous nature of the described individuals, long-term complications may include learning difficulties, developmental delay, and poor growth. There is suspicion that those extraneous findings, such as sensorineural deafness, may be due to other genomic mutations. Furthermore, individuals with the severe GALE deficiency have substantial residual enzyme activity, indicating that they are most likely variants. No evidence of premature ovarian insufficiency has been observed in the women with GALE deficiency, in contrast with GALT deficiency.

GALE deficiency is considered to exist as a continuum disorder that can be categorized in 3 forms: generalized, peripheral, and intermediate forms. The clinical manifestations differ depending on the availability of the enzyme activity in different tissues and organs. In all forms of GALE deficiency, there is reduced activity of the GALE enzyme in red blood cells. However, in the peripheral form of GALE deficiency the enzyme activity is almost in the normal range in other tissues, whereas in the intermediate form enzyme activity is reduced in lymphoblasts. In contrast, generalized GALE deficiency is associated with a systemic significant reduction of enzyme activity in the liver and other organs. Individuals with peripheral and intermediate forms of GALE deficiency are usually identified through newborn screening and are largely asymptomatic when they ingest unlimited amounts of regular milk and dairy products.

Enzyme Defect

GALE is the third enzyme in the Leloir pathway and catalyzes the reversible epimerization of UDPgalactose to UDPglucose and also catalyzes the reversible epimerization of UDP-N-acetylglucosamine to UDP-N-acetylgalactosamine (see **Fig. 1**). UDP-galactose 4'-epimerase requires NAD^+ as a cofactor and functions as a homodimer.

The epimerase enzyme is not only important in the catabolism of dietary galactose, by catalyzing interconversion of UDPgalactose and UDPglucose, but also contributes to endogenous biosynthesis of UDPgalactose as well as UDP-N-acetylgalactosamine, when these important substrates of glycolipid, glycosaminoglycan and glycoprotein biosynthesis are not otherwise available.

Molecular Genetics

The *GALE* gene that encodes GALE is located in short (p) arm of chromosome 1 at position 36.11 (1p36.11). The mode of inheritance for GALE deficiency is autosomal recessive. There are 24 mutations of missense and nonsense origin listed in the Human Gene Mutation Database. The V94M mutation, which was found in the Pakistani individuals with the generalized epimerase deficiency, is associated with absence of the enzyme activity. The effect of various mutations, including G90E and L183P, on enzyme activity has been evaluated in a yeast model.[18]

Treatment

Individuals with generalized GALE deficiency should be treated with a galactose-restricted diet. However, complete elimination of galactose from the diet is not recommended, because galactose deficiency interferes with the ability to form complex carbohydrates and lipids because glucose cannot be converted into galactose when needed. Individuals with peripheral and intermediate form of GALE deficiency are largely asymptomatic, even when they have regular milk and galactose intake. However, unlike individuals with the peripheral form, some individuals with the intermediate type have been placed on dietary therapy because of concomitant problems, such as speech defects and developmental delays.

HEREDITARY FRUCTOSE INTOLERANCE

> **Key points**
>
> - Dietary fructose, sucrose, and sorbitol must be eliminated when hereditary fructose intolerance (HFI) is suspected.
> - The complications associated with HFI are resolved upon complete elimination of fructose from the diet.

Clinical Description

HFI (OMIM 229600) is an autosomal-recessive disorder caused by the deficiency of enzyme aldolase B (**Fig. 2**). The first case of HFI was reported as a 24-year-old woman who complained of vomiting after fruit or sugar intake. It was described as a condition different than benign fructosuria and suspected to be presumably owing to accumulation of a toxic intermediate upstream of fructose-6-phosphate.[19] A similar clinical picture was described in 4 members of a single family and later associated with an aldolase enzyme that failed to break down fructose 1-phosphate in liver biopsy samples.[20-22]

The first signs of HFI are usually observed during weaning from breast milk when fruits and vegetables are started to be consumed by the infant. Newborns with HFI usually do not show any signs while on breast milk, unless they are fed with a sweetened milk formula. The signs and symptoms upon introduction of fructose-containing foods include abdominal pain, nausea, recurrent vomiting, hypoglycemia, and failure to thrive. Besides hypoglycemia, metabolic disturbances such as lactic acidemia,

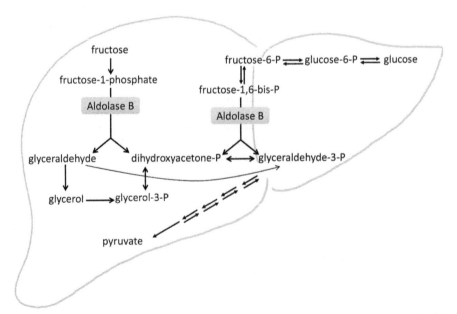

Fig. 2. Fructose metabolism. The enzyme defect in hereditary fructose intolerance (HFI) is aldolase B. The activity of aldolase B for fructose-1-phosphate is greater than for fructose-1,6-bis-phosphate. P, phosphate.

hypophosphatemia, hyperuricemia, hypermagnesemia, and hyperalaninemia are observed in untreated HFI. Prolonged fructose intake leads to poor feeding, vomiting, hepatomegaly, jaundice, hemorrhage, renal Fanconi syndrome, poor growth, and hepatic failure and death.[23] Upon dietary restriction of fructose, symptoms resolve and normal growth and development is achieved. Continuous exposure to fructose, sucrose, and sorbitol might lead to irreversible liver and kidney damage (reviewed by Ali and colleagues[24]). Individuals with HFI who survived to adulthood usually exhibit a self-imposed aversion to sweet foods.

Enzyme Defect

Dietary fructose is phosphorylated by fructokinase into fructose 1-phosphate, which is then cleaved into triose sugars dihydroxyacetonephosphate and glyceraldehyde by aldolase B (fructose 1,6-bisphosphate aldolase; see **Fig. 2**). Aldolase B is present in the liver, kidney, and small intestine, whereas the aldolase A and aldolase C isoforms are found primarily in the muscle and brain, respectively. The expression of aldolase B is not constitutively active, unlike the A and C isoforms, and depends on the dietary control.[25]

The ingestion of large amounts of fructose in individuals with HFI causes rapid accumulation of fructose 1-phosphate, which leads to a sequestration and thereby depletion of inorganic phosphate (hypophosphatemia) and reduced intracellular adenosine triphosphate (ATP) concentrations. Reduced inorganic phosphate causes uric acid formation (hyperuricemia) via the degradation of purine nucleotides because monophosphates lack the phosphate to be converted to their di and triphosphate forms (adenosine monophosphate to ATP). The ATP depletion causes the dissolution of magnesium-ATP complex, which is clinically important, because the release of magnesium ions causes hypermagnesemia, which can be detected on electrolyte analyses. Fructose ingestion in individuals with HFI may cause hypoglycemia by fructose 1-phosphate–induced impairments in glycogenolysis and gluconeogenesis. The impairment in gluconeogenesis in conjunction with an activation of pyruvate kinase by fructose 1-phosphate leads to the accumulation of alanine, lactate, and pyruvate in liver and, thus, to the development of lactic acidemia and hyperalaninemia.

Molecular Genetics

The *Aldolase B* (*ALDOB*) gene is located on chromosome 9q22.3. The mode of inheritance for HFI is autosomal recessive. The incidence is estimated to be 1 in 20,000.[26] There are 65 *ALDOB* mutations listed in the Human Gene Mutation Database; 30 of these are missense or nonsense mutations, 11 splicing substitutions, and 14 small deletions or small deletions or duplications. The most common mutations are A149P, A174D, and N334K. The del4, A337V, R303W, and R59X mutations are also widely distributed.[27] There are no established genotype–phenotype correlations for HFI and the severity of disease manifestations seems to be largely dependent on the affected individual's lack of adherence to a fructose-restricted diet.

Treatment

Individuals with HFI should be treated with a fructose-restricted diet. Dietary fructose, sucrose, and sorbitol must be eliminated when HFI is suspected. Parenteral administration of fructose, sorbitol, or sucrose, that is, invert sugar, may cause death in individuals with HFI and must be avoided. Affected individuals should be aware of the presence of fructose in certain medicinal formulations and such medications should be avoided. Specific ingredients to avoid include fructose, high-fructose corn syrup, honey, agave syrup, sucrose, maple-flavored syrup, molasses, palm or coconut sugar, and sorghum.[28] The complications associated with HFI are resolved upon complete elimination of fructose from the diet and normal growth and development is observed.

TYROSINEMIA

Key points

- Succinylacetone is the pathognomonic marker for tyrosinemia type I and can be found in both blood and urine.
- Plasma amino acid elevations include tyrosine, phenylalanine, and methionine.
- If tyrosinemia type I is diagnosed, nitisinone (NTBC) therapy should be started as soon as possible to minimize the risk of hepatocellular carcinoma development.
- The treatment of tyrosinemia involves life-long dietary therapy.
- Hepatocellular carcinoma is a life-long risk and must be monitored by imaging.
- Indications for liver transplant include treatment failure with NTBC or the development of hepatocellular carcinoma.

Clinical Description

Tyrosinemia refers to elevated plasma tyrosine levels (>120 μmol/L) and can have many causes (immature liver, liver damage, high-protein diet, and total parenteral nutrition), which include the metabolic disorders tyrosinemia types I (OMIM 276700), II (OMIM 276600), and III (OMIM 276710). Only tyrosinemia type I (hepatorenal) causes significant hepatopathy, which is characterized by severe synthetic failure involving vitamin K–resistant coagulopathy with gastrointestinal bleeding, hypoalbuminemia, ascites, jaundice, and cirrhotic change. The development of liver nodules and hepatocellular carcinoma can occur before 6 months of age.[29,30] An α-fetoprotein level is typically elevated with an average of 160,000 ng/mL (normal, <1000 in infants 1–3 months of age) in the neonatal period. Coagulation factors II, VII, IX, XI, and XII are affected most severely, whereas factors V and VIII are spared.[29,31]

Markers of liver damage are only modestly elevated compared with the degree of synthetic failure and decrease with age of presentation. In the more severe neonatal presentation, an average aspartate aminotransferase of 113 U/l, alanine aminotransferase of 64 U/l, and gamma-glutamyl transferase of 158 U/l were associated with an average partial thromboplastin time of 80.5 s in infants presenting before 6 months of age.[30] Pertinent physical examination signs include hepatomegaly that is hard to palpation and a "boiled cabbage odor."[31]

Tyrosinemia type I has 2 separate patterns of presentation, one being an acute neonatal form presenting with liver failure before 6 months of age and a more chronic form presenting after 6 months of age characterized by liver dysfunction, renal tubular dysfunction, hypophosphatemic rickets, and acute porphyria-like neurologic crises, which present with dystonia, peripheral neuropathy, and can lead to respiratory failure. If untreated, the neonatal presentation is often fatal before 2 years of age with the primary cause of death being hepatocellular carcinoma or liver failure in the majority of cases. Before 1992 and the development of nitisinone, also known as NTBC [2-(2-nitro-4-trifluoro-methylbenzyol)-1,3 cyclohexanedione]; the only definitive treatment was liver transplantation because phenylalanine- or tyrosine-deficient dietary therapy, which can be effective in types II and III, generally only slowed progression, with many patients surviving less than 12 years.[29,31]

Enzyme Defect

Tyrosinemia type I is associated with a metabolic defect in fumarylacetoacetase, the most distal enzyme in the tyrosine catabolic pathway, which is responsible for the hydrolysis of fumarylacetoacetate into fumarate and acetoacetate (**Fig. 3**). Its deficiency causes toxic increases in fumarylacetoacetate, maleylacetoacetate, and succinylacetone.[30,32]

Fumarylacetoacetate and maleylacetoacetate are confined to the intracellular compartments where they are generated. The liver (90%) and the kidney (10%) are the principal organs of tyrosine catabolism and are the most affected. Fumarylacetoacetate and maleylacetoacetate act as alkylating agents, disrupt sulfhydryl metabolism, increase oxidative stress, and are carcinogenic.[32] NTBC blocks their production and can reduce risk of hepatocellular carcinoma significantly. Children started on NTBC therapy after 12 months of age are at a 13-fold higher risk of developing hepatocellular carcinoma than children starting in the neonatal period.[30] Succinylacetone is produced from both fumarylacetoacetate and maleylacetoacetate, and is secreted into the blood where it is the pathognomonic serum marker used to establish the diagnosis. Hypermethioninemia is also present owing to an acquired deficit in its conversion into S-adenosylmethionine. Succinylacetone, methionine, and tyrosine levels are markers for tyrosinemia type I in newborn screening.[31]

Succinylacetone is a potent inhibitor of δ-aminolevulinic acid dehydratase and can result in acute intermittent porphyria-like signs such as peripheral neuropathies in affected individuals. Therefore, δ-aminolevulinic acid can also be used as a urine marker for the disease. Succinylacetone is also an inhibitor of 4-hydroxyphenylpyruvate dioxygenase leading to elevated tyrosine levels and the presence of 4-hydroxyphenylpyruvate, 4-hydroxyphenyllactate, and 4-hydroxyphenylacetate in blood and urine.[29]

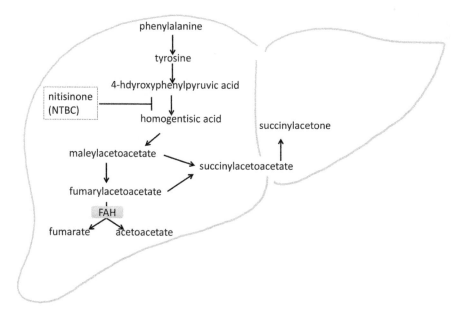

Fig. 3. Tyrosine metabolism. The defective enzyme in tyrosinemia, type 1 is fumarylacetoacetate hydrolase. Treatment is inhibition of 4-hydroxyphenylpyruvic acid dioxygenase by nitisinone (NTBC).

Ironically, it is the more proximal inhibition of 4-hydroxyphenylpyruvate dioxygenase by NTBC that prevents the formation of the more downstream maleylacetoacetate and fumarylacetoacetate, which mediate the hepatotoxicity. A secondary effect of this inhibition is a secondary tyrosinemia, because it induces the metabolic defect associated with tyrosinemia type III. Tyrosine is significantly less toxic than fumarylacetoacetate or succinylacetone, and crystallizes in the skin and eyes when serum concentrations are greater than 800 μmol/L. Dietary restriction of phenylalanine and tyrosine is effective at preventing this effect.[29]

Molecular Genetics

The prevalence of tyrosinemia type I worldwide is 1 in 100,000. There are several geographic areas where the incidence is increased such as the Saguenay Lac–Saint Jean region of Quebec (1:846), Norway (1:74,000) and Finland (1:60,000).[29,31] Tyrosinemia type I is inherited in an autosomal-recessive manner and, although several pathologic mutations in the FAH gene have been identified, there are no genotype–phenotype correlations in terms of severity of presentation. The FAH gene is located at 15q23-q25. The most common mutations are IVS12+5 G→A (French-Canadian/Norway), p.G337S (Norway), p. W262X (Finland), IVS6-1 G→T (southern Europe), and p.P251L (Ashkenazi Jewish).[29–31] The current theory behind phenotypic differences in the severity of disease is the presence of hepatic nodules, which have undergone allelic reversion and do not contain a pathologic variant in the FAH gene. Hepatocytes with this reversion would have a survival advantage over their germline counterparts because they would not be exposed to the toxic metabolites that induce apoptosis and would retain more normal synthetic function.[29]

Treatment

NTBC therapy should be started as soon as tyrosinemia type I is diagnosed through succinylacetone elevation or molecular genetic testing to decrease risk of hepatocellular carcinoma. NTBC is an oral medication. Dosing is 1 mg/kg divided 2 times a day and is therapeutic at 40 to 60 μmol/L. After initiation, succinylacetone levels normalize in 1 to 2 days, liver function in 1 week, prothrombin time and partial thromboplastin time in 1 month, and α-fetoprotein levels in 6 months to 1 year.[29] The response rate is typically 90%. Failure to respond is an indication for liver transplantation. Hepatocellular carcinoma is a lifelong risk and requires routine monitoring. MRI or computed tomography examination is currently recommended yearly with ultrasound examination of the liver every 6 months if nodules are present at time of diagnosis or concerning changes in either imaging or α-fetoprotein levels develop. Nodules present before starting therapy should regress after NTBC therapy. If hepatocellular carcinoma is an indication for liver transplantation, a hepatic biopsy should not be pursued because it may risk seeding the malignancy.[30,31,33,34]

Life-long dietary therapy is indicated and includes 50% to 75% intact protein and 25% to 50% phenylalanine- and tyrosine-deficient formula to prevent tyrosine toxicity (ocular lesions and lesions) with care to avoid the phenylalanine deficiency. The plasma tyrosine concentration should be maintained between 200 and 500 μmol/L, and the phenylalanine concentration should be between 20 and 80 μmol/L.[31] Radiographic examination of the hands is recommended to evaluate for rickets at the time of diagnosis. Routine laboratory monitoring involves plasma amino acids (every 3 months), NTBC and α-fetoprotein (every 6 months), and renal ultrasound imaging and renal tubular function tests initially and as symptomatology dictates. Recommended with age-based intervals are found in more detail in Sniderman King and colleagues.[31]

REFERENCES

1. Venditti CP, Berry G. Inborn errors of metabolism and the liver. In: Walker W, editor. Nutrition in pediatrics. 4th edition. Hamilton (Canada): B.C. Decker, Inc; 2007. p. 513–21.
2. Berry GT. Classic galactosemia and clinical variant galactosemia. In: Pagon RA, Adam MP, Ardinger HH, et al, editors. GeneReviews. Seattle (WA): University of Washington, Seattle; 2014. 1993-2017. Available at: https://www.ncbi.nlm.nih.gov/books/NBK1518/.
3. von Reuss A. Zuckerausscheidung im Sauglingsalter. Wien Med Wochenschr 1908;58:799–801.
4. Goppert F. Galaktosurie Nach Milchzuckergabe Bei Angeborenum. Klin Wochenschr 1917;54:473–7.
5. Mason HH, Turner M. Chronic galactosemia. Am J Dis Child 1935;50:359–63.
6. Isselbacher KJ, Anderson EP, Kurahashi K, et al. Congenital galactosemia, a single enzymatic block in galactose metabolism. Science 1956;123(3198):635–6.
7. Walter JH, Fridovich-Keil JL. Galactosemia. In: Valle D, Beaudet AL, Vogelstein B, et al, editors. The online metabolic and molecular bases of inherited disease. New York: McGraw-Hill; 2014. Available at: http://ommbid.mhmedical.com.ezp-prod1.hul.harvard.edu/content.aspx?bookid=971&sectionid=62672411. Accessed January 03, 2018.
8. Waisbren SE, Potter NL, Gordon CM, et al. The adult galactosemic phenotype. J Inherit Metab Dis 2012;35(2):279–86.
9. Berry GT, Walter JH, Friedovich-Keil J. Disorders of galactose metabolism. In: Saudubray JM, Baumgartner MR, Walter JH, editors. Inborn metabolic diseases – Diagnosis and treatment. 6th edition. New York: Springer-Verlag Inc; 2016. p. 139–47.
10. Fridovich-Keil JL, Gambello MJ, Singh RH, et al. Duarte variant galactosemia. In: Pagon RA, Adam MP, Ardinger HH, et al, editors. GeneReviews. Seattle (WA): University of Washington, Seattle; 2014. 1993-2017. Available at: https://www.ncbi.nlm.nih.gov/books/NBK258640/.
11. McCorvie TJ, Kopec J, Pey AL, et al. Molecular basis of classic galactosemia from the structure of human galactose 1-phosphate uridylyltransferase. Hum Mol Genet 2016;25(11):2234–44.
12. Otaduy MCG, Leite CC, Lacerda MTC, et al. Proton MR spectroscopy and imaging of a galactosemic patient before and after dietary treatment. AJNR Am J Neuroradiol 2006;27(1):204–7.
13. Calderon FRO, Phansalkar AR, Crockett DK, et al. Mutation database for the galactose-1-phosphate uridyltransferase (GALT) gene. Hum Mutat 2007;28(10):939–43.
14. Welling L, Bernstein LE, Berry GT, et al. International clinical guideline for the management of classical galactosemia: diagnosis, treatment, and follow-up. J Inherit Metab Dis 2017;40(2):171–6.
15. Gitzelmann R. Deficiency of uridine diphosphate galactose 4-epimerase in blood cells of an apparently healthy infant. Preliminary communication. Helv Paediatr Acta 1972;27(2):125–30.
16. Holton JB, Gillett MG, MacFaul R, et al. Galactosaemia: a new severe variant due to uridine diphosphate galactose-4-epimerase deficiency. Arch Dis Child 1981;56(11):885–7.
17. Walter JH, Roberts RE, Besley GT, et al. Generalised uridine diphosphate galactose-4-epimerase deficiency. Arch Dis Child 1999;80(4):374–6.
18. Fridovich-Keil J, Bean L, He M, et al. Epimerase deficiency galactosemia. In: Pagon RA, Adam MP, Ardinger HH, et al, editors. GeneReviews. Seattle (WA):

University of Washington, Seattle; 2016. 1993-2017. Available at: https://www. ncbi.nlm.nih.gov/books/NBK51671/.

19. Chambers RA, Pratt RT. Idiosyncrasy to fructose. Lancet 1956;271(6938):340.

20. Froesch ER, Prader A, Labhart A, et al. Die hereditäre Fructoseintoleranz, eine bisher nicht bekannte kongenitale Stoffwechselstörung. Schweiz Med Wochenschr 1957;87(37):1168–71.

21. Hers HG, Joassin G. Anomalie de l'aldolase hépatique dans l'intolérance au fructose. Enzymol Biol Clin 1961;1:4.

22. Froesch ER, Wolf HP, Baitsch H, et al. Hereditary fructose intolerance. An inborn defect of hepatic fructose-1-phosphate splitting aldolase. Am J Med 1963;34: 151–67.

23. Steinmann B, Gitzelmann R, Van den Berghe G. Disorders of fructose metabolism. In: Valle D, Beaudet AL, Vogelstein B, et al, editors. The online metabolic and molecular bases of inherited disease. New York: McGraw-Hill; 2014. Available at: http:// ommbid.mhmedical.com.ezp-prod1.hul.harvard.edu/content.aspx?bookid=971& sectionid=62671933. Accessed January 03, 2018.

24. Ali M, Rellos P, Cox TM. Hereditary fructose intolerance. J Med Genet 1998;35(5): 353–65.

25. Munnich A, Besmond C, Darquy S, et al. Dietary and hormonal regulation of aldolase B gene expression. J Clin Invest 1985;75(3):1045–52.

26. Cross NC, de Franchis R, Sebastio G, et al. Molecular analysis of aldolase B genes in hereditary fructose intolerance. Lancet 1990;335(8685):306–9.

27. James CL, Rellos P, Ali M, et al. Neonatal screening for hereditary fructose intolerance: frequency of the most common mutant aldolase B allele (A149P) in the British population. J Med Genet 1996;33(10):837–41.

28. Baker P II, Ayres L, Gaughan S, et al. Hereditary fructose intolerance. In: Pagon RA, Adam MP, Ardinger HH, et al, editors. GeneReviews. Seattle (WA): University of Washington, Seattle; 2015. 1993-2017. Available at: https://www. ncbi.nlm.nih.gov/books/NBK333439/.

29. Scott CR. The genetic tyrosinemias. Am J Med Genet C Semin Med Genet 2006; 142C(2):121–6.

30. Mayorandan S, Meyer U, Gokcay G, et al. Cross-sectional study of 168 patients with hepatorenal tyrosinaemia and implications for clinical practice. Orphanet J Rare Dis 2014;9(1):107.

31. Sniderman King L, Trahms C, Scott CR. Tyrosinemia type I. In: Pagon RA, Adam MP, Ardinger HH, et al, editors. GeneReviews. Seattle (WA): University of Washington, Seattle; 2014. 1993-2017. Available at: https://www.ncbi.nlm.nih. gov/books/NBK1515/.

32. Lindstedt S, Holme E, Lock EA, et al. Treatment of hereditary tyrosinemia type I by inhibition of 4-hydroxyphenylpyruvate dioxygenase. Lancet 1992;340:813–7.

33. Chakrapani A, Gissen P, McKiernan P. Disorders of tyrosine metabolism. In: Saudubray JM, Baumgartner MR, Walter JH, editors. Inborn metabolic diseases - Diagnosis and treatment. 6th edition. New York: Springer-Verlag Inc; 2016. p. 265–75.

34. de Laet C, Dionisi-Vici C, Leonard JV, et al. Recommendations for the management of tyrosinaemia type 1. Orphanet J Rare Dis 2013;8(1):8.

Inborn Errors of Metabolism Involving Complex Molecules

Lysosomal and Peroxisomal Storage Diseases

Cinzia Maria Bellettato, PhD[a], Leroy Hubert, PhD[b], Maurizio Scarpa, PhD, MD[a,c,d], Michael F. Wangler, MD[b,e,f],*

KEYWORDS

- Peroxisome • Lysosome • Storage disorder • Very long chain fatty acids

KEY POINTS

- Peroxisomes and lysosomes are distinct organelles that are implicated in a range of pediatric metabolic disorders.
- Peroxisomes and lysosomes share the pattern of involvement in complex macromolecule metabolism and a relationship between their functions and diseases.
- Peroxisomal disorders are multisystem diseases due to global or single enzyme loss of peroxisomal function.
- Lysosomal disorders lead to accumulation of storage material in lysosomes in multiple organs.

PEROXISOMES, LYSOSOMES, AND DISEASE

Eukaryotic cells perform several biological processes in organelles, which compartmentalize and organize key functions (**Fig. 1**). Peroxisomes and lysosomes perform distinct metabolic functions; however, they are very similar in size, such that they were discovered around the same time by similar methods of ultracentrifugation by Christian de Duve.[1] Both peroxisomes and lysosomes catalyze several metabolic

[a] Brains for Brains Foundation, Department of Women and Children Health, Via Giustiniani 3, Padova 35128, Italy; [b] Department of Molecular and Human Genetics, Baylor College of Medicine, Houston, TX 77030, USA; [c] Center for Rare Diseases, Department of Pediatric and Adolescent Medicine, Helios Dr. Horst Schmidt Klinik, Ludwig-Erhard-Straße 100, Wiesbaden 65199, Germany; [d] Department of Women and Children Health, University of Padova, Via Giustiniani 3, Padova 35128, Italy; [e] Jan and Dan Duncan Neurological Research Institute, Texas Children's Hospital, Houston, TX 77030, USA; [f] Program in Developmental Biology, Baylor College of Medicine, Houston, TX 77030, USA
* Corresponding author. Department of Molecular and Human Genetics, Baylor College of Medicine, Houston, TX 77030.
E-mail address: michael.wangler@bcm.edu

Pediatr Clin N Am 65 (2018) 353–373
https://doi.org/10.1016/j.pcl.2017.11.011
0031-3955/18/© 2017 Elsevier Inc. All rights reserved.

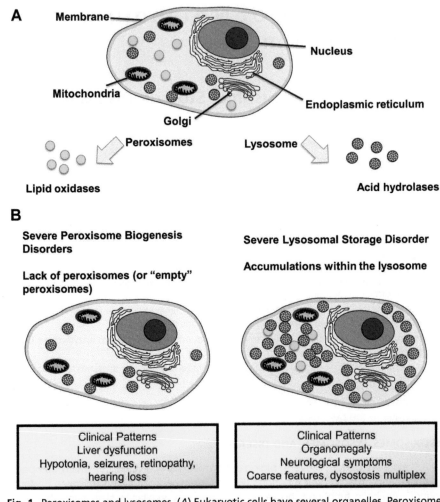

Fig. 1. Peroxisomes and lysosomes. (*A*) Eukaryotic cells have several organelles. Peroxisomes are shown in green and lysosomes are shown in yellow-red. The peroxisomes primarily contain lipid oxidases and perform complex lipid metabolism, whereas lysosomes contain enzymes, including acid hydrolases. (*B*) The most severe peroxisomal and lysosomal disease states. Severe peroxisome biogenesis disorders lead to lack of peroxisomes. The severe peroxisome biogenesis disorders have liver dysfunction, hypotonia, seizure, and retinopathy. Lysosomal storage disorders, in contrast, are characterized by lysosomal enzyme dysfunction and resultant substrate accumulation in the lysosome, resulting in organomegaly, neurologic symptoms, coarse features, and dysostosis multiplex due to bone involvement.

functions indispensable in cell biology. When these organelles are impaired they lead to several distinct pediatric metabolic disorders.[2] Although individually most of these disorders are rare, the careful clinical and cell biology characterization of these disorders has offered insight into the crucial role peroxisomes and lysosomes play in human health.[3–5] In addition, both organelles can produce a range of diseases that affect multiple organ systems, presenting to the pediatrician with an array of clinical presentations. Given the complexity of these disorders and the large number of biochemical pathways implicated, a general framework is needed for recognizing patterns and determining initial screening tests and referrals. Peroxisomes and lyso-somes share in the principle that to understand disease mechanism, insight into cell biology and organelle function is a useful initial step.

Peroxisomes and lysosomes are both made up of a single lipid bilayer and, contained within the organelle, a collection of subspecialized enzymes, particularly acid hydrolases for lysosomes and lipid oxidative enzymes for peroxisomes (see **Fig. 1A**). The organelle brings the enzymes into an environment optimal for their function, which is acidic for lysosomes[6] and highly oxidative for peroxisomes.[7]

Peroxisomal disorders are thought to stem from the biochemical dysfunction that results from absent peroxisomal enzymes.[8] At the extreme of peroxisomal dysfunction are children with severe peroxisome biogenesis disorders (PBDs) in the Zellweger-syndrome disorder (ZSD) spectrum.[8–10] These individuals lack peroxisomes or have empty or ghost peroxisomes, and the result is dramatic global peroxisomal biochemical dysfunction[11] (see **Fig. 1B**). Clinically, these individuals exhibit neurologic disease with hypotonia, epilepsy and polymicrogyria, liver disease with cholestasis and bile acid defects, and other systemic manifestations.[2] Lysosomal disorders also stem from lack of biochemical function of lysosomal enzymes but, at the extreme, result in massive accumulation of substrates within lysosomes (see **Fig. 1B**). The disease pattern for these affected individuals tends to include hepatomegaly; neurologic dysfunction, depending on the substrate; and dysostosis multiplex, a result of a lysosomal accumulative bone disease.

PEROXISOMAL DISORDERS
Peroxisomal Disorders Overview and Classification

Peroxisomal disorders can be broadly categorized as 2 distinct groups: PBDs and single enzyme defects.[2] PBDs are the result of autosomal recessive mutations in the *PEX* genes, encoding the machinery responsible for synthesizing peroxisomes and targeting enzymes to the peroxisome[7,8,12] (**Fig. 2**). In these conditions, global biochemical alterations affecting multiple peroxisomal pathways are apparent, particularly in ZSDs. A range of clinical phenotypes have been reported for PBD-ZSD and are listed in **Box 1**.

In contrast, peroxisomal single enzyme defects result from autosomal recessive (ie, X-linked for adrenoleukodystrophy) mutations in individual peroxisomal components, resulting in specific biochemical defects[18] (see **Fig. 2**).

The peroxisomal biochemical pathways (**Fig. 3A**) include the catabolism or clearance of very long chain fatty acids (VLCFAs), with greater than 22 carbon backbone, branched chain fats, such as phytanic acid, and metabolism of bile acids. Peroxisomes also synthesize several substrates, including the mature bile acids, plasmalogens, which are a unique group of membrane phospholipids with several roles in physiology,[19] and docosahexanoic acid.[20] A central peroxisomal biochemical system is the β-oxidation machinery (**Fig. 3B**). This pathway shares similar enzymatic functions with mitochondrial β-oxidation but is involved in the bile acid, branched chain fatty acid and very long chain fatty acid metabolic pathways.

Peroxisome Biogenesis Disorders Diagnosis and Treatment

The diagnostic strategy for PBD-ZSD involves demonstration of defects in multiple peroxisomal pathways.[9,10] Initial testing for children with neonatal hypotonia, seizures, polymicrogyria, and neonatal cholestasis involves plasma levels.[21] Recently some newborn screening programs incorporated detection of a lysophosphatidylcholine for X-linked adrenoleukodystrophy (X-ALD), a strategy that also uncovers neonates

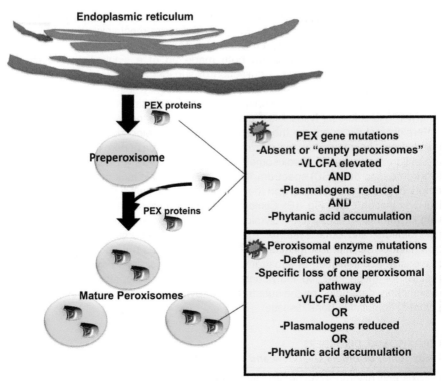

Fig. 2. Peroxisome biogenesis. Peroxisomes (green ovals) are synthesized from membrane derived from the endoplasmic reticulum (blue network) in a process achieved by the PEX proteins (green protein symbols). The peroxisomal enzymes (purple protein symbols) are internalized into the peroxisomes by PEX proteins in which they perform their biochemical functions. Severe mutations in *PEX* genes result in lack of peroxisomal biogenesis and absent or empty peroxisomes, whereas mutations in peroxisomal enzymes can lead to defects in particular peroxisomal biochemical pathways.

with PBD-ZSD.[22,23] For individuals with evidence of elevated VLCFA, red blood cell plasmalogens, if reduced, can provide evidence for a biogenesis disorder as opposed to a peroxisomal fatty acid oxidation defect.[19,24] Guidelines have suggested confirmation in skin fibroblasts by testing the enzymatic functions and the catalase solubility, an assay that detects the function of the peroxisome biogenesis machinery.[9,10]

Traditionally, molecular characterization, starting with the *PEX1* gene, the most common locus for PBD-ZSD, has followed the biochemical workup.[25–27] Next-generation sequencing has increasingly been valuable for diagnosis in PBD.[13,16,28] New methods for metabolic disease diagnosis have also emerged, including global metabolomics profiling,[29,30] and application to peroxisomal disorders remains to be fully explored. The advent of more widespread clinical sequencing, along with these newer methods and the continued effective use of targeted peroxisomal testing, fibroblast studies, and newborn screening, suggest a changing diagnostic landscape in the future for PBD-ZSD (**Fig. 4**).

Given the significant manifestations of PBD-ZSD in multiple systems, and the biochemical defects, some of which can be modified, treatment guidelines are available.[9,10] Multidisciplinary and system-based care is crucial for these individuals. Several management issues for PBD-ZSD are listed in **Box 2**.

Box 1
Clinical phenotypes of peroxisome biogenesis disorders and Zellweger spectrum disorders

Severe PBD-ZSD

- Typically termed Zellweger syndrome in the literature
- Severe neonatal presentation, dysmorphic features, seizures, polymicrogyria, severe hypotonia, and cholestasis of the liver
- Severe biochemical defects due to autosomal recessive mutations in *PEX* loci

Moderate PBD-ZSD

- Typically termed neonatal adrenoleukodystrophy in the literature
- Infantile presentation with hypotonia, feeding problems, leukodystrophy, and cholestasis of the liver
- Moderate biochemical defects due to autosomal recessive mutations in *PEX* loci

Mild PBD-ZSD

- Typically termed infantile Refsum disease in the literature
- Infantile to childhood presentation with hypotonia, hearing loss, retinopathy, and cognitive delay (can be mild)
- Mild-to-moderate biochemical defects due to autosomal recessive mutations in *PEX* loci

Heimler syndrome[13]

- Dental disease and retinopathy
- Adolescent-adult presentation
- *PEX1* or *PEX6* mutations with near normal biochemistry

Ataxia and atypical PBD-ZSD presentations

- Autosomal recessive ataxias
- Reported for *PEX2*,[14] *PEX10*,[15] *PEX16*[16,17]

Peroxisome Single Enzyme Defects

Several peroxisomal single enzyme defects can affect children. As previously noted, these disorders implicate particular peroxisomal pathways.

X-linked adrenoleukodystrophy

X-ALD is an X-linked neurodegenerative condition with adrenal insufficiency due to mutations in the *ABCD1* gene with 3 main clinical presentations[34]:

- Childhood cerebral X-ALD presents in boys between 3 and 10 years, often with a behavioral change progressing to loss of skills, cognitive decline, and neurodegeneration with inflammation
- Adrenomyeloneuropathy presents in adults with distal neuropathy and myelopathy
- Addison disease only represents individuals with isolated adrenal disease due to *ABCD1* mutations.

All affected individuals with X-ALD have elevated VLCFA in plasma. The type of mutation does not correlate to the clinical presentation. Boys with childhood cerebral X-ALD might have maternal uncles with adrenomyeloneuropathy or Addison only. Affected individuals should be monitored and treated for adrenal insufficiency. Boys in the early stage of cerebral X-ALD who undergo hematopoietic stem cell transplantation can have a slowing and eventual cessation of disease progression.[35]

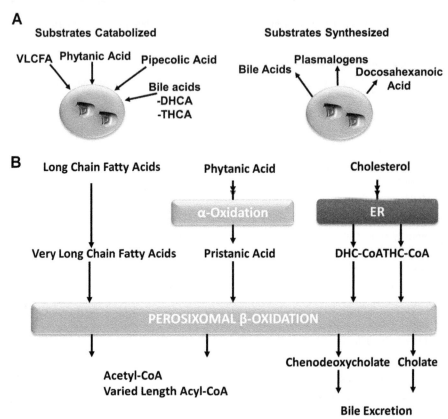

Fig. 3. Peroxisomal biochemistry. (A) Peroxisomes are involved in several metabolic and lipid metabolic pathways. Peroxisomes are required to breakdown very long chain fatty acids (VLCFA), Phytanic acid and pipecolic acid. Bile acid (breakdown of THCA and DHCA) metabolism also depends on peroxisomal oxidation. Biosynthesis also occurs in peroxisomes, and involves plasmalogen, mature bile acids, and docosahexanoic acid (DHA). (B) The peroxisomal β-oxidation pathway is involved in the metabolism of several analytes, including VLCFAs, which depend on β-oxidation for breakdown, branched chain fats such as phytanic acid that depend on α-oxidation in the peroxisome, followed by β-oxidation and bile acid metabolism, which rely on β-oxidation for the oxidation of the toxic bile acid intermediates. ER, endoplasmic reticulum; Acyl-CoA, acyl-coenzyme A.

D-bifunctional protein deficiency and other disorders of peroxisomal fatty acid β-oxidation

Individuals with single enzyme deficits in fatty acid β-oxidation can present with polymicrogyria, hypotonia, retinopathy, and hearing loss.[36] D-bifunctional protein deficiency presents with neonatal hypotonia, seizures, and death within 2 years of life,[37,38] although some individuals with milder manifestations diagnosed by exome sequencing have been recently reported.[39]

LYSOSOMAL DISORDERS
Lysosomal Disorders Overview and Classification

In contrast to peroxisomal disorders in which the biochemical defects lead to accumulations in plasma, lysosomal disorders are generally characterized by accumulation within the lysosome itself. The resulting lysosomal storage diseases (LSDs) represent

PBD-ZSD Diagnosis

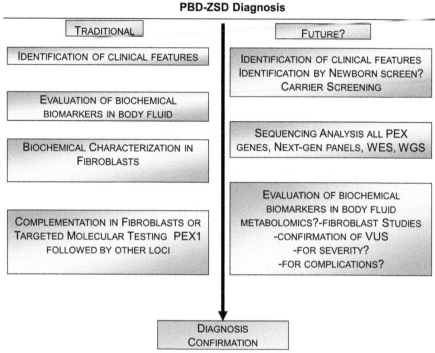

Fig. 4. Peroxisomal disease diagnosis: current and future. The traditional diagnostic paradigm for peroxisomal disorders (*left*) involves identification and clinical features, followed by the assessment of biomarkers such as VLCFA in the plasma or other markers, such as erythrocyte plasmalogen levels. Fibroblast studies, such as catalase localization and enzyme activity, are then undertaken. Molecular confirmation in a targeted manner with *PEX1* mutations being tested first. However, this paradigm for diagnosis is changing (*right*) as options for early detection, such as newborn screening or carrier screening for autosomal recessive disorders, emerge as options for parents. Affected infants are increasingly being identified by molecular studies, such as sequencing analysis, including *PEX* gene panels or whole exome sequencing (WES) or whole genome sequencing (WGS). The evaluation of biomarkers is then undertaken in plasma or fibroblasts and a role for new modalities, such as metabolomics, remains to be explored. These studies are necessary for confirming the pathogenicity of the variants from sequencing studies, and the severity and complications of disease may be correlated to the biochemical markers.

a group of more than 50 distinct rare inherited metabolic and neurodegenerative disorders caused by deficiency of a specific enzyme or lysosomal component. These defects prevent the complete degradation and recycling of specific macromolecules that accumulate inside the endosomal or lysosomal system. This leads to cell enlargement; collapse of the normal cell functions; and, eventually, cell death, giving rise to a progressive and systemic disease commonly affecting multiple organs and tissues, including the central nervous system (CNS)[40] (**Fig. 5**). This effect has been called the cytotoxicity hypothesis.[41–43] Although it was initially thought that clinical phenotypes of LSDs would directly relate to the enzymatic defect, it is now recognized that LSDs are not simply a consequence of pure storage. It is now known that LSDs result from perturbation of complex cell signaling mechanisms downstream of the lysosomal storage. Lysosome involvement in a wide variety of cell functions, including cell signaling, antigen presentation, innate and adaptive immunity,

---

Box 2
General management considerations for individuals with peroxisome biogenesis disorders and Zellweger spectrum disorders

Nutrition and growth

- Fat-soluble vitamin sufficiency and supplementation
- Nutritional and caloric optimization
- Supplementation of docosahexanoic acid (evidence limited)
- Consideration of low phytanic acid diet (evidence limited)

Neurologic

- MRI and electroencephalogram evaluation and monitoring for seizures

Visual

- Visual evaluations and optical coherence tomography

Hearing

- Auditory brainstem evoked responses

Hepatic

- Cholestasis and liver function
- Cholic acid therapy considerations[31,32]

Adrenal

- Evaluation for adrenal insufficiency

Skeletal

- Evaluation for low bone mineral density (dual-energy X-ray absorptiometry [DEXA] scan); bisphosphonate therapy has been used[33]

---

membrane remodeling, cholesterol homeostasis, apoptosis, and synaptic function, are all pleiotropic physiologic consequences resulting from the lysosomal protein defect.

Given the important role of lysosomes, it is clear that the accumulation of primary storage products triggers a complex pathologic cascade responsible for the features of the LSD pathologic and clinical manifestations.[40] The downstream events responsible for the accumulation of secondary storage products (glycosphingolipids, phospholipids, and cholesterol) can be unconnected to the primary protein defect.[44] Therefore, the pathologic consequences go far beyond the primarily affected metabolic pathway.[44]

LSDs can be grouped in 2 different ways[45,46]: (1) based on the biochemical nature of the storage material and (2) by the underlying mechanism causing the disease. In terms of the storage material, LSDs can be divided primarily into 2 major categories: mucopolysaccharidoses (MPSs) and sphingolipidoses (**Table 1**).

Mucopolysaccharidoses

MPSs are a heterogeneous group of inherited metabolic disorders caused by the absence or dysfunction of lysosomal enzymes involved in the degradation of mucopolysaccharides, also called glycosaminoglycans (GAGs). Abnormal GAGs accumulate in various organs and tissues, including the arteries, skeleton, eyes, joints, ears, skin, and/or teeth. Variable accumulations are found in the respiratory system, liver, spleen, CNS, blood, and bone marrow. Neurodegeneration can occur in the advanced

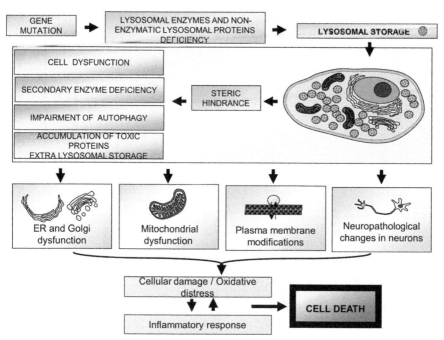

Fig. 5. The cytotoxicity hypothesis of lysosomal storage. Homozygous or compound heterozygous mutations in the genes encoding the lysosomal enzymes and leading to loss-of-function of the enzymatic pathway result in accumulation of lysosomes packed with unmetabolized substrate. This accumulation initiates a cascade involving additional secondary biochemical deficiencies, cell dysfunction, impairment of the recycling autophagy function of the cell, and accumulation of additional toxic proteins both inside and outside the lysosome. This results in dysfunction of the Golgi, ER, mitochondria, and resultant neuropathology due to cell death.

stages of the disease.[47] There are 4 different pathways of lysosomal degradation of GAGs, depending on the molecule to be degraded:

1. Dermatan sulfate, typically found in connective tissue and skin as well as bone, cartilage and tendons, internal organs, blood vessels, and cornea and other tissues
2. Heparan sulfate, a ubiquitous constituent of glycoproteins and the basal membrane
3. Keratan sulfate, a constituent of bone, cartilage, and the cornea
4. Chondroitin sulfate, usually found attached to proteins as part of a proteoglycan.

The stepwise GAGs degradation requires 10 different enzymes: 4 glycosidases, 5 sulfatases, and 1 nonhydrolytic transferase (**Table 2**).

Except MPS II (Hunter syndrome), which is an X-linked disease and affects mostly male patients, all MPSs follow an autosomal-recessive inheritance. Although individually rare, all MPSs account for approximately 1 in 22,000 live births, representing approximately the 35% of all affected individuals with LSDs.[48]

The main manifestations are dwarfism, short neck, coarse face, hepatosplenomegaly, corneal clouding, macroglossia, recurrent infections of ears and upper airways, hernias, cardiac and pulmonary involvement, thoracolumbar kyphoscoliosis, claw hands, joint stiffness and contractures, dysostosis multiplex, and (in some types) neurocognitive impairment; however, symptoms depend on the specific type of stored

Table 1
Classification of lysosomal storage disease according to storage material and molecular defect

Disease Category by Storage Type	Main Storage Material	Disease	Deficiency	Disease Category by Defect
Sphingolipidosis	Glucosylceramide	Gaucher disease	Glucosylceramidase	Primary lysosomal hydrolase defect
	Glucosylceramide	—	Saposin-C activator	
	GM1 ganglioside	GM1 gangliosidosis	β-galactosidase	
	GM2 ganglioside or glycolipid	Tay-Sachs disease	β-hexosaminidase A	
	GM2 ganglioside or glycolipid	Sandhoff disease	β-hexosaminidase A and B	
	Globotriaosylceramide	Fabry disease	α-galactosidase A	
	Sphingomyelin	Niemann-Pick A and B	Sphingomyelinase	
	Galactocerebroside	Krabbe disease	Galactosylceramidase	
	Lipid or mucopolysaccharides	Mucolipidosis II and IIIA	N-acetyl glucosamine Phosphoryl transferase	Trafficking defect in lysosomal enzymes
Mucopolysaccharidosis	Lipid or mucopolysaccharides	Galactosialidosis	Protective protein cathepsin A (β-galactosidase and neuraminidase)	Defect in lysosomal enzyme protection
Sphingolipidosis	GM2 ganglioside or glycolipid	GM2 activator protein deficiency	GM2 activator protein	Defect in soluble nonenzymatic lysosomal protein
	Glycolipids	Sphingolipid activator protein deficiency	Sphingolipid activator protein	
	Subunit c of mitochondrial ATP synthase	Late-infantile NCL	CLN5	
	Cholesterol and sphingolipid	Niemann-Pick C	NPC-1 NPC-2	Transmembrane protein
	Subunit c of mitochondrial ATP synthase	Juvenile NCL	CLN3	
	Sialic acid	Salla disease	Sialin	Others
	Sulphatides	mucosulphatidosis	Multiple sulphatases	
	Sphingolipid activator Proteins A and D	Infantile NCL	PPT1	—
Oligosaccharidosis and glycoproteinosis	Glycogen	Pompe disease	α-glucosidase	—
	Cholesterol esters	Lysosomal acid lipase deficiency	Lysosomal acid lipase	—

Abbreviations: ATP, adenosine triphosphate; CLN5, Ceroid-lipofuscinosis neuronal protein 5; NCL, neuronal ceroid lipofuscinosis.

Data from Futerman AH, van Meer G. The cell biology of lysosomal storage disorders. Nat Rev Mol Cell Biol 2004;5(7):554–65; and Jeyakumar M, Dwek RA, Butters TD, et al. Storage solutions: treating lysosomal disorders of the brain. Nat Rev Neurosci 2005;6(9):713–25.

Table 2
Mucopolysaccharidoses, related enzyme deficits, glycosaminoglycans storage, and main clinical manifestations

MPSs	Enzyme Deficit	GAG Storage	Main Clinical Signs and Symptoms
MPS I (Hurler)	α-L-iduronidase	Heparan sulfate, Dermatan sulfate	Cognitive impairment, developmental delay, severe coarse facies, hearing loss, corneal clouding, macroglossia, hydrocephalus, cardiomyopathy, hepatosplenomegaly, inguinal and umbilical hernia, airway obstruction, dysostosis multiplex, limited joint mobility, death by age 10 y
MPS I (Scheie)	α-L-iduronidase	Heparan sulfate, Dermatan sulfate	Micrognathia, toe walking, moderate coarse facies, possible normal intelligence, death by 20 y
MPS I (Hurler-Scheie)	α-L-iduronidase	Heparan sulfate, Dermatan Sulfate	Aortic valve disease, joint dysostosis, corneal clouding, normal facies, death in decades
MPS II (Hunter)	Iduronate 2-sulfatase	Heparan sulfate, Dermatan Sulfate	In severe forms: no corneal clouding, physical disease similar to MPS I, characteristic skin rash, aggressive behavior and developmental delay, profound neurologic involvement, usually results in death in the first or second decade of life In milder forms: normal or near-normal intelligence
MPS IIIA (Sanfilippo A)	Heparan sulphamidase	Heparan sulfate	Mild somatic disease associated with sleep disturbances and aggressive behavior followed by severe progressive CNS degeneration
MPS IIIB (Sanfilippo B)	Acetyl α-glucosaminidase	Heparan sulfate	
MPS IIIC (Sanfilippo C)	Acetyl Coenzyme A: α-glucosaminide, N-acetyltransferase	Heparan sulfate	
MPS IIID (Sanfilippo D)	N-acetylglucosamine-6-sulphatase	Heparan sulfate	Affected individuals with the attenuated phenotype exhibit a more gradual disease progression with longer survival

(continued on next page)

Table 2
(continued)

MPSs	Enzyme Deficit	GAG Storage	Main Clinical Signs and Symptoms
MPS IVA (Morquio A)	Acetylgalactosamine-6-sulphatase	Keratan sulfate, chondroitin 6-sulphate	The phenotypic spectrum of MPS IVA is a continuum that ranges from a severe and rapidly progressive early-onset form to a slowly progressive later-onset form. The severe form is characterized by skeletal involvement (kyphoscoliosis, genu valgum, and pectus carinatum), short stature, ligamentous laxity, corneal opacities, typically normal intelligence. The slowly progressive form is mainly characterized by hip problems (pain, stiffness, and Legg Perthes disease)
MPS IVB (Morquio B)	β-galactosidase	Keratan sulfate	MPS IV B is much rarer than MPS IV A and the 2 forms are clinically indistinguishable because the severity of symptoms varies in both types
MPS VI (Maroteaux- Lamy)	Arylsulphatase B	Dermatan sulfate	Like MPS I, it presents short stature, hepatosplenomegaly, dysostosis multiplex, stiff joints, corneal clouding, cardiac abnormalities, and facial dysmorphism. No CNS disease (intelligence is usually normal). Death in teens and 20s
MPS VII (Sly)	β-glucuronidase	Dermatan sulfate, heparan sulfate, chondroitin 6-sulphate	Variable intermediate presentation similar to MPS I: coarse facial features, intellectual disability, hepatosplenomegaly, mild skeletal dysostosis in teens. A wide range of clinical variability exists, from the most severe type with hydrops fetalis to a milder phenotype with later onset and normal intelligence
MPS IX (Natowicz)	Hyaluronidase	Hyaluronan	Nodular synovium, popliteal cyst, large joint effusion

GAGs. A pathologic CNS typically causes intellectual disability, progressive neurodegeneration, and premature death. Depending on the subtype, affected individuals may have normal intellect or may be profoundly impaired, may experience developmental delay, or may have severe behavioral problems.

MPSs mostly affect the pediatric population and approximately 70% of all affected individuals present with neurologic involvement. Severe brain involvement characterizes all forms of MPS III, whereas in MPS I, II, and VII a progressive mental delay accompanied by behavioral problems affects the severe forms of these diseases. Finally, MPS IV and VI do not commonly show any significant brain involvement. All MPS disorders affecting dermatan sulfate breakdown show typical progressive morphologic changes that may or may not be associated with mental decline (intelligence is usually normal in MPS VI, Maroteaux-Lamy, and in the nonneuronopathic forms of MPS I and II).[49] In contrast, disorders affecting only heparan sulfate are usually associated with intellectual disability but, as in Sanfilippo disease (MPS type III), do not always show the characteristic morphologic changes. Similarly, in MPS type IV (Morquio disease), the deficient breakdown of keratan sulfate causes a severe skeletal dysplasia but usually is not associated with intellectual disability.[49] It must be highlighted that the degradation of different types of GAGs may include similar lysosomal enzymes (glycosidases and sulfatases), thus the types of degradation products due to single enzyme defect may originate from different types of partially degraded GAGs.[50]

Sphingolipidoses

Sphingolipidoses are a class of lipid storage disorders relating to sphingolipid metabolism. Defects in the degradation of sphingolipids, an essential component of myelin sheaths and neuronal tissue, lead to progressive neurodegeneration, epilepsy, peripheral neuropathy, extrapyramidal symptoms, and characteristic retinal cherry-red spots. The disorders of this group are Gaucher disease (GD), Tay-Sachs disease, Niemann-Pick (NP) disease, Fabry disease (FD), Krabbe disease (KD), and metachromatic leukodystrophy (MLD). They are generally inherited in an autosomal recessive fashion but, notably, FD is X-linked recessive. Taken together, sphingolipidoses have an incidence of approximately 1 in 10,000, but substantially more in certain populations, such as Ashkenazi Jews.

Gaucher disease

GD is the most common sphingolipidosis. It has a prevalence of approximately 1 in 70,000 and is caused by a deficiency of the lysosomal enzyme glucocerebrosidase (ie, acid β-glucosidase), which induces storage of glycolipids in lysosomes, typically inside the cells of the macrophage-monocyte system. Characteristic manifestations include hepatosplenomegaly; severely debilitating bone and hematological disease; and, in the more severe cases, CNS involvement. Three different phenotypes of GD are identified. Type I GD (GDI), the most common, is characterized by splenomegaly, thrombocytopenia, and anemia; it differs from the more severe types II and III GD because it does not have neurologic manifestations.[51] This unique feature has rendered GDI an ideal target for therapeutic industry and, in 1991, enzyme replacement therapy (ERT) for GDI constituted the first breakthrough LSDs therapy in the LSDs commercial treatment.

Niemann-Pick disease

NP is a lipid storage disorder, most commonly affecting infants, which results from the deficiency of acid sphingomyelinase. Three genes (*ASM*, *NPC1*, and *NPC2*), acting on 2 pathways: sphingomyelin hydrolysis and cholesterol transport, underlie NP. The loss of sphingomyelinase activity in NP has a significant impact at the plasma membrane through its effect on ceramide production and lipid raft formation.[52] Defective sphingomyelinase activity can alter apoptotic signaling, leading to Purkinje cell loss in the cerebellum and neurologic manifestation. Sphingomyelin also accumulates at inappropriate sites in neurons, causing defective neuronal survival, synaptic vesicle docking, and (potentially), synaptic function.[52] This further highlights the links between disturbed lipid metabolism, altered lysosomal function, and neuropathology in the lysosomal storage disorders. Two major types exist: type A (the acute infantile form, clinically mainly characterized by failure to thrive) and hepatosplenomegaly, as well as rapidly progressive neurodegenerative disorders. Type B is a milder, less common, chronic, nonneurological form, mainly manifesting with hepatosplenomegaly, growth retardation, and pulmonary infections and dyspnea. A third type of NP is represented by NP type C, which is a biochemically and genetically distinct form of the disease caused by a deficit of cholesterol esterification characterized as visceral, neurologic, and/or psychiatric manifestations, depending on the age of onset: ascites, severe liver disease, and/or respiratory failure in infancy; ataxia, vertical supranuclear gaze palsy, and dementia in childhood; and dementia or psychiatric symptoms in adulthood.

Fabry disease

FD is an X-linked LSD resulting from deficient activity of the enzyme α-galactosidase A. Accumulation of globotriaosylceramide is observed within lysosomes in a variety of cell types, including capillary endothelial, renal (podocytes, tubular cells, glomerular endothelial, mesangial, and interstitial), cardiac (cardiomyocytes and fibroblasts), and nerve cells. In the affected tissue, cellular death, compromised energy metabolism, small vessel injury, calcium-activated potassium (K[Ca]3.1) channel dysfunction in endothelial cells, oxidative stress, and impaired autophagosome maturation are all seen.[53] Tissue ischemia and, importantly, development of irreversible cardiac and renal tissue fibrosis can also occur, further contributing to significant morbidity and mortality. Typically, it affects male patients with symptoms manifesting in childhood or adolescence with acroparesthesia, angiokeratomas, anhidrosis, hypohidrosis, or (rarely) hyperhidrosis, corneal and lenticular opacities, and proteinuria. Some literature suggests that female patients heterozygous for mutations in the α-galactosidase gene are mainly asymptomatic or have mild symptoms.[54] However, recent work with the Fabry Outcome Survey cases suggests that female patients have symptoms more frequently than originally reported.[55]

Gangliosidosis

Gangliosidosis is a subcategory of sphingolipidosis that contains 2 types of lipid storage disorders: GM1 gangliosides and GM2 gangliosidoses. Both types are autosomal recessive diseases caused by the accumulation of lipids known as gangliosides (vital signaling, transport, and regulatory proteins consisting of the neuronal plasma and lysosomal membranes) in the nervous system.

GM1 gangliosidosis is caused by mutations in GLB1, leading to decreased activity of β-galactosidase, a lysosomal hydrolase, which hydrolyzes the terminal β-galactosyl residues from GM1, glycoproteins, and GAGs. GM1 gangliosides, oligosaccharides, and the mucopolysaccharide keratan sulfates (and their derivatives) accumulate.

The term GM2 gangliosidosis includes 3 clinical forms caused by mutations in at least 1 of 3 recessive genes: HEXA, HEXB, and GM2A coding for the alpha subunits of β-hexosaminidase A (Hex A), the beta subunits of Hex A and the subunits of β-hexosaminidase B (Hex B), and the GM2 activator protein, respectively. A deficiency of lysosomal enzyme β-Hex A causes Tay-Sachs disease, whereas a combined defi-ciency of β-Hex A and Hex B causes Sandhoff disease. GM2 gangliosidosis AB variant is characterized by normal Hex A and Hex B but with the inability to form a functional GM2 activator complex due to absence or defects of the hexosaminidase activator.

Gangliosidoses can manifest with severe, extremely variable clinical symptoms in almost any age group, though the most common manifestations are characterized by early infantile onset and a late infantile or juvenile fatal disease, mostly due to CNS involvement.[56] Severity of the progressive neurodegeneration is proportional to the re-sidual enzyme activity. Hallmarks of GM1 gangliosidosis are dysostosis, and coarsening and degeneration of the CNS, in which ganglioside synthesis is the highest,[57] whereas classic infantile GM2 gangliosidoses present with spared systemic involvement, except in the case of the Sandhoff variant, in which organomegaly and bony deformity may occur. Macular cherry-red spots are typical of early onset forms of the gangliosidoses and are less frequently manifested in the less severe, later-onset phenotypes. Macroce-phaly, a marked startle reflex to noise, seizures, cognitive decline, ataxia, and progres-sive muscular atrophy may occur in the different forms of gangliosidosis.[58]

Krabbe disease

KD is an autosomal recessive sphingolipidosis caused by deficient activity of galacto-sylceramide β-galactosidase, also named galactosylceramidase, a lysosomal hydro-lase that degrades galactosylceramide (a major lipid in myelin, kidney, and epithelial cells of the small intestine and colon), and other terminal β-galactose–containing sphingolipids, including psychosine (galactosylsphingosine). Most disease-causing missense mutations result in the production of the galactocerebrosidase enzyme, which is unstable, rapidly degraded, and consequently less active, leading to accumu-lation of incompletely metabolized galactocerebroside and increased psychosine levels, which are responsible of progressive white matter disease and widespread destruction of oligodendroglia in the CNS and to subsequent demyelination. Typically, disease onset is within the first year of life with irritability, severe progressive neurologic deterioration, developmental delay, and vision deficits, as well as early death. Juvenile and adult-onset cases may have less classic presentations with variable psychomotor deterioration and vision loss, making diagnosis difficult and often delayed.[59]

Metachromatic leukodystrophy

MLD is due to the arylsulfatase A deficiency, which is commonly listed in the cate-gories of leukodystrophies, as well as among the sphingolipidoses, because it affects the sphingolipids metabolism. Leukodystrophies affect the growth and/or develop-ment of myelin. In MLD, deficient activity of arylsulfatase A, or lack of a cofactor, cause accumulation of sulfatide in various tissues and diffuse demyelination, with no curative treatment currently available.[60,61]

Three clinical subtypes exist: a late-infantile form, characterized by rapid deteri-oration of motor and neurocognitive function; a juvenile form, manifesting with cognitive and behavioral problems followed by slowly progressing motor decline; and an adult form, mainly presenting as a psychiatric disorder or progressive dementia.

Lysosomal Storage Disease Diagnosis

Timely diagnosis of LSDs is often difficult and demands high clinical suspicion, phys-ical examination, appropriate investigations, and a coordinated approach of many different medical specialists. This is particularly true for individuals with more attenu-ated phenotypes; in these cases, diagnosis is often missed or delayed.

Clinical suspicion should be raised by the by the following clinical findings:

- Presence of dysmorphic features (coarse facies, macroglossia)
- Skeletal radiographic evidence of dysostosis multiplex (joint or skeletal deformities)
- Short stature
- Hepatosplenomegaly
- Presence of umbilical or inguinal hernias
- Abnormal hearing screening results
- Presence of angiokeratoma
- Echocardiographic evidence of cardiac involvement (arrhythmia or cardiomegaly)
- Muscle weakness
- Neurologic deterioration (decline in motor skills or other development, increasing dementia or behavioral or psychiatric abnormalities, and seizures)

Other important laboratory findings include

- Presence of white blood cell vacuoles (granular, fingerprint lipid whorls, zebra bodies, or autophagic vacuoles) in peripheral blood smear
- Elevated excretion of oligosaccharides (oligosaccharidoses) and GAGs (MPSs) from urine test
- Elevated level of blood chitotriosidase (enzymatic marker of macrophage activation).

In suspected cases, final diagnosis is confirmed by measurement of enzymatic activity (by biochemical and/or molecular assay, commonly using cells derived from peripheral blood) and DNA mutation analysis.

Currently, newborn screening offers a potential mechanism for the early detection of these disorders.

Lysosomal Storage Disease Management

Several therapies for treating the LSDs already exist and are commercially available (**Fig. 6**). They can be divided into 2 major groups:

Those restoring lysosomal activity
- ERT consists of the regular intravenous infusions of a recombinant form of the defective enzyme, which is then scavenged by affected cells, endocytosed, and incorporated into lysosomes, restoring functional activity. The first ERT for Gaucher type I went on the market in 1991. ERT is a treatment option for Gaucher type I, Fabry, MPS I, Pompe, MPS II, MPS IV, and MPS VI. Clinical trials studying an investigational ERT (Recombinant human beta-glucuronidase [rhGUS; UX003]) in individuals with MPS VII are ongoing. Unfortunately, ERT does not cross the blood-brain barrier, thus hindering effective treatment of LSDs with CNS involvement. To overcome this problem, direct intrathecal administration of ERT is being investigated in individuals with MPS I, MPS II, and MPS III.
- Bone marrow transplant consists of using donor bone-marrow-derived cells as a source of enzyme. Since the first attempt in the 1980s, it has shown some positive results, especially when performed early in a disease's course.
- Hematopoietic stem cell transplant consists of intravenous transplantation of healthy stem cells (usually from bone marrow, sometimes from cord blood) producing the enzyme, as well as new healthy cells. It has shown to be efficacious in

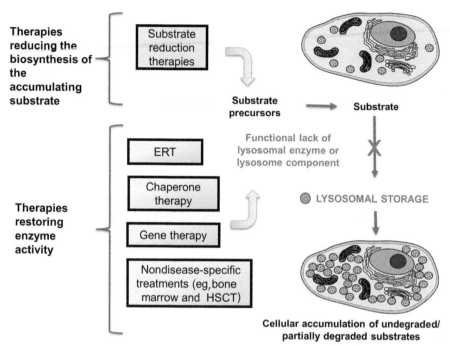

Fig. 6. Therapeutic strategies in lysosomal storage disease. A wide array of therapeutic strategies for LSDs is available and differs in efficacy for the different disorders. However, the rationale for the strategies includes reducing the substrate that is appearing in the lysosome with substrate reduction therapy. Another strategy is to restore function to the lysosome, which can use several approaches, including ERT, chaperones to facilitate folding of misfolded enzymes, gene therapy to rescue the genetic defect, or bone marrow transplantation to allow for clearance of the substrate by donor cells. HSCT, hematopoietic stem cell transplantation.

MPS I if started before the manifestation of neuroregression. It has also been tried in several other LSDs, including MLD, KD, and GD.
- Gene therapy is currently only used in animal models. Multiple viral vectors have been used to accomplish in vivo gene transfer, such as herpesviruses, lentiviruses, adeno-associated viruses, adenoviruses, and others.[62]
- Protein chaperone therapy (PCT) consists of the use of small molecule compounds to assist the folding of mutated enzymes, therefore restoring their catalytic activity. Since 2006, PCT has been in early-stage clinical trials for FD, GDI, and Pompe. Recent data indicate that PCT is a promising strategy for KD.[63,64]

Those reducing the biosynthesis of the accumulating substrate
- Substrate reduction therapy (SRT) consists of the oral administration of a drug capable of inhibiting or reducing the rate of production of the substrate, reducing the metabolic load on the lysosome. The inhibitors Zavesca (miglustat) and Cerdelga (eliglustat) are the only SRT agents available and approved for affected individuals who are unable to tolerate ERT for GD. Indeed, SRT although used for other disorders, is only approved for GD by the US Food and Drug Administration. Clinical trials are ongoing for Niemann-Pick Disease Type C (NPC) FD, GM2, Tay-Sachs, and Sandhoff.

Because more than 70% of individuals with LSDs suffer from different grades of CNS involvement,[40,65] current research efforts are particularly focused on the development of new strategic approaches for enhancing enzyme delivery across the blood-brain barrier. Several clinical trials are ongoing for MPS III A and B, MPS VII, MLD, Neuronal ceroid lipofuscinosis type 2 (CLN2) neuronal ceroid lipofuscinosis, α-mannosidosis deficiency, GM2 gangliosidosis, acid sphingomyelinase deficiency, and MPS II (intrathecal ERT). Additional studies will be required for assessing related efficacy and safety, and for a better comprehension of the mechanisms that drive the drug delivery process.

SUMMARY

Diseases of the peroxisome and lysosome are individually rare in the pediatric population but they collectively make up a substantial burden of metabolic disease. These disorders have defined diagnostic and management strategies that are related to an understanding of the function of the organelle and the pathogenesis of these important disorders.

REFERENCES

1. de Duve C. The lysosome turns fifty. Nat Cell Biol 2005;7(9):847–9.
2. Baumgartner MR, Saudubray JM. Peroxisomal disorders. Semin Neonatol 2002; 7(1):85–94.
3. Delille HK, Bonekamp NA, Schrader M. Peroxisomes and disease - an overview. Int J Biomed Sci 2006;2(4):308–14.
4. Pan T, Kondo S, Le W, et al. The role of autophagy-lysosome pathway in neurodegeneration associated with Parkinson's disease. Brain 2008;131(Pt 8): 1969–78.
5. Lizard G, Rouaud O, Demarquoy J, et al. Potential roles of peroxisomes in Alzheimer's disease and in dementia of the Alzheimer's type. J Alzheimers Dis 2012;29(2):241–54.
6. Sun-Wada GH, Wada Y, Futai M. Lysosome and lysosome-related organelles responsible for specialized functions in higher organisms, with special emphasis on vacuolar-type proton ATPase. Cell Struct Funct 2003;28(5):455–63.
7. Wanders RJ, Waterham HR. Biochemistry of mammalian peroxisomes revisited. Annu Rev Biochem 2006;75:295–332.
8. Wanders RJ, Waterham HR. Peroxisomal disorders I: biochemistry and genetics of peroxisome biogenesis disorders. Clin Genet 2005;67(2):107–33.
9. Braverman NE, Raymond GV, Rizzo WB, et al. Peroxisome biogenesis disorders in the Zellweger spectrum: an overview of current diagnosis, clinical manifestations, and treatment guidelines. Mol Genet Metab 2016;117(3):313–21.
10. Klouwer FC, Berendse K, Ferdinandusse S, et al. Zellweger spectrum disorders: clinical overview and management approach. Orphanet J Rare Dis 2015;10:151.
11. Wanders RJ. Metabolic and molecular basis of peroxisomal disorders: a review. Am J Med Genet 2004;126A(4):355–75.
12. Moser HW. Genotype-phenotype correlations in disorders of peroxisome biogenesis. Mol Genet Metab 1999;68(2):316–27.
13. Ratbi I, Falkenberg KD, Sommen M, et al. Heimler syndrome is caused by hypomorphic mutations in the peroxisome-biogenesis genes PEX1 and PEX6. Am J Hum Genet 2015;97(4):535–45.
14. Gootjes J, Elpeleg O, Eyskens F, et al. Novel mutations in the PEX2 gene of four unrelated patients with a peroxisome biogenesis disorder. Pediatr Res 2004; 55(3):431–6.

15. Regal L, Ebberink MS, Goemans N, et al. Mutations in PEX10 are a cause of autosomal recessive ataxia. Ann Neurol 2010;68(2):259–63.
16. Bacino C, Chao YH, Soto E, et al. A homozygous mutation in identified by whole-exome sequencing ending a diagnostic odyssey. Mol Genet Metab Rep 2015;5:15–8.
17. Ebberink MS, Csanyi B, Chong WK, et al. Identification of an unusual variant peroxisome biogenesis disorder caused by mutations in the PEX16 gene. J Med Genet 2010;47(9):608–15.
18. Van Veldhoven PP. Biochemistry and genetics of inherited disorders of peroxisomal fatty acid metabolism. J Lipid Res 2010;51(10):2863–95.
19. Braverman NE, Moser AB. Functions of plasmalogen lipids in health and disease. Biochim Biophys Acta 2012;1822(9):1442–52.
20. Paker AM, Sunness JS, Brereton NH, et al. Docosahexaenoic acid therapy in peroxisomal diseases: results of a double-blind, randomized trial. Neurology 2010;75(9):826–30.
21. Moser AB, Kreiter N, Bezman L, et al. Plasma very long chain fatty acids in 3,000 peroxisome disease patients and 29,000 controls. Ann Neurol 1999;45(1):100–10.
22. Hubbard WC, Moser AB, Liu AC, et al. Newborn screening for X-linked adrenoleukodystrophy (X-ALD): validation of a combined liquid chromatography-tandem mass spectrometric (LC-MS/MS) method. Mol Genet Metab 2009; 97(3):212–20.
23. Hubbard WC, Moser AB, Tortorelli S, et al. Combined liquid chromatography-tandem mass spectrometry as an analytical method for high throughput screening for X-linked adrenoleukodystrophy and other peroxisomal disorders: preliminary findings. Mol Genet Metab 2006;89(1–2):185–7.
24. Heymans HS, Schutgens RB, Tan R, et al. Severe plasmalogen deficiency in tissues of infants without peroxisomes (Zellweger syndrome). Nature 1983; 306(5938):69–70.
25. Gartner J, Preuss N, Brosius U, et al. Mutations in PEX1 in peroxisome biogenesis disorders: G843D and a mild clinical phenotype. J Inherit Metab Dis 1999;22(3): 311–3.
26. Poll-The BT, Gootjes J, Duran M, et al. Peroxisome biogenesis disorders with prolonged survival: phenotypic expression in a cohort of 31 patients. Am J Med Genet 2004;126A(4):333–8.
27. Walter C, Gootjes J, Mooijer PA, et al. Disorders of peroxisome biogenesis due to mutations in PEX1: phenotypes and PEX1 protein levels. Am J Hum Genet 2001; 69(1):35–48.
28. Ventura MJ, Wheaton D, Xu M, et al. Diagnosis of a mild peroxisomal phenotype with next-generation sequencing. Mol Genet Metab Rep 2016;9:75–8.
29. Donti TR, Cappuccio G, Hubert L, et al. Diagnosis of adenylosuccinate lyase deficiency by metabolomic profiling in plasma reveals a phenotypic spectrum. Mol Genet Metab Rep 2016;8:61–6.
30. Miller MJ, Kennedy AD, Eckhart AD, et al. Untargeted metabolomic analysis for the clinical screening of inborn errors of metabolism. J Inherit Metab Dis 2015; 38(6):1029–39.
31. Berendse K, Klouwer FC, Koot BG, et al. Cholic acid therapy in Zellweger spectrum disorders. J Inherit Metab Dis 2016;39(6):859–68.
32. Setchell KD, Bragetti P, Zimmer-Nechemias L, et al. Oral bile acid treatment and the patient with Zellweger syndrome. Hepatology 1992;15(2):198–207.
33. Rush ET, Goodwin JL, Braverman NE, et al. Low bone mineral density is a common feature of Zellweger spectrum disorders. Mol Genet Metab 2016; 117(1):33–7.

34. Moser HW, Mahmood A, Raymond GV. X-linked adrenoleukodystrophy. Nat Clin Pract Neurol 2007;3(3):140–51.

35. Krivit W, Peters C, Shapiro EG. Bone marrow transplantation as effective treatment of central nervous system disease in globoid cell leukodystrophy, metachromatic leukodystrophy, adrenoleukodystrophy, mannosidosis, fucosidosis, aspartylglucosaminuria, Hurler, Maroteaux-Lamy, and Sly syndromes, and Gaucher disease type III. Curr Opin Neurol 1999;12(2):167–76.

36. Clayton PT. Clinical consequences of defects in peroxisomal beta-oxidation. Biochem Soc Trans 2001;29(Pt 2):298–305.

37. Ferdinandusse S, Denis S, Mooyer PA, et al. Clinical and biochemical spectrum of D-bifunctional protein deficiency. Ann Neurol 2006;59(1):92–104.

38. Ferdinandusse S, Ylianttila MS, Gloerich J, et al. Mutational spectrum of D-bifunctional protein deficiency and structure-based genotype-phenotype analysis. Am J Hum Genet 2006;78(1):112–24.

39. Matsukawa T, Koshi KM, Mitsui J, et al. Slowly progressive d-bifunctional protein deficiency with survival to adulthood diagnosed by whole-exome sequencing. J Neurol Sci 2017;372:6–10.

40. Bellettato CM, Scarpa M. Pathophysiology of neuropathic lysosomal storage disorders. J Inherit Metab Dis 2010;33(4):347–62.

41. Gieselmann V. Lysosomal storage diseases. Biochim Biophys Acta 1995; 1270(2–3):103–36.

42. Cox TM, Cachon-Gonzalez MB. The cellular pathology of lysosomal diseases. J Pathol 2012;226(2):241–54.

43. Desnick RJ, Thorpe SR, Fiddler MB. Toward enzyme therapy for lysosomal storage diseases. Physiol Rev 1976;56(1):57–99.

44. Walkley SU, Vanier MT. Pathomechanisms in Lysosomal Storage Disorders. Biochim Biophys Acta 2009;1793(4):726–36.

45. Ballabio A, Gieselmann V. Lysosomal disorders: from storage to cellular damage. Biochim Biophys Acta 2009;1793(4):684–96.

46. Platt FM, Walkley SU. Lysosomal disorders of the brain: recent advances in molecular and cellular pathogenesis and treatment. New York: Oxford University Press; 2004.

47. Lampe C, Bellettato CM, Karabul N, et al. Mucopolysaccharidoses and other lysosomal storage diseases. Rheum Dis Clin North Am 2013;39(2):431–55.

48. Quiney FRE, Amirfeyz R, Smithson S, et al. The Mucopolysaccharidoses. Orthop Trauma 2012;6(1):60–3.

49. Hoffmann GF, Zschocke J, Nyhan WL. Inherited metabolic diseases: a clinical approach. Springer; 2009.

50. Greiner-Tollersrud OK, Berg T. Lysosomal storage disorders. Madame Curie bioscience database [Internet]. Austin (TX): Landes Bioscience; 2000–2013.

51. Biegstraaten M, van Schaik IN, Aerts JM, et al. 'Non-neuronopathic' Gaucher disease reconsidered. Prevalence of neurological manifestations in a Dutch cohort of type I Gaucher disease patients and a systematic review of the literature. J Inherit Metab Dis 2008;31(3):337–49.

52. Parkinson-Lawrence EJ, Shandala T, Prodoehl M, et al. Lysosomal storage disease: revealing lysosomal function and physiology. Physiology (Bethesda) 2010;25(2):102.

53. Germain DP. Fabry disease. Orphanet J Rare Dis 2010;5:30.

54. Mehta A, Hughes DA. Fabry disease. In: Pagon RA, Adam MP, Ardinger HH, et al, editors. GeneReviews [Internet]. Seattle (WA): Univeristy of Washington, Seattle; 1993–2017. Available from http://www.ncbi.nlm.nih.gove/books/NBK1292/.

55. Deegan PB, Baehner AF, Barba Romero MA, et al. Natural history of Fabry disease in females in the Fabry Outcome Survey. J Med Genet 2006;43(4):347–52.
56. Sandhoff K, Harzer K. Gangliosides and gangliosidoses: principles of molecular and metabolic pathogenesis. J Neurosci 2013;33(25):10195–208.
57. Okada S, O'Brien JS. Generalized gangliosidosis: beta-galactosidase deficiency. Science 1968;160(3831):1002–4.
58. Patterson MC. Gangliosidoses. Handb Clin Neurol 2013;113:1707–8.
59. Pastores GM. Krabbe disease: an overview. Int J Clin Pharmacol Ther 2009; 47(Suppl 1):S75–81.
60. Batzios SP, Zafeiriou DI. Developing treatment options for metachromatic leukodystrophy. Mol Genet Metab 2012;105(1):56–63.
61. Gieselmann V, Krageloh-Mann I. Metachromatic leukodystrophy–an update. Neuropediatrics 2010;41(1):1–6.
62. Sands MS, Davidson BL. Gene therapy for lysosomal storage diseases. Mol Ther 2006;13(5):839–49.
63. Spratley SJ, Deane JE. New therapeutic approaches for Krabbe disease: The potential of pharmacological chaperones. J Neurosci Res 2016;94(11):1203–19.
64. Hughes DA, Nicholls K, Shankar SP, et al. Oral pharmacological chaperone migalastat compared with enzyme replacement therapy in Fabry disease: 18-month results from the randomised phase III ATTRACT study. J Med Genet 2017; 54(4):288–96.
65. Platt FM, Boland B, van der Spoel AC. The cell biology of disease: lysosomal storage disorders: the cellular impact of lysosomal dysfunction. J Cell Biol 2012; 199(5):723–34.

Complex Phenotypes in Inborn Errors of Metabolism

Overlapping Presentations in Congenital Disorders of Glycosylation and Mitochondrial Disorders

Thatjana Gardeitchik, MD[a], Jeroen Wyckmans, MD[b],
Eva Morava, MD, PhD[b,c],*

KEYWORDS

- Glycosylation • Mitochondrial disease • Lactic acid
- Transferrin isoelectric focusing (TIEF) • Stroke-like episodes • Hypoglycemia
- Cutis laxa • Cholestasis

KEY POINTS

- Congenital disorders of glycosylation (CDG) and mitochondrial disorders are multisystem disorders. Both affect the central nervous system and many of their features overlap.
- Coagulation abnormalities, when involving both coagulation and anticoagulation factors, are highly suggestive of CDG and should suggest serum transferrin isoform analysis.
- Abnormal fat distribution and congenital malformations (conotruncal malformation and eye malformations; eg, coloboma) have been described in CDG, but are unique in mitochondrial disease.
- Diabetes and sensorineural deafness are rare in CDG, but common in individuals with mitochondrial diseases.
- Certain disorders affect both the mitochondria and glycosylation, such as NGLY1 deficiency (deglycosylation deficiency) and SLC38A9 defect, leading to Leigh syndrome and type 2 CDG.

INTRODUCTION

Inborn errors of metabolism are frequently divided into disorder groups of (1) intoxication, (2) energy metabolism, and (3) complex molecules. Most intoxication-type disorders affect multiple organ systems. The early, acute, or fluctuating symptoms; and, primarily, central nervous system involvement make identification relatively easy.

[a] Department of Human Genetics, Radboudumc Medical Center, Geert Grooteplein, 6500 HB, Nijmegen, The Netherlands; [b] Department of Pediatrics, University Hospitals Leuven, Leuven, Belgium; [c] Hayward Genetics Center, Tulane University Medical School, New Orleans, LA, USA
* Corresponding author. Hayward Genetics Center, Tulane University Medical School, New Orleans, LA.
E-mail address: emoravakozicz@tulane.edu

Pediatr Clin N Am 65 (2018) 375–388
https://doi.org/10.1016/j.pcl.2017.11.012
0031-3955/18/© 2017 Elsevier Inc. All rights reserved.

pediatric.theclinics.com

Disorders of the energy metabolism also involve multiple organs and, almost always, the central nervous system but usually in a nonacute pattern. Affected individuals show early symptoms of hypotonia, muscle weakness, and developmental delay; and develop learning disabilities and progressive neurologic symptoms. Because the most energy-demanding organs are the brain, skeletal muscle, heart muscle, and liver, these are most severely affected by mitochondrial disease. Some mitochondrial conditions, such as disorders of mitochondrial maintenance, might present with an acute energy failure, similar to the intoxication-type of inborn errors of metabolism. These individuals show early-onset profound metabolic acidosis, frequently with fatal evolvement.[1]

Congenital disorders of glycosylation (CDG) are disorders of complex molecule synthesis. Due to the essential role of glycosylation in posttranslational protein-modification, CDG can involve any organ or organ system, and mimic any given disease.[2] For the practicing clinician, these inborn errors of metabolism could be significantly overlapping clinically, causing a diagnostic challenge, especially in the early stage of the disease. This article compares the different aspects of mitochondrial disease and CDG, with a focus on overlapping phenotypes and on giving a practical guide for the differential diagnosis.

GLYCOSYLATION

Glycosylation is an essential process for the posttranslational modification of many functional proteins. Examples include hormones and endocrine regulators, such as TSH, TBG, FSH, LH, ACTH, or IGFBP3; or important transport proteins, such as transferrin, ceruloplasmin, or proteins involved cholesterol metabolism. Other factors in coagulation, such as factor IX and XI or antithrombin III, are also glycosylated.[3] Not only secretory proteins but also many cell membrane proteins are heavily glycosylated, playing a role in cell–cell interaction, cellular immunity, and even in cell migration during fetal development. Obviously, due to its ubiquitous presence in the human body and because of the various functions in which glycosylated proteins are involved, abnormal glycosylation has major implications for human health.

Glycosylation involves three cellular compartments. On activating monosaccharides and phosphorylating dolichol as an acceptor for nucleotide sugars, the glycan chain is built in a stepwise enzymatic process in the cytoplasm and then flips into the endoplasmatic reticulum. The dolichol-linked oligosaccharides are transferred to the acceptor protein and transported to the Golgi for final processing. This includes cutting back of mannose residues; importing monosaccharides, such as fucose, galactose, or sialic acid, to the Golgi; adding it to the oligosaccharide chain on the protein; and exporting the molecule to the secretory vesicles.[4]

Congenital Disorders of Glycosylation

CDG are a disease family with more than 100 different members. CDG were defined by Jaeken and colleagues[5] in 1980. CDG types have been divided into four different groups, including defects in N-linked glycosylation, O-linked glycosylation, lipid-linked glycosylation, and combined glycosylation pathways.[2] For the clinician in general practice, the most frequent, important type is the group of N-linked glycosylation defects. The names of the different CDG are composed from the name of the gene hyphenated with CDG (eg, PMM2-CDG).The most common form is PMM2-CDG, which has more than 700 reported individuals. The second most common type is ALG6-CDG. Both disorders have a recognizable phenotype. In most cases, individuals with PMM2-CDG show hypotonia, strabismus, abnormal fat distribution,

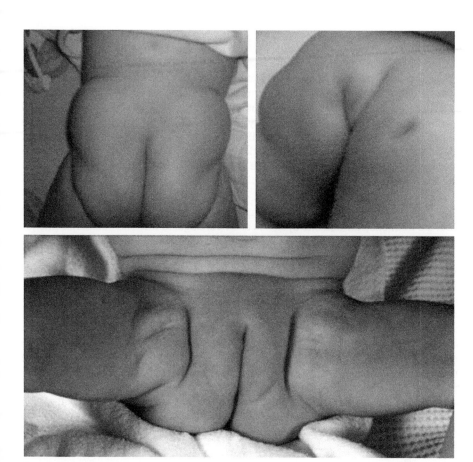

Fig. 1. Abnormal fat distribution is a characteristic sign in PMM2-CDG but not present in all affected individuals.

inverted nipples (**Fig. 1**), feeding difficulties, and ataxia. Individuals with ALG6-CDG have hypotonia; seizures; proximal muscle weakness; and frequent, mostly subtle, finger malformations. These two CDG types are associated with the longest survival (some of the initially diagnosed individuals are currently older than 40 years of age).[6]

Diagnostics

N-glycosylation got its name from the glycan linked to the N-group of an asparagine amino acid. In O-linked glycosylation, the specific glycan is linked to the O-group of a serine or threonine. Both N-linked glycosylation defects and the combined N-linked and O-linked glycosylation abnormalities can be diagnosed by routine biochemical assays in plasma, serum, and (in special cases) in urine. Glycans carry sialic acid residues at the terminal ends, giving the glycans a negative charge. The degree of missing negative charges in individuals with CDG, or the difference in charge, has been used in diagnostics, especially in the traditional test called transferrin isoelectric focusing (TIEF).[7,8] Other diagnostic methods include mass spectrometry, or matrix assisted laser desorption/ionisation time-of-flight analyzer (MALDI-TOF) glycan analysis. According to the origin of glycosylation abnormalities in the endoplasmic reticulum (ER), or Golgi-related defects, the authors divide N-linked CDG into CDG-I and CDG-II, respectively.

Direct enzyme analysis is only available in a few CDG-I (PMM- and MPI-CDG) and in the mixed type PGM1 deficiency. Lipid-linked oligosaccharide analysis is available in fibroblasts for several ER defects. Genetic testing is the confirmatory diagnosis in all CDG.[9]

An example for secretory type of O-linked glycosylation is the O-mucin type of glycosylation. Secretory O-glycosylation abnormalities can be screened by a specific method called apolipoprotein C-III isoelectric focussing (apoClII IEF). This is especially helpful in N-linked multiple glycosylation pathway defects. So far, no isolated mucin type O-glycosylation defects have been described.[10] Most O-glycosylation disorders known so far, such as O-linked mannosylation defects (different alpha-dystroglycanopathies) or the multiple exostosis syndromes, are tissue-specific and their diagnosis is based on either histochemistry or direct genetic analysis (**Fig. 2**).

Clinical Presentation

CDG are frequently divided into systemic and neurologic forms. The neurologic phenotype includes developmental delay, muscle weakness, ataxia, neuropathy, pyramidal syndrome, dystonia, stroke-like episodes, visual or hearing loss, and frequent seizures. Speech delay is very common and many individuals with CDG develop intellectual disability.[11] The multisystemic form affects the heart, liver, gastrointestinal tract, endocrine and immune system, and coagulation system and skeleton, in addition to the central nervous system. Pathognomonic findings are abnormal fat distribution and inverted nipples; however, these are not present in all individuals with PMM2-CDG. The clinician should also consider the diagnosis of CDG in the presence of bizarre laboratory abnormalities. For instance, individuals with PMM2-CDG can have several different endocrine abnormalities at once, or a bleeding disorder parallel with thrombotic events. Specific malformations described in different CDG include congenital cardiac abnormalities, such as aortic valve defect, ventricle septum defect (VSD), and tetralogy of Fallot; vermis hypoplasia; Dandy-Walker malformation; cobblestone brain dysgenesis; eye coloboma and cataract; glaucoma; cleft palate; skeletal dysplasias, especially metaphyseal and chondrodysplasia; limb malformations; and cutis laxa.[12]

Clinical suspicion of mitochondrial disorder versus CDG

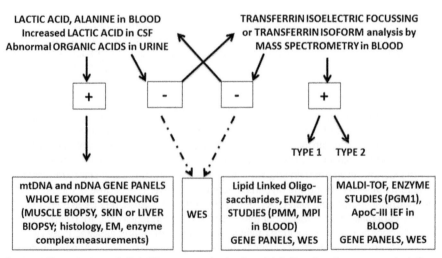

Fig. 2. Differentiation of clinically suspected mitochondrial disorders from congenital disorders of glycosylation. CSF, cerebrospinal fluid; WES, whole exome sequencing.

MITOCHONDRIAL FUNCTION
Pathomechanism

Mitochondria are elongated cell structures surrounded by a double membrane. Mitochondrial function is essential for the aerobic energy metabolism of the cell. Fundamental energy-providing pathways in the mitochondria localized in the mitochondrial matrix or embedded in the mitochondrial membrane include the respiratory chain, fatty acid β-oxidation, the pyruvate dehydrogenase complex (PDHc), and the tricarboxylic acid cycle. Additionally, several essential pathways (eg, amino acid metabolism, an important part of the urea cycle) are also localized in the mitochondria. The respiratory chain consists of five multisubunit enzyme complexes: complexes I to V. Most of these complexes have subunits coded by both nuclear and mitochondrial DNA (mtDNA), except for complex II. The supercomplexes work together on passing electrons in the intermembrane space and creating a proton gradient across the membrane, which is then turned in to adenosine triphosphate (ATP) production in the final step by complex V.[13]

Human cells contain hundreds of mitochondria, especially those with high energy demand, such as neurons and skeletal muscle cells. Mitochondria are unique in that they are controlled by their own genome and the nuclear genome of the cell. Defects in either genome can cause mitochondrial disease. The mtDNA controls 13 essential proteins of the respiratory chain and there are more than 300 nuclear genes known to code for mitochondrial proteins. Mitochondria and their genome are only inherited from the mother. The genetic code is different in the mitochondrial genome than in the nuclear genome. There is no repair mechanism in mtDNA and thus a higher mutation rate. Each mitochondrion has multiple copies of its genome, which can be heteroplasmic or homoplasmic. If 2 or more sequence variants exist in a single mitochondrion, it is considered heteroplasmic. Mitochondria are capable of connecting with other mitochondria (fusion or fission) and shuffling their genetic material.[1]

Mitochondrial Disorders

Mitochondrial disorders are a group of disorders caused by a disturbance in metabolic pathways localized in the mitochondria. The occurrence of mitochondrial disease is approximately 1 in 8500 individuals. Per definition, classic mitochondrial diseases involve a disruption of the respiratory chain or oxidative phosphorylation, with a single enzyme deficiency or a mitochondrial multicomplex deficiency. Since the initial definition of mitochondrial disease, however, there is an emerging group of other types of mitochondrial defects, frequently in association with profound energy depletion, affecting mitochondrial transcription, translation, maintenance, fusion or fission, or mtDNA synthesis.

There are different mtDNA changes that can result in disease. Large mtDNA deletions, but point mutations in genes, transfer (t)RNA, or ribosomal (r)RNA encoding regions, and could be maternally inherited or occur de novo. A growing number of nuclear mutations cause mtDNA depletion syndromes. Mutations in genes coding structural proteins and mutations that affect intergenomic communication between the nucleus and mitochondria also result in mitochondrial dysfunction.[1]

In cases of mtDNA mutations, the threshold effect is also in play and, as long as sufficient normal mtDNA is present, the effects of mutant mtDNA are covered up. If the critical threshold is exceeded, the respiratory chain function will be impaired. The mtDNA goes through continuous semiautonomous replication even in nondividing cells. If mutant and wild-type mtDNA replicate at different rates, heteroplasmy can be increased in nondividing mitochondria. In dividing mitochondria, daughter cells are not partitioned equally and can cause nonuniform distribution of mutant mtDNA.

All of these unique properties of mitochondria cause the variability seen in mitochondrial disease phenotypes.

Mitochondrial disorders affect many organ systems across the body. The most affected tissues and organs are those that have a high-energy demand, such as the brain, heart, muscle, and liver. Endocrine function, growth, the gastrointestinal tract, and the bone marrow are also often affected.[14]

Diagnostics

The traditional way to diagnose mitochondrial disease, based on a clinical and biochemical suspicion, is by muscle biopsy. Clinical suspicion relies mostly on the phenotypic involvement of the central nervous system, the presence of muscle disease, and eventual multisystem presentation. Chronically elevated lactate levels; increased alanine concentration in blood; and urine organic acids showing elevated levels of Krebs' cycle intermediates, 3-methyl-glutaconic acid, ethyl-malonic acid or lactate are highly suggestive of abnormal mitochondrial function. A muscle biopsy for histology; immune staining, especially in the presence of ragged red fibers; or abnormal complex staining can be used for establishing the diagnosis; however, this is highly invasive approach. PDHc deficiency and severe homoplasmic or nuclear complex I deficiency are also reliably measurable in skin fibroblasts. Mitochondrial oxidative phosphorylation measurements are frequently reliable in liver biopsy, especially in mtDNA depletion syndromes. Some mitochondrial phenotypes are clinically recognizable, making direct mutation analysis possible. Stroke-like episodes or Leigh syndrome on neuroimaging can also warrant direct genetic diagnostics. In the last 10 years, the diagnostic approach has been shifting away from invasive techniques toward an increased use of massive parallel sequencing and next-generation sequencing techniques[15] (see **Fig. 2**).

Clinical Presentation

Most individuals with mitochondrial diseases show multisystem involvement. The central nervous system is rarely unaffected. Neurologic regression is very common. Global developmental delay, muscle hypotonia, muscle weakness, seizures, ataxia, dystonia, and spasticity are characteristic features. Cardiac manifestations include cardiomyopathy and rhythm disturbances, but rarely congenital heart defects. Liver failure is suggestive of mtDNA depletion defects. The gastrointestinal system and growth are almost always involved in mitochondrial diseases. Endocrine involvement mostly affects glucose homeostasis (diabetes or recurrent hypoglycemia), growth, and thyroid and parathyroid function. The bone marrow function could be also profoundly affected. Renal involvement is less common, mostly involving the renal tubuli.

The most common recognizable mitochondrial phenotypes are Kearns-Sayre Syndrome (KSS) with progressive ophthalmoplegia, ptosis, myopathy, short stature and cardiac rhythm anomalies, endocrine features, or myoclonic epilepsy ragged red fiber (MERRF) syndrome, associated with gastrointestinal motility problems, muscle pain, lipomas, and seizures. Individuals with mitochondrial encephalopathy, lactic acidemia, and stroke-like episodes (MELAS) are said to be in the MELAS syndrome spectrum. They have a high percentage of mtDNA mutation heteroplasmy, typically associated with failure to thrive, abnormal cardiac function, neurologic regression, psychopathology, and (especially) depression; however, individuals with lower heteroplasmy might present with only recurrent migraines or diabetes-deafness syndrome. Different phenotypes are associated with *POLG* mutations, including Alpers syndrome with intractable seizures, whereas other affected individuals have neurologic regression and life-threatening liver failure suggestive of *POLG*-related disease.[16]

OVERLAPPING PHENOTYPES IN CONGENITAL DISORDERS OF GLYCOSYLATION AND MITOCHONDRIAL DISEASE
Cutis Laxa with Developmental and Growth Delay

Cutis laxa is a condition characterized by wrinkled, inelastic, sagging skin frequently associated with vascular, pulmonary, and vesicourinary involvement (autosomal recessive cutis laxa [ARCL] type I), or skeletomuscular and central nervous system involvement (ACRL type II [ARCL2] and ACRL III [ARCL3], respectively). Several ARCL syndromes, especially ARCL2 and ARCL3, have an underlying metabolic pathologic factor.[17,18] The first metabolic cutis laxa ARCL2 was described decades ago as a multiple congenital anomaly syndrome and recently redefined as a CDG. This glycosylation disorder is caused by pathogenic variants in the *ATP6V0A2* gene (ARCL2A) affecting the membrane subunit of the vesicular ATPase, responsible for the proton gradient in the Golgi and secretory vesicles. This abnormal proton gradient leads to an insufficient glycosylation of glycoproteins throughout the Golgi and abnormal glycosylation of oligosaccharide transferases. There is a delayed maturation of proelastin and related elastic fibers, leading to both cutis laxa and CDG. ATP6V0A2-CDG presents with generalized cutis laxa, short stature, joint laxity, muscle weakness, and developmental delay.[19]

Other glycosylation disorders associated with cutis laxa include COG7-CDG; however, that phenotype is distinctive, due to the severe dwarfism, failure to thrive, adducted thumbs, and VSD in affected individuals.

Recently, two additional cutis laxa phenotypes with glycosylation defects have been described: ATP6V1A-CDG and ATP6V1E1-CDG.[20] These disorders show similar features to the *ATP6V0A2* defect, including generalized skin involvement, growth, and developmental delay. They involve cardiopulmonary function (even congenital cardiac defects have been observed) and they are also associated with hypercholesterolemia.[20]

PYCR1 is located in the mitochondria. PYCR1 is involved in mitochondrial proline synthesis and PYCR1 deficiency leads to altered mitochondrial morphology, membrane potential, and increased apoptosis rate on oxidative stress, in association with cutis laxa. The clinical symptoms in individuals with pathogenic variants in *PYCR1* (ARCL2B and ARCL3B) can fully imitate those of ATP6V0A2-CDG, including generalized skin involvement, growth and developmental delay, joint dislocations, and intellectual disability. ARCL types related to glycosylation or mitochondrial defects, specifically ATP6V0A2-CDG, show spontaneous improvement of the skin abnormalities with aging. Transferrin isoform analysis (eg, TIEF) is the recommended diagnostic approach to discriminate between the two conditions; however, clinicians should be aware that TIEF in infants younger than six weeks old may be false-negative. Abnormal Apo CIII IEF supports the diagnosis, demonstrating the associated O-mucin type of glycosylation defect. Histology (elastin staining) is not discriminative between the two types of cutis laxa because both ARCL types lead to abnormal elastin synthesis. Sequence analysis confirms the diagnosis.

Epilepsy with Proximal Myopathy, Ataxia, and Developmental Delay

Individuals with ALG6-CDG always present with hypotonia and developmental delay. More than 90% of children develop epilepsy, ataxia, and proximal muscle weakness due to pathogenic mutations in the *ALG6* gene. Cyclic behavioral changes, with autistic features or depressive episodes, are frequent complaints. The characteristic, common symptoms are quite unspecific and could fit a glycosylation disease but also many mitochondrial disorders. Several individuals with MELAS, MERRF, KSS, mitochondrial neurogastrointestinal encephalomyopathu (MNGIE) and Alpers syndrome have been described with a very similar phenotype. In young affected individuals with recurrent seizures or refractory epilepsy, the lactic acid levels are frequently unreliable. The clinical diagnosis of ALG6-CDG is not so straightforward, because CDG-specific coagulation anomalies are only present in half of the cases, without spontaneous bleedings. Facial dysmorphism is rare, and only a few affected individuals show missing phalanges and brachydactyly, raising the possibility of a complex molecule synthesis defect, such as CDG, and discriminating the phenotype from other CDG.[21] When the clinician suspects CDG, biochemical testing for glycosylation is always diagnostic. To date, the TIEF analysis has been abnormal in all reported ALG6-CDG cases. Further diagnosis can be either through lipid-linked oligosaccharide analysis in fibroblasts, or by the use of genetic panels for massive parallel sequencing.

Cholestasis with Liver Failure

Liver involvement, a common feature in childhood mitochondrial hepatopathies, mostly presents as neonatal acute liver failure or cholestasis.[22] Some affected individuals develop slowly progressive chronic liver failure, leading to fibrosis or liver cirrhosis. Several specific molecular defects (pathogenic variants in nuclear genes; eg, *POLG, DGUOK, MPV17, SCO1, BCS1L,* and *EARS2*; or deletions of mtDNA) have been identified as underlying severe mitochondrial liver disease.

Although severe liver involvement is present in only in about one-quarter of the reported CDG types, it can be progressive and even life-threatening.[23] CDG types with predominant, or isolated, liver involvement include MPI-CDG, TMEM199-CDG,[24] CCDC115-CDG,[25] and ATP6AP1-CDG.[26] Some of the CDG with multisystem involvement and significant liver disease include ALG1-CDG, ALG3-CDG, ALG8-CDG, COG-CDG, and PGM1-CDG. This type is well known to cause significant liver abnormalities in young individuals, including cholestasis; however, in more than 20% of the cases it can progress to cirrhosis and liver failure. In TMEM199-CDG, CCDC115-CDG, and ATP6AP1-CDG additional abnormalities, including hypercholesterolemia, high alkaline phosphatase levels, or decreased ceruloplasmin, can facilitate early recognition and diagnosis of CDG. In PGM1-CDG, the presence of midline malformations or cardiomyopathy is suggestive of PGM1 deficiency; however, in the absence of cleft palate the clinical features highly imitate those of mitochondrial disease.[15] Lactic acid elevations have been observed in ALG1-CDG and COG-CDG; however, in PGM1-CDG the lactate level is decreased, especially when fasting samples are evaluated. Coagulation factors are not as helpful because abnormal clotting factor and antithrombotic factor production can occur in liver failure, independent of the metabolic origin.

In mitochondrial disease-related cholestasis and fibrosis there are usually significant neuromuscular symptoms, multisystem involvement, and lactic acidemia, somewhat overlapping with COG-CDG and some ALG-CDG. The liver disease is usually progressive.

Diagnosis in liver failure includes TIEF to screen for CDG, lactic acid and alanine measurements for mitochondrial function, and (in most cases) direct sequencing.

Liver transplantation has been a debated issue in both disorder groups. A few individuals with CDG underwent successful liver transplantation and recovered from their metabolic conditions (MPI-CDG, CCDC115-CDG).[27] Interestingly, the individuals with MPI-CDG who have been successfully transplanted experienced improvement even in gastrointestinal function, not just in hepatic-related glycosylation abnormalities.[27]

The role of liver transplantation in individuals with mitochondrial liver failure is questioned because of the systemic nature of the disease. In specific individuals with organ specific manifestation, however, this can be overweighed, even in mitochondrial disease.

Cardiomyopathy, Short Stature, and Normal Intellectual Development

PGM1-CDG was previously defined as glycogen storage disorder type XIV,[28] presenting with dilated cardiomyopathy, short stature, and recurrent hypoglycemia in most affected individuals.[29] An array of midline malformations have been observed from cleft palate to bifid uvula. Some affected individuals also show significant or progressive liver disease, in addition to low blood sugar levels. These features are thought to be related to abnormal glycogen metabolism. Individuals with PGM1-CDG have no central nervous system involvement. Similar presentation of dilated cardiomyopathy, short stature, and normal intelligence has been observed in children with DOLK-CDG (see also DK1-CDG[30]). The latter type necessitated cardiac transplantation in several cases; some of which were successful.[31,32]

Cardiac muscles are among the highest energy-demanding tissues of the body and cardiomyopathies are among the most frequent cardiac manifestations in mitochondrial disease. Hypertrophic cardiomyopathy is the most common type, occurring in almost 20% of individuals with mitochondrial defects; however, only in the minority of cases presenting as dilated cardiomyopathies.[33] Dilated cardiomyopathy has been observed in structural complex subunit and assembly factors defects, mitochondrial transfer RNAs, ribosomal RNAs, ribosomal proteins, translation factors, mtDNA maintenance, and coenzyme Q10 synthesis.

Among the recognizable mitochondrial diseases with cardiomyopathies is TMEM70-CDG mitochondrial complex V deficiency. This disorder is common in the Roma population (common mutation c.317-2A > G), associated with short stature (89%), nonprogressive cardiomyopathy (89%), recurrent liver dysfunction with poor feeding, and 3-methylglutaconic aciduria, which are characteristic for the disease.[34] Less than half of the affected individuals have normal or low-normal intelligence. Hyperammonemic episodes respond well to glucose infusion and ammonia scavengers. Individuals with TMEM70 deficiency might have a milder disease course and long survival. Recurrent metabolic decompensations and hyperammonemic episodes help to differentiate affected individuals from those with similar phenotype due to a glycosylation defect.

In individuals with dilated cardiomyopathy and normal intelligence, the clinician should always screen for glycosylation abnormalities (TIEF analysis in serum), measure lactate and ammonia, and screen for 3-methylglutaconic aciduria by urine organic acid analysis. Although muscle biopsy can be helpful in a *TMEM70* defect, in most cases based on the recognizable phenotype, the authors advise direct sequence analysis in the diagnostics.

Vermis Hypoplasia and Severe Neurologic Impairment

Pontocerebellar hypoplasia is a group of autosomal recessive neurodegenerative disorders with abnormal cerebellar and vermis development already in the intrauterine period. Cerebellar hypoplasia can evolve further to cerebellar atrophy and is commonly associated with cortical atrophy, ventriculomegaly, and microcephaly.[35] Congenital cerebellar vermis hypoplasia is among the most common symptoms of CDG, especially PMM2-CDG, which is a recessive disease also associated with cerebellar and cortical atrophy during the course of the disease. In many cases, it presents with only developmental delay, ataxia, and speech delay, lacking of the classic multisystem presentation. Another type of CDG that can present as pontocerebellar hypoplasia is SRD5A3-CDG, in which affected individuals have diverse associated eye malformations (coloboma, cataract, glaucoma). One-third of the affected individuals also have severe ichthyosis. Interestingly, several affected individuals have been described with no abnormalities of transferrin isoform analysis (normal TIEF), making the diagnosis very difficult.[36]

Several mitochondrial disorders are known with similar phenotype, especially pathogenic variants in the transfer RNA splicing endonuclease subunit genes (*TSEN54*, *TSEN2*, *TSEN34*) and the mitochondrial transfer RNA arginyl synthetase gene (*RARS2*). In these disorders, the cerebellar vermis is abnormal but relatively spared compared with CDG. Mutations in *TSEN54* are clinically associated with dyskinesia and/or dystonia and variable degrees of spasticity, which is rare in PMM2-CDG but was observed in individuals with SRD5A3-CDG. Lactic acidosis is not always present in mitochondrial pontocerebellar hypoplasias; however, elevated cerebrospinal fluid (CSF) lactate might be diagnostic in individuals with pathogenic variants of the *RARS2* gene.

In individuals with pontocerebellar hypoplasia, the clinician should recommend a detailed eye examination; followed by TIFF; lactate measurements in both blood and CSF; and, because TIEF can be false-negative, gene panel sequencing.

Stroke-Like Episodes

Stroke-like episodes have been observed in association with different mtDNA point mutations (MELAS syndrome) and are considered highly suggestive of mitochondrial disease. However, it is a relatively frequent complication in CDG, especially PMM2-CDG. The underlying pathomechanism seems to be different, including abnormal vascular reaction and metabolic energy failure in mitochondrial defects, and mostly coagulation and perfusion abnormality-related strokes in CDG; however, the symptoms and the MRI picture can be indistinguishable.

Individuals with mitochondrial diseases who have stroke-like episodes have almost always elevated lactate levels in blood and CSF. TIEF is reliable in most children with PMM2-CDG, in whom stroke-like episodes are the most frequent. Early diagnosis of the underlying type of metabolic condition is very important because further episodes might be preventable with oral L-arginine therapy, hydration, and prevention of hypercoagulability.[6]

MITOCHONDRIAL DYSFUNCTION IN GLYCOSYLATION DEFECTS

Signs of abnormal mitochondrial function were described in different CDG. Individuals with COG7 defects have been described with ethylmalonic aciduria and lactate elevations.[37] Abnormal mitochondrial complex activity and lactic acidemia was described in COG8-CDG, originally misdiagnosed as a primary mitochondrial defect.[38] Individuals with ALG1-CDG also showed recurrent lactate elevations.[37] The origin of mitochondrial dysfunction in these cases is not yet understood. TIEF analysis is reliable in both ALG1-CDG and ALG8-CDG, and also in COG7-CDG in serum.

Manganese transporter defect (due to pathogenic variants in *SLC39A8*) was originally reported as a severe neurologic condition with basal ganglion involvement, seizures, and developmental delay. The disorder was subsequently rediscovered as a glycosylation disease (SLC39A8-CDG), with abnormal function of manganese-dependent glycosyltransferases, showing a skeletal dysplasia phenotype, in addition to the previously described primarily central nervous system disease.[39] Surprisingly, the same gene defect was also redefined as a mitochondrial disease in association with Leigh syndrome and lactic acidosis and cerebral lactic acidemia, with mitochondrial abnormalities in muscle and liver biopsies, due to secondary superoxide dismutase deficiency.[40] Individuals with SLC39A8 deficiency, therefore, show both abnormal TIEF and lactic acid elevation, even cerebral lactic acidemia, and can be diagnosed by direct sequencing.

Pathogenic variants in *NGLY1* cause glycosylation defects, but not classic CDG. The abnormal glycosylation in the *NGLY1*-related phenotype is due to a deglycosyla-tion defect, leading to an insufficient breakdown of abnormally synthesized glycans and an increase in the concentration of abnormal glycans in the ER, associated with normal transferrin isoform analysis, including a normal TIEF. Affected individuals do have a CDG-like phenotype but also some features overlapping with mitochondrial disease (eg, developmental delay, seizures, ataxia, muscle weakness, dystonia, spas-ticity) and frequent elevation of lactic acid, which might point to the wrong diagnosis. A pathognomic clinical feature is the presence of alacrimia, or hypolacrimia (but not in all cases). In these cases, increased ER stress might lead to lactic acid elevations in affected individuals.[32] The diagnosis in NGLY1 deficiency is by direct sequencing, based on the suspected phenotype, in the lack of a specific biochemical marker.

SUMMARY

The phenotype in glycosylation defects sometimes overlaps with the clinical features of mitochondrial disease and could be difficult to distinguish based on just the clinical presentation. The classic CDG signs, abnormal fat distribution and inverted nipples, are only present in less than 20% of all individuals with CDG.[41] Many nonspecific neurologic features overlap, including developmental, speech delay, ataxia, hypoto-nia, muscle weakness, and visual loss or seizures. Even MRI signs could be very similar (pontocerebellar hypoplasia, stroke-like disease). Cardiomyopathy and liver involvement (cholestasis, fibrosis) might be an early sign in both disorders.

Coagulation abnormalities, however, when present, involve both coagulation factors and anticoagulation factors, such as antithrombin-III in CDG, diagnostic for glycosylation abnormalities in the absence of liver failure. Although hypoglycemia is present in both disorders, hyperinsulinism is common in CDG, but unique in mitochon-drial disease. The same way diabetes and sensorineural deafness are very rare in CDG but common in mitochondrial disease. Congenital eye abnormalities, such as colo-boma, and cardiac defects, such as conotruncal malformations, have been described in different CDG but are unique in disorders of energy metabolism. Lateral ophthalmo-plegia and psychiatric disorders, especially depression and schizophrenia, are sug-gestive of a mitochondrial disease.

Lactic acid elevations have been observed in several individuals with CDG but not consistently and without cerebral lactic academia, except for SLC38A9-CDG.

Serum transferrin isoform analysis is diagnostic in most secretory CDG types; however, the clinician has to be aware of the possibility of normal TIEF in neonates with CDG (eg, PMM2-CDG, ATP6V0A2-CDG) and some older individuals with PMM2-CDG, SRD5A3-CDG, ALG13-CDG, and nonsecretory forms of CDG.[8,42]

OUTCOME AND DIETARY THERAPY

Recent statistics show that about 10% to 20% of individuals with either mitochondrial disease or CDG die in the first 2 to 4 years of life.[41] Most affected individuals with a high mortality have the multisystem phenotype present from birth. Early cardiac or liver involvement, hydrops, pericardial fluid collection, ascites, and severe feeding dif-ficulties in the neonatal period are significant adverse prognostic factors. The best prognosis is to be expected in the sole neurologic form, which is rare in both disorders. Unfortunately, most types of CDG and most mitochondrial disorders do not yet have an effective form of treatment other than supportive therapy.

The known treatable type is MPI-CDG. In MPI-CDG an alternate pathway can activate mannose molecules and bypass the enzymatic defect, leading to an improvement of the coagulation anomalies and malabsorption and protein-losing enteropathy (mannose in the dose of 1 g/kg/d, divided to 3–5 doses[43]). Affected individuals still can develop liver fibrosis during the course of disease. Another treatable CDG is PGM1-CDG. Affected individuals treated with D-galactose improve their liver function tests and anticoagulation parameters. A galactose dosage of 0.5 to 1 g/kg/d is recommended to alleviate symptoms.[44] Other possible treatable CDG types that react to monosaccharide intervention include SLC35A2-CDG (galactose), SLC35C1 (fucose), and SL39A8-CDG (galactose supplementation).

Dietary intervention has been proven successful in a few types of mitochondrial disorders, including coenzyme Q in coenzyme Q deficiency, riboflavin in *ACAD9* defect, and biotin and thiamin in their respective transporter defects, in addition to the classic thiamin treatment in thiamin-sensitive PDHc deficiency.

For most individuals with mitochondrial diseases, and with CDG, supportive care is the cornerstone of therapy. This includes adequate feeding, eventual use of tube feeding, or the use of elementary formulas. Ketogenic diet has been used in PDHc deficiency with success and in a few individuals with both glycosylation and energy disorders for seizure treatment; however, this treatment approach can significantly increase hypoglycemic episodes in mitochondrial defects and CDG. Early diagnosis of CDG and the specific form of mitochondrial disease can be essential for adequate treatment and the long-term survival of affected individuals.

REFERENCES

1. Pearce S, Nezich CL, Spinazzola A. Mitochondrial diseases: translation matters. Mol Cell Neurosci 2013;55:1–12.
2. Jaeken J. Congenital disorders of glycosylation. Ann N Y Acad Sci 2010;1214: 190–8.
3. Linssen M, Mohamed M, Wevers RA, et al. Thrombotic complications in patients with PMM2-CDG. Mol Genet Metab 2013;109(1):107–11.
4. Freeze HH. Understanding human glycosylation disorders: biochemistry leads the charge. J Biol Chem 2013;288(10):6936–45.
5. Jaeken J, van Eijk HG, van der Heul C, et al. Sialic acid-deficient serum and cerebrospinal fluid transferrin in a newly recognized genetic syndrome. Clin Chim Acta 1984;144(2–3):245–7.
6. Scott K, Gadomski T, Kozicz T, et al. Congenital disorders of glycosylation: new defects and still counting. J Inherit Metab Dis 2014;37(4):609–17.
7. Babovic-Vuksanovic D, O'Brien JF. Laboratory diagnosis of congenital disorders of glycosylation type I by analysis of transferrin glycoforms. Mol Diagn Ther 2007; 11(5):303–11.
8. Lefeber DJ, Morava E, Jaeken J. How to find and diagnose a CDG due to defective N-glycosylation. J Inherit Metab Dis 2011;34(4):849–52.
9. van Scherpenzeel M, Steenbergen G, Morava E, et al. High-resolution mass spectrometry glycoprofiling of intact transferrin for diagnosis and subtype identification in the congenital disorders of glycosylation. Transl Res 2015;166(6): 639–49.e1.
10. Jaeken J. CDG what's new. J Inherit Metab Dis 2017.
11. Freeze HH, Eklund EA, Ng BG, et al. Neurological aspects of human glycosylation disorders. Annu Rev Neurosci 2015;38:105–25.
12. Morava E, Wevers RA, Cantagrel V, et al. A novel cerebello-ocular syndrome with abnormal glycosylation due to abnormalities in dolichol metabolism. Brain 2010; 133(11):3210–20.

13. Koopman WJ, Willems PH, Smeitink JA. Monogenic mitochondrial disorders. N Engl J Med 2012;366(12):1132–41.

14. Morava E, van den Heuvel L, Hol F, et al. Mitochondrial disease criteria: diagnostic applications in children. Neurology 2006;67(10):1823–6.

15. Morava E, Wong S, Lefeber D. Disease severity and clinical outcome in phosphosglucomutase deficiency. J Inherit Metab Dis 2015;38(2):207–9.

16. de Vries MC, Rodenburg RJ, Morava E, et al. Multiple oxidative phosphorylation deficiencies in severe childhood multi-system disorders due to polymerase gamma (POLG1) mutations. Eur J Pediatr 2007;166(3):229–34.

17. Dimopoulou A, Fischer B, Gardeitchik T, et al. Genotype-phenotype spectrum of PYCR1-related autosomal recessive cutis laxa. Mol Genet Metab 2013;110(3):352–61.

18. Fischer B, Callewaert B, Schröter P, et al. Severe congenital cutis laxa with cardiovascular manifestations due to homozygous deletions in ALDH18A1. Mol Genet Metab 2014;112(4):310–6.

19. Hucthagowder V, Morava E, Kornak U, et al. Loss-of-function mutations in ATP6V0A2 impair vesicular trafficking, tropoelastin secretion and cell survival. Hum Mol Genet 2009;18(12):2149–65.

20. Van Damme T, Gardeitchik T, Mohamed M, et al. Mutations in ATP6V1E1 or ATP6V1A cause autosomal-recessive cutis laxa. Am J Hum Genet 2017;100(2):216–27.

21. Morava E, Tiemes V, Thiel C, et al. ALG6-CDG: a recognizable phenotype with epilepsy, proximal muscle weakness, ataxia and behavioral and limb anomalies. J Inherit Metab Dis 2016;39(5):713–23.

22. Lee WS, Sokol RJ. Mitochondrial hepatopathies: advances in genetics, therapeutic approaches, and outcomes. J Pediatr 2013;163(4):942–8.

23. Marques-da-Silva D, Dos Reis Ferreira V, Monticelli M, et al. Liver involvement in congenital disorders of glycosylation (CDG). A systematic review of the literature. J Inherit Metab Dis 2017;40(2):195–207.

24. Jansen JC, Timal S, van Scherpenzeel M, et al. TMEM199 deficiency is a disorder of golgi homeostasis characterized by elevated aminotransferases, alkaline phosphatase, and cholesterol and abnormal glycosylation. Am J Hum Genet 2016;98(2):322–30.

25. Jansen JC, Cirak S, van Scherpenzeel M, et al. CCDC115 Deficiency causes a disorder of golgi homeostasis with abnormal protein glycosylation. Am J Hum Genet 2016;98(2):310–21.

26. Jansen EJ, Timal S, Ryan M, et al. ATP6AP1 deficiency causes an immunodeficiency with hepatopathy, cognitive impairment and abnormal protein glycosylation. Nat Commun 2016;7:11600.

27. Janssen MC, de Kleine RH, van den Berg AP, et al. Successful liver transplantation and long-term follow-up in a patient with MPI-CDG. Pediatrics 2014;134(1):e279–83.

28. Tegtmeyer LC, Rust S, van Scherpenzeel M, et al. Multiple phenotypes in phosphoglucomutase 1 deficiency. N Engl J Med 2014;370(6):533–42.

29. Wong SY, Beamer LJ, Gadomski T, et al. Defining the phenotype and assessing severity in phosphoglucomutase-1 deficiency. J Pediatr 2016;175:130–6.e8.

30. Kapusta L, Zucker N, Frenckel G, et al. From discrete dilated cardiomyopathy to successful cardiac transplantation in congenital disorders of glycosylation due to dolichol kinase deficiency (DK1-CDG). Heart Fail Rev 2013;18(2):187–96.

31. Lefeber DJ, de Brouwer AP, Morava E, et al. Autosomal recessive dilated cardiomyopathy due to DOLK mutations results from abnormal dystroglycan O-mannosylation. PLoS Genet 2011;7(12):e1002427.

32. Wolfe LA, Morava E, He M, et al. Heritable disorders in the metabolism of the dolichols: a bridge from sterol biosynthesis to molecular glycosylation. Am J Med Genet C Semin Med Genet 2012;160c(4):322–8.

33. El-Hattab AW, Scaglia F. Mitochondrial cardiomyopathies. Front Cardiovasc Med 2016;3:25.

34. Magner M, Dvorakova V, Tesarova M, et al. TMEM70 deficiency: long-term outcome of 48 patients. J Inherit Metab Dis 2015;38(3):417–26.

35. Namavar Y, Barth PG, Kasher PR, et al. Clinical, neuroradiological and genetic findings in pontocerebellar hypoplasia. Brain 2011;134(Pt 1):143–56.

36. Cantagrel V, Lefeber DJ. From glycosylation disorders to dolichol biosynthesis defects: a new class of metabolic diseases. J Inherit Metab Dis 2011;34(4): 859–67.

37. Morava E, Vodopiutz J, Lefeber DJ, et al. Defining the phenotype in congenital disorder of glycosylation due to ALG1 mutations. Pediatrics 2012;130(4): e1034–9.

38. Foulquier F, Ungar D, Reynders E, et al. A new inborn error of glycosylation due to a Cog8 deficiency reveals a critical role for the Cog1-Cog8 interaction in COG complex formation. Hum Mol Genet 2007;16(7):717–30.

39. Park JH, Hogrebe M, Grüneberg M, et al. SLC39A8 deficiency: a disorder of manganese transport and glycosylation. Am J Hum Genet 2015;97(6):894–903.

40. Riley LG, Cowley MJ, Gayevskiy V, et al. A SLC39A8 variant causes manganese deficiency, and glycosylation and mitochondrial disorders. J Inherit Metab Dis 2017;40(2):261–9.

41. Funke S, Gardeitchik T, Kouwenberg D, et al. Perinatal and early infantile symptoms in congenital disorders of glycosylation. Am J Med Genet A 2013;161a(3): 578–84.

42. Vermeer S, Kremer HP, Leijten QH, et al. Cerebellar ataxia and congenital disorder of glycosylation Ia (CDG-Ia) with normal routine CDG screening. J Neurol 2007;254(10):1356–8.

43. de Lonlay P, Seta N. The clinical spectrum of phosphomannose isomerase deficiency, with an evaluation of mannose treatment for CDG-Ib. Biochim Biophys Acta 2009;1792(9):841–3.

44. Morava E. Galactose supplementation in phosphoglucomutase-1 deficiency; review and outlook for a novel treatable CDG. Mol Genet Metab 2014;112(4):275–9.

Newborn Screening
History, Current Status, and Future Directions

Ayman W. El-Hattab, MD[a], Mohammed Almannai, MD[b],
V. Reid Sutton, MD[b],*

KEYWORDS

- Inborn errors of metabolism • Newborn screening • Tandem mass spectroscopy

KEY POINTS

- Newborn screening aims to achieve presymptomatic diagnosis of treatable disorders to allow for early initiation of medical care to prevent or reduce significant morbidity and mortality related to the screened disorders.
- Many of the conditions tested in the newborn screening are inborn errors of metabolism; however, a wide variety of other nonmetabolic disorders may be included.
- In the United States, the Advisory Committee on Heritable Disorders in Newborn and Children (ACHDNC) provides recommendations regarding conditions to be included in newborn screening program panels; however, the final decision of which disorders to be added to the newborn screening is typically made by each individual state.
- Newborn screening tests are not designed to be diagnostic. Therefore, further diagnostic tests are needed to confirm or exclude the suspected diagnosis.
- Further advancement in technology is expected to allow continuous expansion of newborn screening with reduction in cost, shorter turnaround time, and more accurate results.

INTRODUCTION

Newborn screening aims to achieve early presymptomatic diagnosis of treatable disorders for which timely intervention is critical to improve the outcome. Many of the conditions included in the newborn screening panels are inborn errors of metabolism; however, screening for endocrine, hematologic, immunologic, and cardiovascular diseases, and hearing loss is also included in many panels. Newborn screening includes point-of-care tests (eg, hearing test) and blood analysis of samples collected on filter

Declaration of Conflict of Interests: The authors declare that there is no conflict of interest.
[a] Division of Clinical Genetics and Metabolic Disorders, Pediatrics Department, Tawam Hospital, Tawam Roundabout, Al-Ain 15258, United Arab Emirates; [b] Department of Molecular and Human Genetics, Baylor College of Medicine, Texas Children's Hospital, One Baylor Plaza, Houston, TX 77030, USA
* Corresponding author.
E-mail address: vrsutton@texaschildrens.org

Pediatr Clin N Am 65 (2018) 389–405
https://doi.org/10.1016/j.pcl.2017.11.013
0031-3955/18/© 2017 Elsevier Inc. All rights reserved.

pediatric.theclinics.com

paper spots between 24 and 48 hours of age. Tests in newborn screening are not designed to be diagnostic. Therefore, abnormal newborn screen results should prompt the initiation of further diagnostic testing, neonate evaluation, and consideration of treatment initiation while waiting for the diagnostic test results.[1–3] This article focuses on newborn screening for inborn errors of metabolism. The goals and history of newborn screening are discussed. Then how disorders are selected for inclusion in newborn screening and how to optimize its results are explained. Logistics, factors affecting newborn screening results, and confirmation process are then presented. Finally, future directions of newborn screening are discussed.

GOALS OF NEWBORN SCREENING

Newborn screening aims to achieve presymptomatic and rapid diagnosis of treatable disorders for which timely intervention is critical to improve the outcome. These conditions are typically not evident at birth and if not diagnosed and treated could result in disability or death. Therefore, the goal of newborn screening is the prevention or reduction of significant morbidity and mortality related to various disorders. Newborn screening programs have enabled early diagnosis and initiation of medical care for the screened diseases, which has modified the outcome for many disorders that were previously associated with high morbidity (eg, inborn errors of metabolism, cystic fibrosis, and primary immunodeficiencies) or with significant neurodevelopmental disabilities (eg, phenylketonuria and congenital hypothyroidism). Improving the outcome for affected children is productive for society and the individual child.[2–4]

Because early diagnosis by newborn screening facilitates early intervention, the outcome of newborn screening programs has been favorable. Several studies of long-term follow-up of individuals ascertained by newborn screening indicated significant improvement in morbidity and mortality for all diseases that have been studied including fatty acid oxidations defects, urea cycle disorders, severe combined immunodeficiency, cystic fibrosis, and sickle cell disease.[5–9]

HISTORY OF NEWBORN SCREENING

The establishment of newborn screening was based on early work in the management of phenylketonuria. The importance of early diagnosis for phenylketonuria emerged when it was observed that individuals with phenylketonuria had improvement in their clinical status when given formulas modified to restrict phenylalanine intake, and such restriction can typically prevent intellectual disability associated with phenylketonuria if started early in life.[10,11] In 1963 Guthrie and Susi[12] reported a simple method for detecting phenylketonuria in large populations of newborns. Not different from today's sampling method, the blood for this test was collected from newborns on filter paper. The analysis method, which is known as bacterial inhibition assay, depended on placing a small punch from the filter paper on an ager plate containing a heavy inoculum of Bacillus subtilis bacteria and β_2-thienylalanine, which is an inhibitor of bacterial growth that is counteracted by any significant excess of phenylalanine in the blood sample. Elevated phenylalanine in phenylketonuria reverses the effect of the inhibitor, and the extent of bacteria growth surrounding the filter paper disk is correlated with phenylalanine level in the blood spot.[12] In the same year, Massachusetts began universal mandatory screening for phenylketonuria, and rapidly, other states started establishing newborn screening programs.

Screening tests for other inborn errors of metabolism were subsequently developed. The bacterial inhibition assay was used to detect other inborn errors of metabolism, such as galactosemia, maple syrup urine disease, and homocystinuria, although they were not as widely adopted as screening for phenylketonuria. Enzyme assays for newborn screening blood spots were then developed for galactosemia in 1968 and biotinidase deficiency in 1984.[13,14] In 1980s fluorimetric assays were developed and replaced bacterial inhibition assays for analyte analysis. In 1990 tandem mass spectroscopy, which had been used clinically to measure urine acylcarnitines, was demonstrated to be amenable to the detection of analytes in newborn screening blood spots.[15] This methodology is highly automated; allows the detection of large number of analytes simultaneously in a single assay; and has high speed of sample preparation, assay, and analysis. Therefore, the adoption of this methodology has revolutionized newborn screening by allowing rapid expansion of the number of diseases included in newborn screening with reduction of cost and turnaround time for testing.

In the United States, the Newborn Screening Saves Lives Act of 2007 was passed by the Congress and signed into law in 2008. Subsequently, seven Regional Genetics and Newborn Screening Service Collaboratives and a National Coordinating Center for the Collaboratives were established to facilitate improvements in education, training, screening technology, and follow-up strategies. This law also established programs for newborn screening improvement, quality assurance, and activities coordination.[16]

SELECTION OF DISORDERS INCLUDED IN NEWBORN SCREENING

Wilson and Jungner[17] published 10 principles that could be used for inclusion of a condition in newborn screening in 1986 (**Box 1**). However, over time a broad and disparate profile of screening targets emerged because each state determines what disorders should be included for screening.

In 2006, the Maternal and Child Health Bureau of the Health Resources and Services Administration and the American College of Medical Genetics and Genomics published practice guidelines for newborn screening to standardize a panel that would be used nationwide. In these guidelines three minimal criteria were used to include a disease as a primary target in newborn screening (**Box 2**), and disorders were evaluated based on their clinical characteristics (eg, incidence, burden of disease if not

---

Box 1
Wilson and Jungner principles for including a disease in newborn screening

1. The condition sought should be an important health problem.

2. There should be an accepted treatment for patients with recognized diseases.

3. Facilities for diagnosis and treatment should be available.

4. There should be a recognizable latent or early symptomatic stage.

5. There should be a suitable test or examination.

6. The test should be acceptable to the population.

7. The natural history of the condition, including development from latent to declared disease, should be adequately understood.

8. There should be an agreed policy on whom to treat as patients.

9. The cost of case-finding (including diagnosis and treatment of patients diagnosed) should be economically balanced in relation to possible expenditure on medical care as a whole.

10. Case-finding should be a continuing process and not a "once and for all" project.

Box 2
The American College of Medical Genetics and Genomics minimal criteria for a condition to be included as a primary target in newborn screening

1. It can be identified at a time (24–48 hours after birth) at which it would not ordinarily be detected clinically

2. A test with appropriate sensitivity and specificity is available for it

3. There are demonstrated benefits of early detection, timely intervention, and efficacious treatment of the condition.

---

treated, and phenotype in the newborn); analytical characteristics of the screening test (eg, availability and features of the platform); and availability of health professionals experienced in diagnosis, treatment, and management to come to a recommended panel for screening. Disorders were scored and those with high scores, treatment availability, and well-understood natural history were included in the core panel. Other conditions with potential clinical significance but that did not fulfill the criteria to be in the core panels were included as secondary targets. Twenty-nine conditions were assigned to the core panel including nine organic acidemias, five fatty acids oxidation disorders, six aminoacidopathies, two other inborn errors of metabolism, two endocrinopathies, three hemoglobinopathies, hearing loss, and cystic fibrosis. The secondary targets included 25 disorders, most of which could be detected through the same analytes used for primary core disorders (**Table 1**).[1]

The Newborn Screening Saves Lives Act recommended the uniform screening panel with primary and secondary conditions. Shortly after this act, screening for the primary conditions on the recommended uniform screening panel was available to all infants born in the United States.[16] The Newborn Screening Saves Lives Act also gave the Advisory Committee on Heritable Disorders in Newborn and Children (ACHDNC) the authority to provide recommendations regarding potential additions to the recommended uniform screening. The committee follows an evidence-based process and on agreement by the committee, recommendations are made. Application to nominate a condition is submitted to the committee by physician, researchers, or advocacy groups. To date, the committee has approved recommendations for addition of screening for glycogen storage disease type II (Pompe disease), severe combined immunodeficiencies, T-cell-related lymphocyte deficiencies, and pulse oximetry for critical congenital heart diseases (see **Table 1**).[18] Although the ACHDNC makes recommendations of conditions to be added to newborn screening, the final decision of which disorders to be added to the newborn screening is usually made by each individual state. This decision is affected by population differences, technological competence, financial burden, and political environment that vary from state to state. Currently all US states provide testing for the original 29 recommended primary conditions. Some states have adopted testing for the additional disorders recommended by ACHDNC and some have included disorders not yet recommended by ACHDNC.[19]

OPTIMIZING NEWBORN SCREENING RESULTS

Tests in newborn screening are not designed to be diagnostic. Therefore, abnormal newborn screen results should prompt the initiation of further diagnostic testing. The follow-up diagnostic tests can confirm the disease suspected by the newborn screening and in this case the newborn screen is considered true positive. In contrast,

Table 1
Conditions included in newborn screening

ACMG core panel (29 primary conditions)

Organic Acidemia	Fatty Acid Oxidation Defects	Aminoacidopathies	Other Inborn Errors of Metabolism	Endocrinopathies	Hemoglobinopathies	Others
1. Isovaleric acidemia	1. Medium-chain acyl-CoA dehydrogenase deficiency	1. Phenylketonuria	1. Biotinidase deficiency	1. Congenital hypothyroidism	1. Sickle cell anemia	1. Hearing loss
2. Propionic acidemia	2. Very-long-chain acyl-CoA dehydrogenase deficiency	2. Maple syrup urine disease	2. Classic galactosemia	2. Congenital adrenal hyperplasia	2. Hemoglobin S/β-thalassemia	2. Cystic fibrosis
3. Methylmalonic acidemia	3. Long-chain hydroxyacyl-CoA dehydrogenase deficiency	3. Homocystinuria			3. Hemoglobin S/C disease	
4. Glutaric acidemia type I	4. Trifunctional protein deficiency	4. CIT I				
5. Multiple carboxylase deficiency	5. Carnitine uptake defect	5. Argininosuccinic acidemia				
6. Cobalamin A and B disorders		6. TYR I				
7. 3-Hydroxy-3-methylglutaric aciduria						
8. 3-Methylcrotonyl-CoA carboxylase deficiency						
9. β-Ketothiolase deficiency						

(continued on next page)

Table 1
(continued)

Organic Acidemia	Fatty Acid Oxidation Defects	Aminoacidopathies	Other Inborn Errors of Metabolism	Endocrinopathies	Hemoglobinopathies	Others
ACMG secondary targets (25 secondary conditions)						
1. Cobalamin C and D disorders	1. Short-chain acyl-CoA dehydrogenase deficiency	1. Argininemia	1. Galactokinase deficiency		1. Variant hemoglobinopathies (including hemoglobin E)	
2. Malonic acidemia	2. Medium/short-chain L-3-hydroxyacyl-CoA dehydrogenase deficiency	2. CIT II	2. Galactose epimerase deficiency			
3. Isobutyryl-CoA dehydrogenase deficiency	3. Glutaric acidemia type II	3. TYR II				
4. 2-Methyl-3-hydroxybutyric aciduria	4. Medium-chain ketoacyl-CoA thiolase deficiency	4. TYR III				
5. 2-Methylbutyryl-CoA dehydrogenase deficiency	5. Dienoyl-CoA reductase deficiency	5. Hyperphenylalaninemia				
6. 3-Methylglutaconic aciduria	6. CPT IA	6. Hypermethioninemia				
	7. CPT II	7. Defects of biopterin cofactor biosynthesis				
	8. Carnitine/acylcarnitine translocase deficiency	8. Defects of biopterin cofactor regeneration				

Additional conditions recommended by ACHDNC

1. Glycogen storage disease type II (Pompe disease)
2. Critical congenital heart diseases
3. Severe combined immunodeficiencies
4. T-cell-related lymphocyte deficiencies

Abbreviations: ACHDNC, Advisory Committee on Heritable Disorders in Newborn and Children; ACMG, American College of Medical Genetics and Genomics; CIT, citrullinemia type I or II; CPT, carnitine palmitoyltransferase type I or II; TYR, tyrosinemia type I or II.

the follow-up diagnostic tests can be normal, excluding the disease suspected by the newborn screen and in this case the newborn screen is considered false positive. The newborn screen is considered false negative when an individual with the disease has a normal newborn screening result for that disease.[20]

In contrast to other clinical tests that have normal range out of which the test is reported to be abnormal, newborn screening tests have cutoff values that are used to determine whether tests are normal (not requiring further testing) or abnormal (requiring further testing). The cutoff value could be either above (high) or below (low) the normal population. The high target value is set in the interval between the 99th percentile of the normal population and the lowest 5th percentile of the affected individual range. However, the low target value is set in the interval between the highest 99th percentile of affected individual range and the 1st percentile of the normal population. Each screening program determines where to set cutoff values for each test aiming for low false-positive and false-negative rates. However, when there is overlap between normal and affected individuals, newborn screening programs typically elect to set the cutoff values that minimize the false-negative rates, which may lead to a higher false-positive rate.[20]

Because abnormal newborn screening results not only carry the consequences of burden of follow-up clinical evaluation and its cost, but can also cause significant parental anxiety,[21–23] efforts have been made to optimize the cutoff points to minimize the false-positive rate while maintaining low false-negative rate. Traditionally, each newborn screening program set its own cutoff values based mainly on normal population results. Once cutoff values selected in this manner are implemented, negative feedback from the follow-up system (too many false positives) or the dreaded occurrence of a false negative case may lead to abrupt changes on the cutoff. Significant improvement in cutoff value determination was achieved by an international collaboration that collected millions of normal and true-positive newborn screening results and determined the percentiles for both populations. The cutoff target ranges of analytes were then defined as the interval between selected percentiles of the two populations.[24]

Other than cutoff points optimization, different approaches have been implemented to reduce the false-positive and -negative rates. First, secondary analytes have been typically used to improve sensitivity and reduce false-positive rate. Second, for some disorders with abnormal results on initial screen, a reflex to a more specific test is done to support a diagnosis and decrease the false-positive rate for a particular test. This second-tier reflex testing can be a measurement of additional metabolites (eg, steroid profiling in congenital adrenal hyperplasia and succinylacetone in tyrosinemia type I), or it can be DNA sequencing to detect common pathogenic variants (eg, cystic fibrosis, medium-chain acyl-CoA dehydrogenase deficiency, and galactosemia).[25–27] Third, a computational approach, that has proved its utility, depends on multivariate pattern recognition software that generates tools integrating multiple clinically significant results into a single score. Retrospective evaluation of past cases suggested that these tools could have avoided significant percentage of the false-positive and could have prevented most of known false-negative events.[28]

LOGISTICS AND FOLLOW-UP

Newborn screening is a system rather than an event in which a test is simply performed. This system includes preanalytical, testing, and postanalytical phases. The preanalytical phase typically takes place at the birth hospital where demographic data are collected and documented, blood sampling is obtained, and filter paper cards are shipped. The testing phase occurs at designated department of health laboratories and includes samples preparation, test conduction, results interpretation, and report issuing. The final and most important phase is the postanalytical phase where results for newborn screening requiring further testing are communicated and confirmed, treatment is initiated, and long-term follow-up is monitored. During this entire process, timeliness of sample transport, test performance, results transmission, and availability of confirmatory testing and treatment are critical to ensure the success of newborn screening programs. Continuous quality assurance for the performed tests, easy access to health care, and system evaluation are also critical for the success of this system.[3,29]

Good communication is an essential part of any successful newborn screening program. Department of health laboratories performing the newborn screening tests, primary health care providers, metabolic centers, and families should all communicate effectively to ensure a timely evaluation and management of newborns whose newborn screening test indicates that further testing is required. Typically, the laboratory reports newborn screening results to the primary health care provider listed on the newborn screening card, who will subsequently notify the family of the results and perform the recommended follow-up evaluation, or refer the infant to a metabolic specialist. In certain urgent cases, the laboratory may also contact the metabolic specialist and the family directly.[21,30] Abnormal newborn screening results requiring further testing do not only carry the consequences of burden of follow-up clinical evaluation and its cost, but can also cause significant parental anxiety. Expectedly, parents who are well-informed by their primary care physician typically feel less stress about the results compared with parents who are not educated. Therefore, parents should be appropriately counseled with regard to the nature of newborn screening, the results in their child, and the possible clinical implication. Particularly, it should be emphasized that results of newborn screening indicate that the infant may be at risk to be affected with a condition, and further testing is needed, but newborn screening results do not indicate definitive diagnoses.[2,21–23]

FACTORS AFFECTING NEWBORN SCREENING RESULTS

Several factors can affect the newborn screening results including the timing of blood sampling. Newborn screening test needs to be done between 24 and 48 hours of life. Some states require a second newborn screen that is usually performed between 7 and 14 days of life. It is important to adhere to the recommend timeframe for obtaining newborn screening tests because the cutoff values for screening analytes are set to reflect values expected at this age range. Obtaining a newborn screening earlier than 24 hours of life can decrease the sensitivity of testing. Beyond the neonatal period, there are no well-established cutoff values.[31,32] In addition, the level of analytes measured in newborn screening is affected by nutrition (parental nutrition vs infant formula or breastfeeding), underlying sickness, gestational age, and birth weight.[33] All of these factors should be taken into consideration when interpreting the results and newborn screening programs typically include this information in the required demographic information of newborn being screened.

For sick newborns in neonatal intensive care units, blood transfusion may affect certain newborn screening results because of the mixture of the transfused blood in the neonate's bloodstream. Newborn screening enzyme tests for galactosemia and biotinidase deficiency, and hemoglobinopathies do not produce accurate results after transfusion; therefore, to permit screening for these conditions it is generally recommended to collect the newborn screening samples before the transfusion starts, if possible, even if this takes place earlier than the usual time frame for obtaining the newborn screening. If the newborn screening is obtained at an earlier time because transfusion is needed, the neonate should still have another newborn screening for detection of disorders not affected by transfusion at the standard time frames.[3] In addition, the newborn screening enzyme tests for biotinidase deficiency and galacto-semia is affected by environmental factors, such as temperature and humidity.[34]

Finally, a mother with an inborn error of metabolism may transmit abnormal metab-olites to her offspring, confounding the infant's newborn screening results. Many cases of abnormal newborn screening for healthy infants of women with carnitine up-take defect, very-long-chain acyl-CoA dehydrogenase deficiency, 3-methylcrotonyl-CoA carboxylase deficiency, and others have been described.[35–37]

CONFIRMATION OF NEWBORN SCREENING RESULTS

Many of the conditions tested in the newborn screening are rare; therefore, the primary health care provider may not be familiar with the nature of the condition and the diag-nostic work-up that needs to be done. A set of action (ACT) sheets that provides the information and guidelines of care for each condition in the newborn screen has been developed collaboratively by the American College of Medical Genetics and Geno-mics and the American Academy of Pediatrics.[38] For most inborn errors of meta-bolism, the initial follow-up testing involves the determination of different metabolites in urine and blood using such tests as plasma amino acids, urine organic acids, and acylcarnitine profile. When the results of the initial follow-up tests are abnormal or equivocal, further testing including enzyme assay and gene sequencing may be used for definitive diagnosis (**Table 2**).

FUTURE DIRECTIONS

Newborn screening will continue to expand by the addition of disorders for which early intervention can significantly modify the outcome. This expansion is driven by the development of new therapies for larger number of inborn errors of metabolism and the advancement in testing methodologies.

With the advancement in enzyme-replacement therapy development for lysosomal storage disorders, these diseases have been considered for inclusion in newborn screening.[39–41] A few states have begun screening for Krabbe, adrenoleukodystorphy, Fabry, Gaucher, Niemann-Pick, and Hurler, although these diseases have not yet been recommended by ACHDNC because of the lack of evidence of the efficacy of screening.[42,43] Besides storage diseases, other conditions have been evaluated for in-clusion in newborn screening, such as guanidinoacetoacetate methyltransferase defi-ciency, cerebrotendinous xanthomatosis, biliary atresia, and Duchenne muscular dystrophy.[44–47]

Although advancements in the utility of tandem mass spectrometry methodology have allowed for expanding the newborn screening,[48] other methodologies have been also considered. With the advancement of next-generation sequencing technol-ogy targeted gene panel and whole exome sequencing have been considered as first-tier or second-tier genetic testing in newborn screening. However, the high costs, prolonged turnaround time, and the detection of variants of uncertain clinical signifi-cance are currently significant limitations for the use of this methodology for newborn screening.[49–53] In contrast to biochemical profiling, molecular testing are time-independent and therefore can be performed earlier than 24 hours of life. In fact, mo-lecular testing can be performed even before birth during fetal life if samples can be obtained noninvasively. Currently, great advancements have been achieved in

Table 2
Follow-up testing for abnormal newborn screening

		Follow-up Tests											Additional Confirmatory Testing
		Initial Testing											
Abnormal Newborn Screen Analytes		Plasma Amino Acids	Urine Organic Acids	Acylcarnitine Profile	Total and Free Carnitine	Urine Acylglycines	Urine Orotic Acid	Total Plasma Homocysteine	Plasma Phenylalanine	Plasma Methylmalonic Acid	Urine Methylmalonic Acid	Succinylacetone	
Organic acidemia													
Propionic acidemia	↑ C3 (propionylcarnitine)	—	X	X	—	X	—	—	—	—	—	—	Enzyme assay in fibroblast or leukocytes; *PCCA, PCCB* gene sequencing
Methylmalonic acidemia	↑ C3	—	X	X	—	X	—	—	—	X	—	—	Enzyme assay in fibroblast; *MUT* gene sequencing
Cobalamin disorders	↑ C3	—	X	X	—	X	—	X	—	X	—	—	Cobalamin complementation studies in fibroblast; *MMAA, MMAB, MMACHC* gene sequencing
Malonic acidemia	↑ C3-DC (malonylcarnitine)	—	X	X	—	—	—	—	—	X	—	—	*MLYCD* gene sequencing
Isobutyryl-CoA dehydrogenase deficiency	↑ C4 (isobutyrylcarnitine)	—	—	X	—	X	—	—	—	—	—	—	*ACAD8* gene sequencing
Isovaleric acidemia	↑ C5 (isovalerylcarnitine/methylbutyrylcarnitine)	—	X	X	—	X	—	—	—	—	—	—	*IVD* gene sequencing
2-Methylbutyryl-CoA dehydrogenase deficiency	↑ C5	—	X	X	—	X	—	—	—	—	—	—	*ACADSB* gene sequencing
Glutaric acidemia type I	↑ C5-DC (glutarylcarnitine)	—	X	X	—	—	—	—	—	—	—	—	Enzyme assay in fibroblast; *GDCH* gene sequencing
Biotinidase deficiency	↑ C5-OH (hydroxy-isovalerylcarnitine/methyl-hydroxybutyrylcarnitine)	—	X	X	—	X	—	—	—	—	—	—	Biotinidase enzyme assay in serum; *BTD* gene sequencing
Multiple carboxylase deficiency	↑ C5-OH	—	X	X	—	X	—	—	—	—	—	—	Enzyme testing in fibroblast, leukocytes; *HLCS* gene sequencing

Disorder	Marker								Confirmatory testing
3-Methylcrotonyl-CoA carboxylase deficiency	↑ C5-OH	X	X	—	—	—	—	X	Enzyme testing in fibroblast, leukocytes; *MCCC1*, *MCCC2* gene sequencing
Hydroxy-3-methylglutaric aciduria	↑ C5-OH	X	X	—	—	—	—	X	*HMGCL* gene sequencing
3-Methylglutaconic aciduria	↑ C5-OH	X	X	—	—	—	—	X	Enzyme assay in fibroblasts; *AUH* gene sequencing
β-Ketothiolase deficiency	↑ C5-OH	X	X	—	—	—	—	—	Enzyme assay in fibroblasts; *ACAT1* gene sequencing
2-Methyl-3-hydroxybutyric aciduria	↑ C5-OH	X	X	—	—	—	—	—	Enzyme assay in fibroblasts; *HSD17B10* gene sequencing
Fatty acid oxidation defects									
Carnitine uptake defect	↓ C0 (free carnitine)	—	—	X	—	—	—	—	Carnitine transport assay in fibroblasts; *OCTN2* gene sequencing
CPT IA	↑ C0	X	X	X	—	—	—	—	CPT assay in fibroblasts; *CPT1A* gene sequencing
Short-chain acyl-CoA dehydrogenase deficiency	↑ C4 (butyrylcarnitine)	X	X	—	—	—	—	X	*ACADS* gene sequencing
Glutaric acidemia type II	↑ C4	X	X	—	—	—	—	X	*ETFA, ETFB, ETFDH* gene sequencing
Medium/short-chain L-3-hydroxyacyl-CoA dehydrogenase deficiency	C4-OH (3-hydroxy-butyrylcarnitine)	X	X	—	—	—	—	X	*HADH* gene sequencing
Medium-chain acyl-CoA dehydrogenase deficiency	↑ C8 (octanoylcarnitine)	X	X	—	—	—	—	X	*ACADM* gene sequencing
Very-long-chain acyl-CoA dehydrogenase deficiency	↑ C14:1 (tetradecenoylcarnitine)	X	—	—	—	—	—	X	*ACADVL* gene sequencing
CPT II	↑ C16 (hexadecanoylcarnitine)	X	—	—	—	—	—	X	*CPT2* gene sequencing

(continued on next page)

Table 2 (continued)

Abnormal Newborn Screen Analytes	Initial Testing							Follow-up Tests			Additional Confirmatory Testing
	Plasma Amino Acids	Urine Organic Acids	Acylcarnitine Profile	Total and Free Carnitine	Urine Acylglycines	Urine Orotic Acid	Total Plasma Homocysteine	Plasma Phenylalanine	Plasma Methylmalonic Acid	Urine Succinylacetone	
Carnitine/acylcarnitine translocase deficiency — ↑ C16	—	—	X	—	—	—	—	—	—	—	SLC25A20 gene sequencing
Long-chain hydroxyacyl-CoA dehydrogenase deficiency — ↑ C16-OH (hydroxyl-hexadecanoylcarnitine)	—	—	X	—	—	—	—	—	—	—	HADHA gene sequencing
Trifunctional protein deficiency — ↑ C16-OH	—	—	X	—	—	—	—	—	—	—	HADHA, HADHB gene sequencing
Aminoacidopathies											
Phenylketonuria — ↑ Phenylalanine	—	—	—	—	—	—	—	X	—	—	PAH gene sequencing
Defects of biopterin cofactor metabolism — ↑ Phenylalanine	—	—	—	—	—	—	—	X	—	—	Urine pterins; CSF neurotransmitters; enzyme assay in erythrocytes; GCH1, PTS, or QDPR gene sequencing
Maple syrup urine disease — ↑ Leucine	X	X	—	—	—	—	—	—	—	—	Enzyme assay in lymphoblast or fibroblast; BCKDHA, BCKDHB, DBT gene sequencing
Homocystinuria — ↑ Methionine	X	—	—	—	—	—	X	—	—	—	CBS gene sequencing
Hypermethioninemia — ↑ Methionine	X	—	—	—	—	—	X	—	—	—	Plasma S-adenosylhomocysteine and S-adenosylmethionine; MAT1A gene sequencing
Argininemia — ↑ Arginine	X	—	—	—	—	X	—	—	—	—	Enzyme assay in erythrocytes or liver; ARG1 gene sequencing

Disorder	Marker							Confirmatory testing
Argininosuccinic acidemia	↑ Citrulline	X	—	—	—	—	—	Enzyme assay in erythrocytes, fibroblast, or liver; ASL gene sequencing
CIT I	↑ Citrulline	X	—	—	—	—	—	Enzyme assay in fibroblast or liver; ASS1 gene sequencing
CIT II	↑ Citrulline	X	—	—	—	—	—	SLC25A13 gene sequencing
TYR I	↑ Succinylacetone	X	—	—	—	—	X	FAH gene sequencing
TYR II	↑ Tyrosine	X	—	—	—	—	—	TAT gene sequencing
TYR III	↑ Tyrosine	X	—	—	—	—	—	HPD gene sequencing
Endocrinopathies								
Congenital hypothyroidism	↑ Thyroid-stimulating hormone	Serum free T4 and thyroid-stimulating hormone	—	—	—	—	—	—
Congenital adrenal hyperplasia (21-hydroxylase deficiency)	↑ 17-OHP (17-hydroxyprogesterone)	Serum 17-OHP, electrolytes, and glucose	—	—	—	—	—	Adrenocorticotropic hormone stimulation test; steroid profile; CYP21A2 gene sequencing
Hemoglobinopathies								
Sickle cell anemia	+HbS	CBC, reticulocyte count, and hemoglobin electrophoresis	—	—	—	—	—	HBB gene sequencing
Hemoglobin S/β-thalassemia	+HbS	CBC, reticulocyte count, and hemoglobin electrophoresis	—	—	—	—	—	HBB gene sequencing
Hemoglobin S/C disease	+HbS	CBC, reticulocyte count, and hemoglobin electrophoresis	—	—	—	—	—	HBB gene sequencing
Cystic fibrosis	↑ Immunoreactive trypsinogen	Sweat chloride and CFTR gene sequencing	—	—	—	—	—	—

Abbreviations: CBC, complete blood count; CIT, citrullinemia type I or II; CPT, carnitine palmitoyltransferase type I or II; TYR, tyrosinemia type I or II.

noninvasive prenatal diagnosis through the extraction of cell-free fetal DNA from maternal blood for the detection of aneuploidy and genome-wide copy number variation.[54] With more advancement in this field, reliable sequencing data can be obtained from such methodology, which can open the doors for the potentials of doing molecular screening during fetal life.

Another approach that can be potentially used in newborn screening is global metabolomic profiling, which is a mass spectrometry–based method that allows the detection of huge numbers of small molecules in body fluids, and can be applied for the screening of a large number of inborn errors of metabolism.[55–57]

An integrated approach combining the molecular data from next-generation sequencing and biochemical data from global metabolimics can potentially produce robust results. The metabolic profiles can provide a functional readout to assess the penetrance of gene mutations identified by next-generation sequencing. Conversely, metabolic abnormalities can uncover potential damaging mutations that were previously unappreciated by sequencing.[58] Although such an approach has not been considered for newborn screening, it can be of potential utility in the future with more advancement in technologies.

Therefore, further advancement in technology is expected to allow continuous expansion of conditions detected by newborn screening with reduction in cost, shorter turnaround time, and more accurate results with low false-positive and false-negative results.

SUMMARY

Newborn screening aims to achieve early diagnosis of treatable disorders to allow for early initiation of medical care to prevent or reduce significant morbidity and mortality related to these disorders. Many of the conditions tested in newborn screening are inborn errors of metabolism; however, it also tests for some other endocrine, hematologic, and immunologic diseases. Newborn screening tests are not diagnostic. Therefore, abnormal newborn screen results require follow-up tests to confirm or exclude the suspected diagnosis. Further advancement in technology is expected to allow continuous expansion of newborn screening.

REFERENCES

1. American College of Medical Genetics Newborn Screening Expert Group. Newborn screening: toward a uniform screening panel and system–executive summary. Pediatrics 2006;117(5 Pt 2):S296–307.
2. Almannai M, Marom R, Sutton VR. Newborn screening: a review of history, recent advancements, and future perspectives in the era of next generation sequencing. Curr Opin Pediatr 2016;28(6):694–9.
3. Berry SA. Newborn screening. Clin Perinatol 2015;42(2):441–53, x.
4. Grosse SD. Does newborn screening save money? The difference between cost-effective and cost-saving interventions. J Pediatr 2005;146(2):168–70.
5. Pena LDM, van Calcar SC, Hansen J, et al. Outcomes and genotype-phenotype correlations in 52 individuals with VLCAD deficiency diagnosed by NBS and enrolled in the IBEM-IS database. Mol Genet Metab 2016;118(4):272–81.
6. Posset R, Garcia-Cazorla A, Valayannopoulos V, et al. Age at disease onset and peak ammonium level rather than interventional variables predict the neurological outcome in urea cycle disorders. J Inherit Metab Dis 2016; 39(5):661–72.

7. Ding Y, Thompson JD, Kobrynski L, et al. Cost-effectiveness/cost-benefit analysis of newborn screening for severe combined immune deficiency in Washington state. J Pediatr 2016;172;127–35.

8. Castellani C, Massie J, Sontag M, et al. Newborn screening for cystic fibrosis. Lancet Respir Med 2016;4(8):653–61.

9. Chaturvedi S, DeBaun MR. Evolution of sickle cell disease from a life-threatening disease of children to a chronic disease of adults: the last 40 years. Am J Hematol 2016;91(1):5–14.

10. Bickel H, Gerrard J, Hickmans EM. Influence of phenylalanine intake on phenyl-ketonuria. Lancet 1953;265(6790):812–3.

11. Horner FA, Streamer CW. Effect of a phenylalanine-restricted diet on patients with phenylketonuria; clinical observations in three cases. J Am Med Assoc 1956; 161(17):1628–30.

12. Guthrie R, Susi A. A simple phenylalanine method for detecting phenylketonuria in large populations of newborn infants. Pediatrics 1963;32:338–43.

13. Heard GS, Secor McVoy JR, Wolf B. A screening method for biotinidase deficiency in newborns. Clin Chem 1984;30(1):125–7.

14. Beutler E, Baluda M, Donnell GN. A new method for the detection of galactoxemia and its carrier state. J Lab Clin Med 1964;64:694–705.

15. Millington DS, Kodo N, Norwood DL, et al. Tandem mass spectrometry: a new method for acylcarnitine profiling with potential for neonatal screening for inborn errors of metabolism. J Inherit Metab Dis 1990;13(3):321–4.

16. Public Law 110-204-Newborn screening saves lives act of 2007. Available at: https://www.gpo.gov/fdsys/pkg/PLAW-110publ204/content-detail.html. Accessed November 15, 2016.

17. Wilson J, Jungner J. Principles and practices of screening for disease. Geneva (Switzerland): World Health Organization; Public Health Papers; 1968. p. 34.

18. Recommended Uniform Screening Panel. Available at: http://www.hrsa.gov/advisorycommittees/mchbadvisory/heritabledisorders/recommendedpanel/index.html. Accessed November 16, 2016.

19. Screening Programs | National Newborn Screening and Global Resource Center. Available at: http://genes-r-us.uthscsa.edu/screening. Accessed November 15, 2016.

20. Sutton VR, Graham BH. Newborn screening for inborn errors of metabolism, introduction and approaches for confirmation. In: Lee B, Scaglia F, editors. Inborn errors of metabolism, from neonatal screening to metabolic pathways. New York: Oxford University Press; 2015. p. 3–34.

21. Davis TC, Humiston SG, Arnold CL, et al. Recommendations for effective newborn screening communication: results of focus groups with parents, providers, and experts. Pediatrics 2006;117(5 Pt 2):S326–40.

22. Gurian EA, Kinnamon DD, Henry JJ, et al. Expanded newborn screening for biochemical disorders: the effect of a false-positive result. Pediatrics 2006; 117(6):1915–21.

23. Schmidt JL, Castellanos-Brown K, Childress S, et al. The impact of false-positive newborn screening results on families: a qualitative study. Genet Med 2012;14(1):76–80.

24. McHugh DMS, Cameron CA, Abdenur JE, et al. Clinical validation of cutoff target ranges in newborn screening of metabolic disorders by tandem mass spectrometry: a worldwide collaborative project. Genet Med 2011;13(3):230–54.

25. Lacey JM, Minutti CZ, Magera MJ, et al. Improved specificity of newborn screening for congenital adrenal hyperplasia by second-tier steroid profiling using tandem mass spectrometry. Clin Chem 2004;50(3):621–5.

26. Magera MJ, Gunawardena ND, Hahn SH, et al. Quantitative determination of succinylacetone in dried blood spots for newborn screening of tyrosinemia type I. Mol Genet Metab 2006;88(1):16–21.

27. Baker MW, Groose M, Hoffman G, et al. Optimal DNA tier for the IRT/DNA algorithm determined by CFTR mutation results over 14 years of newborn screening. J Cyst Fibros 2011;10(4):278–81.

28. Marquardt G, Currier R, McHugh DMS, et al. Enhanced interpretation of newborn screening results without analyte cutoff values. Genet Med 2012;14(7):648–55.

29. Centers for Disease Control and Prevention (CDC). CDC grand rounds: newborn screening and improved outcomes. MMWR Morb Mortal Wkly Rep 2012;61(21): 390–3.

30. Kim S, Lloyd-Puryear MA, Tonniges TF. Examination of the communication practices between state newborn screening programs and the medical home. Pediatrics 2003;111(2):E120–6.

31. Walter JH, Patterson A, Till J, et al. Bloodspot acylcarnitine and amino acid analysis in cord blood samples: efficacy and reference data from a large cohort study. J Inherit Metab Dis 2009;32(1):95–101.

32. Tang H, Feuchtbaum L, Neogi P, et al. Damaged goods?: an empirical cohort study of blood specimens collected 12 to 23 hours after birth in newborn screening in California. Genet Med 2016;18(3):259–64.

33. Clark RH, Kelleher AS, Chace DH, et al. Gestational age and age at sampling influence metabolic profiles in premature infants. Pediatrics 2014;134(1):e37–46.

34. Adam BW, Hall EM, Sternberg M, et al. The stability of markers in dried-blood spots for recommended newborn screening disorders in the United States. Clin Biochem 2011;44(17–18):1445–50.

35. McGoey RR, Marble M. Positive newborn screen in a normal infant of a mother with asymptomatic very long-chain Acyl-CoA dehydrogenase deficiency. J Pediatr 2011;158(6):1031–2.

36. El-Hattab AW, Li F-Y, Shen J, et al. Maternal systemic primary carnitine deficiency uncovered by newborn screening: clinical, biochemical, and molecular aspects. Genet Med 2010;12(1):19–24.

37. Kör D, Mungan NÖ, Yılmaz BŞ, et al. An asymptomatic mother diagnosed with 3-methylcrotonyl-CoA carboxylase deficiency after newborn screening. J Pediatr Endocrinol Metab 2015;28(5–6):669–71.

38. Information NC for B, Pike USNL of M 8600 R, MD B, USA 20894. Newborn screening ACT sheets and confirmatory algorithms. American College of Medical Genetics. 2001. Available at: https://www.ncbi.nlm.nih.gov/books/NBK55827/. Accessed November 16, 2016.

39. Kumar AB, Masi S, Ghomashchi F, et al. Tandem mass spectrometry has a larger analytical range than fluorescence assays of lysosomal enzymes: application to newborn screening and diagnosis of mucopolysaccharidoses types II, IVA, and VI. Clin Chem 2015;61(11):1363–71.

40. Matern D, Gavrilov D, Oglesbee D, et al. Newborn screening for lysosomal storage disorders. Semin Perinatol 2015;39(3):206–16.

41. Elliott S, Buroker N, Cournoyer JJ, et al. Pilot study of newborn screening for six lysosomal storage diseases using tandem mass spectrometry. Mol Genet Metab 2016;118(4):304–9.

42. Wasserstein MP, Andriola M, Arnold G, et al. Clinical outcomes of children with abnormal newborn screening results for Krabbe disease in New York State. Genet Med 2016;18(12):1235–43.
43. Kemper AR, Brosco J, Comeau AM, et al. Newborn screening for X-linked adrenoleukodystrophy: evidence summary and advisory committee recommendation. Genet Med 2017;19(1):121–6.
44. Wang KS. Section on surgery, committee on fetus and newborn, childhood liver disease research network. Newborn screening for biliary atresia. Pediatrics 2015;136(6):e1663–9.
45. Bleyle L, Huidekoper HH, Vaz FM, et al. Update on newborn dried bloodspot testing for cerebrotendinous xanthomatosis: an available high-throughput liquid-chromatography tandem mass spectrometry method. Mol Genet Metab Rep 2016;7:11–5.
46. Gatheridge MA, Kwon JM, Mendell JM, et al. Identifying non-Duchenne muscular dystrophy-positive and false negative results in prior Duchenne muscular dystrophy newborn screening programs: a review. JAMA Neurol 2016;73(1):111–6.
47. Pasquali M, Schwarz E, Jensen M, et al. Feasibility of newborn screening for guanidinoacetate methyltransferase (GAMT) deficiency. J Inherit Metab Dis 2014; 37(2):231–6.
48. Ombrone D, Giocaliere E, Forni G, et al. Expanded newborn screening by mass spectrometry: new tests, future perspectives. Mass Spectrom Rev 2016;35(1): 71–84.
49. Bhattacharjee A, Sokolsky T, Wyman SK, et al. Development of DNA confirmatory and high-risk diagnostic testing for newborns using targeted next-generation DNA sequencing. Genet Med 2015;17(5):337–47.
50. Poulsen JB, Lescai F, Grove J, et al. High-quality exome sequencing of whole-genome amplified neonatal dried blood spot DNA. PLoS One 2016;11(4): e0153253.
51. Botkin JR, Rothwell E. Whole genome sequencing and newborn screening. Curr Genet Med Rep 2016;4(1):1–6.
52. Wu C-C, Tsai C-H, Hung C-C, et al. Newborn genetic screening for hearing impairment: a population-based longitudinal study. Genet Med 2017;19(1):6–12.
53. Narravula A, Garber KB, Askree SH, et al. Variants of uncertain significance in newborn screening disorders: implications for large-scale genomic sequencing. Genet Med 2017;19(1):77–82.
54. Kølvraa S, Singh R, Normand EA, et al. Genome-wide copy number analysis on DNA from fetal cells isolated from the blood of pregnant women. Prenat Diagn 2016;36(12):1127–34.
55. Goodacre R, Vaidyanathan S, Dunn WB, et al. Metabolomics by numbers: acquiring and understanding global metabolite data. Trends Biotechnol 2004; 22(5):245–52.
56. Miller MJ, Kennedy AD, Eckhart AD, et al. Untargeted metabolomic analysis for the clinical screening of inborn errors of metabolism. J Inherit Metab Dis 2015; 38(6):1029–39.
57. Dénes J, Szabó E, Robinette SL, et al. Metabonomics of newborn screening dried blood spot samples: a novel approach in the screening and diagnostics of inborn errors of metabolism. Anal Chem 2012;84(22):10113–20.
58. Guo L, Milburn MV, Ryals JA, et al. Plasma metabolomic profiles enhance precision medicine for volunteers of normal health. Proc Natl Acad Sci U S A 2015; 112(35):E4901–10.

Printed and bound by CPI Group (UK) Ltd, Croydon, CR0 4YY

07/10/2024

01040500-0007